Magnetic Surgery

Michel Gagner
Editor

Magnetic Surgery

Springer

Editor
Michel Gagner
Hôpital du Sacré-Cœur de Montréal
Montréal, QC
Canada

ISBN 978-3-030-73946-1 ISBN 978-3-030-73947-8 (eBook)
https://doi.org/10.1007/978-3-030-73947-8

This Springer imprint is published by the registered company Springer Nature Switzerland AG
The registered company address is: Gewerbestrasse 11, 6330 Cham, Switzerland

I dedicate this book to my children, Xavier, Guillaume, and Maxime, and spouse, France, for all their moral support during the COVID-19 pandemic.

Foreword

From idea to reality, Professor Michel Gagner does it again. In the quest for more and more minimally invasive access, surgeons have imagined harnessing magnetic energy. Powerful magnets can be swallowed, inserted thru ports intraabdominally, or placed on the skin surface. Considering the potential is only limited by your imagination.

The World Congress of Laparoscopy, hosted by SAGES in 2018, offered a panel session entitled "Magnet Surgery: What's the Attraction?" co-chaired by Michel Gagner of Canada and Marcos Berry of Chile (Fig. 1). Topics pre-

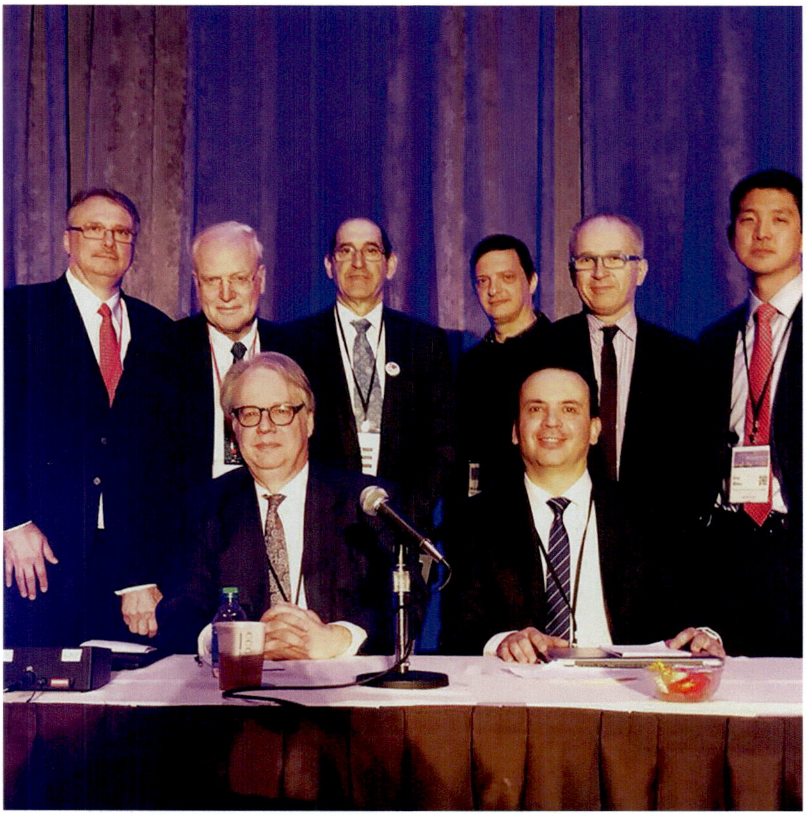

Fig. 1 Speakers of the World Congress of Laparoscopy, hosted by SAGES in 2018, panel session entitled "Magnet Surgery: What's the Attraction?". From left to right, back row: Dr John J Vargo, Dr Michael Harrison, Dr David W Ratner, Dr Galvao Neto, Dr Homero Rivas and Dr Eric G Sheu. Front row: Dr Michel Gagner and Dr Marcos Berry

sented included physical properties and toxicity of magnets, magnetic rings for reflux, magnets for birth defects in pediatric surgery, use of magnets in flexible endoscopy, magnetic retraction, laparoendoscopic GI anastomosis, and endoscopic bowel anastomosis. The session was well attended by surgeon innovators.

On the heels of the panel, Dr. Gagner embarked on the textbook *Magnetic Surgery*. The contributors include visionary surgeons from around the world: Marcos Berry, Eric Sheu, Luigi Bonavina, Homero Rivas, and Galvo Neto. Topics focus on endoluminal and laparoscopic operations, techniques from vascular and GI anastomosis. The book demonstrates the use of magnets to treat a variety of diseases such as reflux, back pain, and fecal incontinence. The reader will learn how to retract and gain exposure, dissect tissue planes, achieve hemostasis, and create anastomosis in a totally different way. Physical properties of external surface and internal magnets are discussed. The authors emphasize the importance of partnering with industry leaders to develop novel surgical tools.

Professor Gagner has been a pioneer in MIS surgery. He has many firsts and was an early adopter of laparoscopies Whipple, endoscopic parathyroidectomy, MIS adrenalectomy, and sleeve gastrectomy. With tiny incisions, patients have experienced less pain, smaller scars, and faster recuperation. In 2017, Dr. Gagner was recognized with the SAGES George Berci Lifetime Achievement Award for Innovation in Surgery. Having advanced surgery from open to laparoscopy, to micro-laparoscopy, to SILS, NOTES, and robotic surgery, Dr. Gagner reimagines surgery now with magnets.

Magnetic Surgery is a glimpse today into what is possible with a little imagination, curiosity, and persistence. Magnets will surely enable tomorrow's surgery in ways we have yet to conceive.

Daniel B. Jones
Professor of Surgery, Harvard Medical School
Boston, MA, USA

Preface

Magnetic surgery is not new, but it is an expression that will be used more frequently in the next several decades. Indeed, China has taken this field very seriously and arranged the first international conference on magnetic surgery in Xian, China, also known as Chang'an or Eternal Peace, a famous imperial city, which had the largest palace on Earth [1]. The scientific committee was comprised of mainly Chinese nationals like Bo Wang, Jianhui Li, Jigang Bai, Rongqian Wu, Shiqi Liu, Xiaopeng Yan, Xin Zhang, Xufeng Zhang, Xuemin Liu, and Truman Cheng; Claire Elizabeth Graves and Mario F. Zaritzky from the USA; Catherine Sim Co from the Philippines; Ibrahim Uygun from Turkey; Luzia Toselli from Argentina; Tim Helge Fass from Ireland; and Vitalii Zablotskii from the Czech Republic.

Their goals are to commence regular international conferences to be held worldwide, that a Magnetic Surgery Alliance (MSA) be recognized for clinical and experimental advancements, and a book "Magnetic Surgery" discoursing the latest progresses and outlook of magnetic surgery be outlined and published. This last desideratum is fulfilled by my book *Magnetic Surgery*. This idea of a book encompassing the different concepts and designs using magnets for surgical purposes has been in my mind for several years and certainly began to materialize before the SAGES conference in Seattle, which took place at the same time as the 16th World Endoscopic Surgery met.

Dr. John H. Marks, the program chair of SAGES 2018, had contacted me to propose an innovative session of 90 minutes for SAGES 2018. This had probably been discussed during the program committee hearings in Houston, March 2017, when Jon C. Gould was chairing that group with Sallie Matthews, the SAGES executive director, and I had made suggestions to attract an international audience at the meeting. Dr. Marks had asked me to propose an innovative session, being a member of the SAGES program committee for a very long time, and I wanted to do a full session on magnetic surgery and assemble the innovators accomplishing this.

On March 26, 2017, I invited Dr. Marcos Berry from Chile to participate and be my co-moderator for that innovative session, as he was a user of magnets for laparoscopic assistance. We, in fact, had already conferred about it during SAGES 2017 in Houston, and envisioned some additional topics/speakers. So, the same day, March 26, 2017, wasting no time, I sent to Dr. Marks a first draft of the proposed session, called "All About Magnets." There was no question in my mind that all teams working on these concepts had to be invited to the table to present, foster a super discussion, and hopefully stimulate the audience about what is coming. It was Richard A. Hruska from Springer, Executive Editor of Clinical Medicine, based in New York, who officially invited me to make this book project a reality on March 20, 2018. He was involved with other SAGES books, which are great successes, and had perused the SAGES program ahead of time and was intrigued about our session. He could not join us in Seattle for the meeting, where our session took place on April 11, 2018. He suggested that as an outstanding clinician as well as a dedicated researcher and educator, I was clearly the ideal authority to be editor of such a volume and would very much like to discuss either a project developing from that session or one developing from my recent work in the field. Hence, the book was born.

SAGES 2018 was special, because the 16th World Congress of Endoscopic Surgery also took place, and had a mega audience, under the auspices of President Dr. Daniel B. Jones from Harvard Medical School. The World Congress, at the Washington State Convention Center from April 11–14, hosted surgeons from over 16 international societies, representing 6 continents, and over 80 countries. The proposed session was one of the very first morning sessions of the meeting and had a full large room audience. The final program was delivered to SAGES on August 2, 2017, with the final title [2] "Magnets in Surgery: What's the Attraction?" After the two co-moderators welcomed the audience, the session began with a talk on "Physical Properties and Toxicity of Magnets Used for Surgical Applications" by Eric G. Sheu, MD, Boston, MA, followed by "Magnetic Rings for Reflux" from David W Rattner, MD, Boston, MA. Then we shifted to compression anastomosis with "Magnets for Birth Defects in Pediatric Surgery" by emeritus professor Michael Harrison, MD, San Francisco, CA; "Use of Magnets in Flexible Endoscopy" by John J. Vargo, MD, from the Cleveland Clinic, Cleveland, OH (with whom I had the privilege to work with while I was an attending there); followed by "Magnetic Retraction for Laparoscopic Cholecystectomy" by Homero Rivas, MD, Stanford, CA; and a similar topic on "Magnetic Retraction for Laparoscopic Sleeve Gastrectomy" by my co-moderator Marcos Berry, MD, Santiago, Chile. I presented on the topic and first patents that I have been working on since 2007, in "Laparo-endoscopic GI Anastomosis." "Endoscopic Bowel Anastomosis" by Galvao Neto, MD, Sao Paulo, Brazil, well known in advanced bariatric endoscopic procedures, closed the session.

Strong from this base, though the session would not allow more speakers (in my mind it could have been a whole day symposium with other subjects and topics), I decided to welcome more authors on additional interesting applications of magnets in other fields of surgery, because concepts can be cross-linked easily if we all talk about them. I have been involved as co-editor on many books, but this is the first time, apart from my Ph.D. thesis, in which I am the sole editor.

I think this book, the very first of its kind, will be a breakthrough, a leap forward in a new field of surgery, to harness the power of attraction, the energy and might of magnets, a force of nature, to realize health improvements to benefit millions of patients worldwide.

Montréal, QC, Canada Michel Gagner

References

1. Lv Y, Shi Y. Scientic committee of the first international conference of magnetic surgery. Xi'an consensus on magnetic surgery. Hepatobiliary Surg Nutr. 2019;8(2):177–8.
2. SAGES & CAGS Host the 16th World Congress of Endoscopic Surgery. SAGES 2018 Program Information. April 11–14, 2018 | Washington State Convention Center, Seattle, WA. https://www.sages2018.org/program/.

Contents

Editor and Contributors

About the Editor

Michel Gagner is a well-respected surgeon known for his contributions to laparoscopic and bariatric surgery. Born in Montreal, Quebec, Canada, he first studied at the Séminaire de Sherbrooke where he obtained a Quebec college diploma in 1978 followed by an M.D. from Université de Sherbrooke in 1982. Completing his residency in general surgery at McGill University in Montreal, during which time he conducted research studies on human lipolysis in sepsis, he went to Paris, France, to complete a fellowship in liver surgery, and he endured a second fellowship in pancreas and complex GI surgery at the Lahey Clinic in Massachusetts.

In 1990, Dr. Gagner accepted his first teaching appointment at the Université de Montréal School of Medicine as an assistant professor of surgery (Hotel-Dieu de Montreal), during which time he introduced his skills in laparoscopic surgery. As a pioneer of robot-assisted surgery, world's first laparoscopic removal of the adrenal glands, the liver, bile duct, and pancreas, he eventually made his way to the USA to practice at the Cleveland Clinic Foundation in Ohio where he co-founded the Minimally Invasive Surgery Center. There he pioneered the use of endoscopic surgery for parathyroid and thyroid tumors in humans. He then became the director of the Minimally Invasive Surgery Center at Mount Sinai School of Medicine in New York, chair of the laparoscopic division, and earned the title Franz W. Sichel Professor of Surgery. There he pioneered telesurgery with Professor Marescaux and Leroy of Strasbourg, the first transatlantic robot-assisted surgery, published in Nature in 2001. Dr. Gagner later became head of the laparoscopic and bariatric surgery section at Cornell University's Weill Medical College (New York City).

After his tenure as chief surgeon at Mount Sinai Hospital in Miami and professor of surgery at Florida International University, Dr. Gagner is now working at Sacré-Coeur Hospital, affiliated to Université de Montréal, as a professor of surgery and senior consultant. He also owns the Westmount Square Surgical Center, a private clinic specialized in bariatric surgery for weight loss and metabolic surgery for type-2 diabetes.

World renowned in laparoscopic and bariatric surgery for weight loss, the clinic of Dr. Gagner, which is located in Montreal, specializes in the laparoscopic sleeve gastrectomy, which he pioneered in 2000, as well as laparoscopic duodenal switch, which he was the first to perform in 1999, and various new innovative endoscopic treatments for obesity, type-2 diabetes, and gastro-intestinal tract disorders.

The author and co-author of more than 400 publications and 11 books, including the *Atlas of Hepato- Pancreatico-Biliary Surgery*, *Endocrine Surgery* (second edition), and *Perfect Sleeve Gastrectomy*, Dr. Gagner is also a patentee in his field, especially on new methods to treat obesity and GI anastomosis. An elected fellow of the American College of Surgeons, the Royal College of Surgeons (Canada), and the American Society for Metabolic and Bariatric Surgery (ASMBS), he is also a honorary member of the Academie Nationale de Chirurgie de France, the Association Francaise de Chirurgie, the Mexican Laparoscopic Surgery Society, the Colombian Surgical Society, the Brazilian Surgical College, the Peruvian Surgical Society, and the European Association for Endoscopic Surgery.

Dr. Gagner received a medal from the city of Marseille, France, in 2017, SAGES Pioneer in Surgical Endoscopy Award (2017), 21st Oliver H. Beahrs Professorship (Mayo Clinic 2016), Surgical innovation award from the ASMBS (2016), a 2011 Excel Award by the Society of Laparoendoscopic Surgeons, a 2010–2011 French National Assembly Award, and Medal of the City of Bordeaux, Nice, and Sete, France. He has been highlighted in many editions of Who's Who in America, Who's Who in Medicine and Healthcare, Who's Who in Science and Engineering, Who's Who in the South and Southwest, and Who's Who in the World. Married to France Lapointe, Dr. Gagner has three children (Xavier, Guillaume, and Maxime).

Reference

https://www.24-7pressrelease.com/press-release/449817/michel-gagner-md-presented-with-the-albert-nelson-marquis-lifetime-achievement-award-by-marquis-whos-who

Contributors

Juan Pablo Barros, MD Department of Surgery, Hospital Regional de Copiapó, Copiapó, Atacama, Chile

Marcos Berry, MD Bariatric Surgery, Department of Surgery, Clinica Las Condes, Santiago, Chile

Luigi Bonavina, MD, FACS Division of General and Foregut Surgery, Department of Biomedical Sciences for Health, University of Milano School of Medicine, IRCCS Policlinico San Donato, Milan, Italy

Mauro Bortolotti, MD Gut Motility Laboratory, Section of Pathophysiology of Digestion, Internal Medicine and Gastroenterology, S.Orsola-Malpighi Polyclinic, University of Bologna, Bologna, Italy

Vitor Ottoboni Brunaldi, MD, MSc Gastrointestinal Endoscopy Unit, Gastroenterology Department, University of São Paulo Medical School, São Paulo, Brazil

Samuel Engle, BA Business Development, Synectic Medical Product Development, Woodbridge, CT, USA

Michel Gagner, MD, FRCSC. FACS, FASMBS, FASSO Hôpital du Sacré-Cœur de Montréal, Montréal, QC, Canada

Chief of Surgery, Westmount Square Surgical Center, Westmount, QC, Canada

Manoel Galvão Neto, MD, MSc Surgery Department, Florida International University, Miami, FL, USA

Katherine Kendrick, MD Department of Internal Medicine, Navicent Health/Mercer University School of Medicine, Macon, GA, USA

Reiko Kumano, MD Department of Radiology, St. Marianna University Yokohama Seibu Hospital, Yokohama City, Kanagawa-ken, Japan

Sheng-Chiang Lee, PhD Appetec INC, Macon, GA, USA

James N. Luo, MD Department of Surgery, Brigham and Women's Hospital, Harvard Medical School, Boston, MA, USA

Rodrigo Lynch, MD Surgery Department, Hospital San Jose de Melipilla, Santiago, Chile

Hironori Ohdaira, MD, PhD Department of Surgery, International University of Health and Welfare Hospital, Nasushiobara-shi, Tochigi-ken, Japan

Marie-Claire Rassweiler-Seyfried, Dr. med. Department of Urology and Urosurgery, University Medical Center Mannheim, Medical Faculty Mannheim, University of Heidelberg, Mannheim, Germany

Homero Rivas, MD, MBA, FACS, FASMBS Department of Surgery, Innovation and the Future, Mohammed Bin Rashid University of Medicine and Healthcare Sciences, Dubai, United Arab Emirates

Shahriar Sedghi, MD, AGAF Appetec INC, Gastroenterology Associates of Central Georgia, Macon, GA, USA

Eric G. Sheu, MD, DPhil Department of Surgery, Brigham and Women's Hospital, Harvard Medical School, Boston, MA, USA

C. Roberto Simons-Linares, MD, MSc Gastroenterology, Hepatology and Nutrition Department, Cleveland Clinic, Cleveland, OH, USA

Bethany Slater, MD Department of Pediatric Surgery, University of Chicago Medicine, Chicago, IL, USA

Betsy Smith, PhD Department of Internal Medicine, Mercer University School of Medicine, Macon, GA, USA

Yutaka Suzuki, MD, PhD Department of Surgery, International University of Health and Welfare Hospital, Nasushiobara-shi, Tochigi-ken, Japan

Lionel Urrutia, MD Department of Surgery, Clinica Las Condes, Santiago, Chile

John J. Vargo, MD, MPH Enterprise Endoscopy Operations, Endoscopic Research and Innovation, Section of Therapeutic, Gastroenterology, Hepatology and Nutrition, Cleveland Clinic, Cleveland, OH, USA

Russell K. Woo, MD Department of Surgery, Division of Pediatric Surgery, University of Hawaii, John A. Burns School of Medicine, Honolulu, HI, USA

Zhongfa Xu, MD Department of Gastrointestinal Surgery, The Third Affiliated Hospital of Shandong First Medical University (Affiliated Hospital of Shandong Academy of Medical Sciences), Jinan, Shandong, People's Republic of China

Eigoro Yamanouchi, MD, PhD Department of Radiology, International University of Health and Welfare Hospital, Nasushiobara-shi, Tochigi-ken, Japan

Kenji Yoshida, BS Clinical/Research, Gastroenterology Associates of Central Georgia, Macon, GA, USA

Ya'nan Zhen, MD Department of Gastrointestinal Surgery, The Third Affiliated Hospital of Shandong First Medical University (Affiliated Hospital of Shandong Academy of Medical Sciences), Jinan, Shandong, People's Republic of China

1 Introduction: Ideas and People Leading to Successful Products for Patient Care Leading to Magnetic Surgery

Michel Gagner

> There is nothing more powerful in the world than the idea that came in time.
>
> Victor Hugo (1802–1855)

Compression anastomosis has come and gone in the last century, and apart from sutures and staples, there has been nothing innovative and fresh, yet we are capable of much progress. Those efforts today, are "en phase" with the movement of minimally invasive surgery that took off at the end of the eighties in the last century, especially with laparoscopic cholecystectomies between 1985 and 1988, from pioneers like Erich Muhe from Boblingen Germany, Francois Dubois from Paris, Philippe Mouret of Lyon, Jacques Perissat from Bordeaux France, Barry McKernan and William Saye in Marietta Georgia, and Eddie Joe Reddick from Nashville, USA [1]. After a year at the Lahey Clinic in complex biliary and pancreatic surgeries, I left Burlington Massachusetts for a short mini-fellowship in laparoscopic surgery with Drs Reddick, Doug Olsen, and Al Spaw from Nashville, in the hot and humid heat wave of July 1990. After my return to Montreal, I became interested in fashioning anastomosis laparoscopically in early fall of 1990, at the Hotel-Dieu de Montreal, the historic hospital affiliated with the University of Montreal, while I started my career as a young surgical attending and teaching enthusiastically, almost religiously, laparoscopic cholecystectomy to many surgeons from Eastern Canada and New England [2]. When I tried a colonic resection but was unable to make any connection with the two segments and had to exteriorize them to make a conventional anastomosis outside the abdominal wall, I was unaware that Moises Jacob and his team from Miami were also working on something similar, mainly exteriorizing the bowel segments outside the patient abdominal wall and making a hand-sewn or stapled conventional anastomosis [3]. The major inconvenience of this "laparoscopic assistance," of course, was the incision needed, decreasing the advantage of laparoscopy for the patient, causing pain, infection, and hernia risks, and possibly higher dehiscence, slower recovery, and worse cosmesis. In order to continue with the "pure" laparoscopic surgical concept and not involve open surgery, I had to do mostly left-sided colon lesion, trying to remove the specimen transanally and creating the anastomosis with laparoscopic endoloops, putting the anvil of an EEA in the proximal colon (delivered again transanally) and another endoloop closing the distal bowel, trying to make an anastomosis that would be full thickness without any parts slipping and requiring intracorporeal suturing, as needle drivers and efforts to do so were in their infancy. This prompted efforts to do compression anastomosis using the "open" BAR Valtrac device, which I worked on in a porcine model. Laparoscopic staplers were not

M. Gagner (✉)
Hôpital du Sacré-Cœur de Montréal, Montréal, QC, Canada

Chief of Surgery, Westmount Square Surgical Center, Westmount, QC, Canada

M. Gagner (ed.), *Magnetic Surgery*, https://doi.org/10.1007/978-3-030-73947-8_1

available in the first years of 1990s, and nobody was doing any sort of stapled intracorporeal anastomosis until 1991–1992, except for transanal EEA end-to-end anastomosis with the circular stapler. The innovation of the laparoscopic stapler by US Surgical, led by Leon Hirsch, kind of killed the ongoing efforts of compression anastomosis at that time and put it on the backburner.

On the commercial development of the traditional open stapler and the laparoscopic form, one man stands out, Leon C. Hirsch. "Lee Hirsch" was born July 20, 1927, grew up in the Bronx, and had made his business apprenticeship in advertising, eventually creating his own company in 1948, the Lebow, Hirsch, and Windley. Several other companies followed in the 1950s, until the Soviet Union's surgical staplers were trying to make an entry in the USA market, which led to the establishment of United States Surgical Corporation in 1963, a Connecticut-based medical technology company, where Mr. Hirsch was the Founder, Chairman, and CEO of the corporation.

Since their development in 1908, surgical staplers have been utilized as a process of "mechanical suturing" in efforts to partition hollow visceral organs and fashion anastomoses in an effective and sterile methodology [4]. The concept for the surgical stapler was first exploited by Humér Hultl, a Hungarian surgeon and professor, and reconceived by Victor Fischer, a savvy Hungarian businessman and creator of surgical instruments. The design was highly praised. Nevertheless, it was too large, awkward, and costly to produce [4]. Aladár Petz, a student of Hultl, integrated two innovations to the Fischer-Hultl stapler to generate a lightweight model in 1920, which was named the "Petz clamp" [5]. Then in 1934, Friedrich of Ulm Germany fabricated the next generation of the modern-day linear stapler. In parallel, Russian staplers began to emerge in the 1950s, and one ended up on the desk of Leon C. Hirsch [4, 6].

Indeed, on a 1958 trip to the Soviet Union, Mark Ravitch learned that Russia had made headway in perfecting the surgical stapler. Ravitch had worked with and visited Russian colleagues, including Pavel Iosifovich Androsov, and then conferring with and working to convince Leon C. Hirsch. Dr. Mark Ravitch was Professor of Surgery at Johns Hopkins University, and they thought that a cartridge could be created with the Russian stapler to make it simple to use for daily gastrointestinal surgeries. Pavel Iosifovich Androsov and Alexey Alexeevich Strekopytov, both from Moscow, USSR, filed this patent on Christmas Eve December 24, 1962, 2 months after the Cuban missiles crisis, published in the gazette on May 24, 1966 and given the number 3,252, 643 for a surgical stapler that is now reminiscent of the full metal TA [7–11].

After Hirsch made an initial investment of $50,000 to make prototypes, Zanvyl Kreiger, part owner of the Baltimore Orioles baseball team and major donor to Johns Hopkins University, agreed to contribute more than $2 million in loans to the company. It took more than 3 years and $3 million to develop the first series of AUTO SUTURE staplers, which came to market in 1967. In 1967, in its first year as an operating business, USSC posted sales of just over $350,000. Fourteen years later, annual sales surpassed $100 million, and revenues reached $1 billion in 1992. In 1990, USSC launched the world's first laparoscopic clip applier, which I was happy to use for many patients, making possible a revolutionary new laparoscopic technique for gallbladder removal. The inventors Henry Bolanos, David T. Green, Lisa M. Heaton, Richard A. Mcgarry, Keith Ratcliff, and Wayne P. Young deposited the laparoscopic clip applier patent on the 18th of July 1989, with a Priority number of US07/381,265 on behalf of USSC. Most members of this team will be seen again later, for the laparoscopic stapler invention [12].

The benefits of this procedure were so dramatic that, without a randomized control trial, approximately 90% of the 600,000 gallbladder removals accomplished annually in the USA were converted to laparoscopy. Under Mr. Hirsch's leadership, USSC sales nurtured from $350,000 in its first year of sales (1967) to $1.5 billion in 1998. Zanvyl Krieger made a fortune and became a major benefactor for medicine, science, and arts in Baltimore. Ultimately USSC was acquired by Tyco International for $3.3 billion.

Certainly, in the world of compression anastomosis, the "Valtrac" by American Cyanamid, was successful. It began with Davis & Geck, a surgical/medical device company founded in 1909 by Charles T. Davis and Fred A. Geck in Brooklyn, NY, dedicated to surgical sutures, wound closure devices, and care. In 1930, during the great US Depression, the company was sold to American Cyanamid but continued as a division, later moving to Danbury, Connecticut, in the 1950s. Its most significant contribution to the surgical arena was the invention of the synthetic absorbable suture, including the Dexon (1970s), made with polyglycolic acid.

American Cyanamid, founded by Frank Washburn in 1907, was part of the Fortune 500 in the 1970s and 1980s and finally merged with American Home product in 1994, after a series of litigations for tetracycline problems and environmental damages from its manufacturing. Many of its subsidiaries ended in the hands of Pfizer, BASF, and Procter and Gamble. The Davis & Geck products and materials were sold to Sherwood, renamed Sherwood-Davis and Geck, and thereafter the CEO, David Low, tripled the sales to 1 billion dollars and retired in 1997. Tyco Corporation bought Sherwood-Davis on Dec. 22, 1997 for $1.7 billion. In an acquisition spree, Tyco International Ltd. also acquired US Surgical Corp. from Leon C. Hirsch, a maker of disposable medical sutures and staples, for nearly 3.3 billion in stock. The combination led to the creation of Covidien later in 2007, and Tyco Corporation renamed the suture line from Sherwood-Davis as Syneture. Tyco eventually decided to sell its healthcare division and Covidien, Ltd. to Medtronic plc in 2015.

The patent for the biodegradable anastomosis ring (BAR), sold under the name of Valtrac, was awarded to Thomas G. Hardy of Columbus Ohio, who had a similar nonabsorbable design, reminiscent of the Murphy button, a few years back. He was aided by Alan L. Kaganov from Danbury, Connecticut, and W. G. Pace of Columbus, Ohio, on behalf of the American Cyanamid Company, Stamford, Conn.; Appl. No. 287,500, filed on July 27, 1981 [13]. According to the patent description, the special anastomotic device was characterized by engageable locking slots supplied by mating prongs and a multiplicity of pawls carried by separate prongs which connect two ring members and retain it in a preselected position after being closed from the open position.

The Valtrac BAR accommodated different thicknesses of tissue and therefore could be used in a variety of circumstances and with pomp! The ring members and pinned prongs are so designed that they consist of a single unit that can be injection molded. The invention developed met the constraints of anastomotic surgery and provided a safe, reasonably economical, easy to use anastomotic device and was disintegratable! It was very successful for two decades but abruptly fell off after Leon C. Hirsch laparoscopic stapler developments were completed by USSC engineers. The irony is that both finally ended with the Medtronic family. The patent was called "Apparatus and method for placing staples in laparoscopic or endoscopic procedures," by inventors David T. Green of Westport, Henry Bolanos of East Norwalk, Daniel E. Alesi of New Fairfield, Keith Ratcliff of Sandy Hook, and Charles R. Sherts of Southport, all from Connecticut. This was assigned to United States Surgical Corporation of Norwalk, Connecticut with the application no. 358,64,622, filed on May 26, 1989, and issued a patent number 5,040,715 on August 20, 1991 [14]. The rest is history and led to an explosion of laparoscopic and robotic-assisted procedures for three decades [15].

The book initiates a dialog on the development of magnetic anastomosis, which is an extension of previous compression anastomosis. It is in fact an extension of the 16th World Congress of Endoscopic Surgery, SAGES, in Seattle April 11–14, 2018, during a special symposium I chaired called "Magnets In Surgery: What's The Attraction?" Many authors of the present book were presenters at that particular innovative and inaugural program. History and physical properties of using magnets are discussed in the first chapters, following with specific applications in the body. Some are simple and some are intricate. Some have led to successful companies like the development of magnet collar for gastroesophageal reflux. Indeed, I was presented with the first prototype by Pete McNerney who was the lead investor of Capital Venture, which supported the development efforts of Torax, the company that successfully led clinical trials of LINX.

Pete McNerney has over 30 years of healthcare operating and venture capital experience. He co-founded Thomas, McNerney & Partners, and Coral Ventures and has been involved with The Kensington Group, Memtec North America, and Baxter Healthcare Corporation, as a certified accountant, and has a B.A. from Yale and an M.B.A. from Stanford University.

Torax Medical was founded in 2002 by Sanderling Ventures, Mayo Medical Ventures, and veteran medtech entrepreneur Todd Berg. Dr. Timothy Mills was the managing director Sanderling Ventures and chairman and co-founder of Torax Medical, headquartered in St. Paul, Minnesota. Torax matured and promoted products conceived to treat sphincter disorders utilizing its technology proposal, a sort of magnetic sphincter enhancement [16, 17]. Torax Medical was marketing the LINX® Reflux Management System for the treatment of GERD in both the USA and Europe. Previously, it raised a total of $3.5 million in Series A financing from Sanderling Ventures and Mayo Medical Ventures, and in 2005, Torax Medical Inc. had completed a $10 million Series B round of financing, led by Thomas, McNerney & Partners, Minneapolis, Minn.; Sanderling Ventures, San Mateo, California; and Mayo Medical Ventures, Rochester, Minnesota.

Torax became very successful and was acquired by Ethicon EndoSurgery, a division of Johnson and Johnson in March 2017, for an additional 102.2 million. Torax had estimated annual revenues of $15.9 million, according to a report by the Cincinnati Business Courier. The company announced that it had completed a $25 million round of Series E financing before the J&J acquisition. Other investors included Sanderling Ventures, Thomas McNerney & Partners, Accuitive Medical Ventures, Kaiser Permanente Ventures, Piper Jaffray Companies, and Mayo Clinic Ventures.

My involvement with McNerney goes back to 12 years ago, when he had invested in EndoMetabolic Solutions Inc., a company I co-founded in Minneapolis with Dave Blaeser and the late Dale Spencer, in 2007, after both were extremely successful with ev3, Inc. Interestingly enough, Covidien had acquired this company in 2010 for 2.6 billion dollars. EndoMetabolic Solutions (obesity treatment devices) had closed a $3.8 million Series A round through five investors including myself, Thomas McNerney & Partners, 3 years after it had invested in Torax. Unfortunately, Dale Spencer passed away in November 2016. Dale Spencer had been chairman of ev3, Inc., and the former CEO of SciMed Life Systems Inc., a mechanical engineer from the University of Maine by training. He was a real leader at SciMed Life Systems until the merger with Boston Scientific in 1995, and the founder of eV3, which is now a part of global medical device leader Medtronic. As a start-up mentor for me, we liked to discuss mountaineering, which we both did separately in the South American Andes. Dave Blaeser, named CEO of EndoMetabolic Solutions, has been an active leader in the medical device industry for 35 years, steering teams at Boston Scientific, Velocimed, Nidus, Endometabolic Solutions-EMS, Libra Medical, and ZIFT Medical. Most recently, he was Founder and CEO of Ideal Medical Solutions, a medical device-consulting firm, and is the new CEO of Minneapolis-based medical device company, Resolution Medical, as of May 2020. EMS was ahead of its time in terms of having the right intellectual property, but the surgical field was not mature enough and ready for its IP. A very hard "great" recession in 2008, triggered by the housing bubble, with the collapse of several US banks, unemployment from 4.7% to 10%, made a difficult environment for a multitude of start-ups at the time, causing VCs to demand more equity for valuations down by 25–50%, and the expensive costs of raising capital made it very difficult for the next round for the large human clinical trial necessary for FDA approval.

Magnets used externally on the skin surface are used for laparoscopic retraction and surgical manoeuvring inside the abdominal cavity and are successfully sold by Levita Magnetics from San Mateo California. The person behind Levita is Dr. Albert Rodriguez-Navarro, Founder and CEO, is a minimally invasive general surgeon with more than 10 years of clinical involvement and was an Assistant Professor of Medicine at the Universidad de Chile. As a medical inventor, he has multiple patents and has published in international journals, especially in the field of post-operatory pain. Levita Magnetics is evolving minimally invasive surgery by reducing the number of incisions and improving surgical outcomes, with a technology platform that will enable magnetic surgery across an array of minimally invasive surgical procedures. Levita Magnetics was founded in Chile in 2012, has been solely funded by Chilean investors and CORFO, and is currently based in Silicon Valley. The company has a robust IP portfolio and is expecting both US and European regulatory clearances for commercialization. Greg Liu, a BS and MS in Mechanical Engineering from Stanford University, has helped Dr. Rodriguez-Navarro as their Chief Operations Officer; he has 25 years of product development and operations experience. Before this appointment, he held leadership roles at Luma Therapeutics, Acclarent, Google, and Google (x) and was a founding member of Verily Life Sciences (Google).

The very interesting endoscopic developments initiated by Endometabolic Solutions of Minneapolis is continued with GI Windows of West Bridgewater, Massachusetts, and by GT Metabolic Solutions from San Jose, California. Concerning GI Windows, it is now led by Brian Tinkham CEO, and according to the company's website, he is a leader in innovation and entrepreneurship, with significant prior roles at Medtronic as Vice President of Sales and New Technologies for the GI & Hepatology division. He was the co-founder of Beacon Endoscopic (acquired by Covidien 2014) and held global marketing and sales leadership positions at Boston Scientific. He apparently replaced James Wright, the first President and CEO of GI Windows, who led the company's first clinical series data presentation in May 2016. This company is aided by Marvin Ryou, M.D., the Chief Medical Officer and co-founder of GI Windows, who is an Assistant Professor of Medicine at Harvard Medical School and Associate Physician in the Division of Gastroenterology, Hepatology, and Endoscopy at Brigham and Women's Hospital and Director of Endoscopic Innovation and Education. He is the partner of Dr. Christopher Thompson who has been also on the board of this company. Very recently, on December 12, 2019, GI Windows had announced a $14.6 million Series A financing. Asia-focused healthcare investment firm GT Healthcare Capital Partners led this financing and Silicon Valley-based Sonder Capital. Dr. Galvao Neto's chapter will be discussing their initial efforts.

Concerning GT Metabolic Solutions, the company based in San José California, was co-founded by Dr. Michel Gagner and Thierry Thaure, in May 2020. It is a rebirth of EMS with its initial IP. Michel Gagner is the Chief Medical Officer and has spent 15 years in the USA as chief of laparoscopy or/and bariatric surgery at the Cleveland clinic, Mount Sinai School of Medicine, Weil Cornell in NYC, and chief of surgery at Mount Sinai Miami. He has more than 500 publications and 15 books in surgery and is an honorary member of the Academie Nationale de Chirurgie de France, the Association Francaise de Chirurgie, the Mexican Laparoscopic Surgery Society, the Colombian Surgical Society, the Brazilian Surgical College, the Peruvian Surgical Society, and the European Association for Endoscopic Surgery. Dr. Gagner also has received a 2017 City of Marseille, France, Medal, SAGES Pioneer in Surgical Endoscopy Award (2017), 21st Oliver H. Beahrs Professorship (Mayo Clinic 2016), Surgical innovation award from the ASMBS (2016), a 2011 Excel Award by the Society of Laparoendoscopic Surgeons, a 2010–2011 French National Assembly Award, and Medal of the City of Bordeaux, Nice and Sete, France.

Concerning Thierry Thaure, the Chief Executive Officer, who has over 35 years experience in medtech, is an entrepreneur and CEO. He demonstrated repeated successes in building businesses with disruptive technologies and driving their market expansions. He was previously CEO & Co-founder of Cephea Valve Technologies –

purchased by Abbott in 2020 for $200 M, CEO of EndoGastric Solutions, a private company leader in NOTES, launched technology SVP of Accuray, a leader in radiosurgery had taken them public, and was the founding VP of Sales & Marketing of Intuitive Surgical, a leader in surgical robotic, and had a key management roles at Guidant, Origin Medsystems, and Edwards Life Science. The company is also supported by key engineers like Hal Heitzmann, the Chief Technical Officer and previously Senior VP, R&D & Engineering, and Distinguished Scientist at Glaukos Corporation (GKOS, NYSE). He also held positions as Sr. Distinguished Engineer at Edwards Lifesciences and as VP, R&D at four medical device start-ups. He holds over 100 US and International patents and applications. He holds a Ph.D. in Molecular Biophysics and Biochemistry from Yale University. Todd Krinke is the VP Development and Lead Engineer; he held Principal and Senior Engineering positions at Conventus Orthopaedics, Travanti Pharma, St. Jude Medical, and Hutchinson Technology; he holds a Bachelor of Science, Aerospace Engineering & Mechanics, from University of Minnesota – Twin Cities. The initial team is extremely promising, "on ne change pas une equipe qui gagne."

With this book my hope is that the reader will be inspired about the future of surgery, pushing boundaries in the mid twenty-first century and beyond, all to create more minimally invasive procedures and interventions than we did with laparoscopic surgery at the end of the twentieth century. It appears that the surgical gestures of creating anastomosis will be delayed (I call this "DAT" for delayed anastomosis technologies), while creating a positive new tunnelling will disperse the negative effects of creating connections in the body, with fewer acute leaks, infections, strictures, and ulcerations and with a reduced inflammatory response. This is occurring with gradual wound healing, a slow and steady connection permitting optimal collagen deposition, and creating strength without foreign body reaction; that is DAT!

> Until you spread your wings, you'll have no idea how far you can fly.
>
> Napoleon Bonaparte

References

1. Reynolds W Jr. The first laparoscopic cholecystectomy. JSLS. 2001;5(1):89–94.
2. https://en.wikipedia.org/wiki/Hôtel-Dieu_de_Montréal.
3. Jacobs M, Verdeja JC, Goldstein HS. Minimally invasive colon resection (laparoscopic colectomy). Surg Laparosc Endosc. 1991;1(3):144–50.
4. Gaidry AD, Tremblay L, Nakayama D, Ignacio RC Jr. The history of surgical staplers: a combination of Hungarian, Russian, and American innovation. Am Surg. 2019;85(6):563–6.
5. Oláh A, Dézsi CA. Aladár Petz (1888–1956) and his world-renowned invention: the gastric stapler. Dig Surg. 2002;19:393–9.
6. Robicsek F. The birth of the surgical stapler. Surg Gynecol Obstet. 1980;150(4):579–83.
7. Ravitch MM, Steichen FM, Fishbein RH, Knowles PW, Weil P. Clinical experiences with the Soviet mechanical bronchus stapler (UKB-25). J Thorac Cardiovasc Surg. 1964;47:446–54.
8. Steichen FM. The use of staplers in anatomical side-to-side and functional end-to-end enteroanastomoses. Surgery. 1968;64(5):948–53.
9. Steichen FM. Clinical experience with autosuture instruments. Surgery. 1971;69(4):609–16.
10. Ravitch MM, Steichen FM. Technics of staple suturing in the gastrointestinal tract. Ann Surg. 1972;175(6):815–37.
11. https://patents.google.com/patent/US3252643.
12. https://patents.google.com/patent/US5084057.
13. Hardy et al. United States Patent, Number: 4,467,804. Aug. 28, 1984.
14. https://patents.google.com/patent/US5040715B1/en.
15. Daniell JF, Gurley LD, Kurtz BR, Chambers JF. The use of an automatic stapling device for laparoscopic appendectomy. Obstet Gynecol. 1991;78(4):721–3.
16. Ganz RA, Edmundowicz SA, Taiganides PA, Lipham JC, Smith CD, DeVault KR, Horgan S, Jacobsen G, Luketich JD, Smith CC, Schlack-Haerer SC, Kothari SN, Dunst CM, Watson TJ, Peters J, Oelschlager BK, Perry KA, Melvin S, Bemelman WA, Smout AJ, Dunn D. Long-term outcomes of patients receiving a magnetic sphincter augmentation device for gastroesophageal reflux. Clin Gastroenterol Hepatol. 2016;14(5):671–7.
17. Reynolds JL, Zehetner J, Wu P, Shah S, Bildzukewicz N, Lipham JC. Laparoscopic magnetic sphincter augmentation vs. laparoscopic Nissen fundoplication: a matched-pair analysis of 100 patients. J Am Coll Surg. 2015;221:123–8.

Physical Properties, Toxicity, and Physiological Effects of Magnets

2

James N. Luo and Eric G. Sheu

Brief History of Magnets

Magnets have been a part of human civilization for millennia. The ancient Greeks described the magnetic lodestone as early as the sixth century B.C. According to legend, a Greek shepherd named Magnes, while living in the region of Magnesia, first noticed that metallic debris and even the tip of his staff were attracted to the rock on which he was standing. He then dug up what is perhaps the earliest recorded example of lodestone. The term "lodestone" itself is believed to have derived from the Anglo-Saxon meaning "leading stone." The Greek region of Magnesia, where the shepherd is said to have first found the lodestone, also gives root to the modern term magnet.

The ancient Chinese first made reference to lodestone around the fourth century B.C., where they described lodestone's ability to attract iron and other metallic objects to itself. These early civilizations continued to experiment with this mysterious material. By the twelfth century, the Chinese began to use the lodestone for navigation when they realized that one end of the object reliably points toward one direction (north) [1]. The industrial usefulness of the magnet continued to expand in the subsequent centuries, and today, it is an indispensable part of modern society.

Lodestone, or magnetite, is a class of substance collectively known as ferrites. Ferrites have the characteristic of being ferromagnetic, which includes the ability for spontaneous magnetization. Unlike other ferromagnetic metals, ferrites have relatively low electrical conductivity. This low electrical conductivity allows them to become an important part of the electronic industry.

What Is a Magnet?

Broadly, and intuitively defined, a magnet is a material that exerts an attractive or repulsive force on another object. The scale of this magnetic force ranges from the subatomic to the intergalactic. Individual subatomic particles exert a magnetic force and in turn experiences a magnetic force exerted by a neighboring particle [2]. The earth itself can be viewed as a magnet, and it is the largest magnet with which we come into daily contact [3].

In order to appreciate the important role that magnets play in the modern life, and in modern medicine, several basic principles of magnetism must be noted. The magnetic properties of an object derive from the magnetic properties of its constituent atoms. A substance is said to

J. N. Luo · E. G. Sheu (✉)
Department of Surgery, Brigham and Women's Hospital, Harvard Medical School, Boston, MA, USA
e-mail: esheu@bwh.harvard.edu

M. Gagner (ed.), *Magnetic Surgery*, https://doi.org/10.1007/978-3-030-73947-8_2

be *diamagnetic* if its constituent atoms do not possess free magnetic dipole moments [4]. These substances have a negative magnetic susceptibility that is independent of the strength of any external magnetic field or of temperature. On the other hand, a substance is said to be *paramagnetic* if its constituent atoms have free magnetic dipole moments [4]. Even in these paramagnetic atoms, their magnetic dipole moments are normally oriented randomly, and thus they have no net magnetization. When in the presence of an external magnetic field, these dipole moments no longer orient randomly and are instead oriented toward or away from the external magnetic source, and a net positive magnetization is produced. These substances in turn have a positive magnetic susceptibility.

Whether a potentially magnetic substance exhibits macroscopic magnetic properties depends on the arrangement of the atomic magnetic dipoles. If the atomic dipoles align in parallel throughout a large volume of any matter, then these net magnetic dipole moments will be additive, and the substance will exhibit *ferromagnetism* [5]. However, if nearly equal numbers of atomic magnetic dipole moments of similar magnitude align themselves in opposite orientation, and thus cancelling each other out, then the substance will have no permanent macroscopic magnetic property. These substances are referred to as *antiferromagnetic* [5]. Therefore, a ferromagnetic material is any material that contains *permanent atomic magnetic dipole moments* that spontaneously orient themselves in a *parallel* fashion even in the absence of an external magnetic field.

All magnets, from the smallest magnetic dipole moment to the household refrigerator magnet to the earth itself, have an inherent directionality, or pole. A given magnetic material has its strongest magnetic forces at the poles. Traditionally, because the earth's magnetic poles are located north and south, thereby attracting the corresponding poles of other magnets, the two magnetic poles are grossly referred to as *north* and *south* [6] (Fig. 2.1).

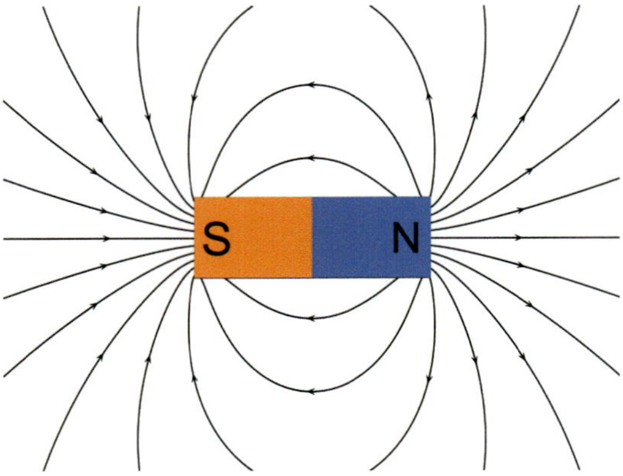

Fig. 2.1 Magnetic field lines. All magnetic objects have an inherent directionality, with the strongest forces at the poles. Traditionally, because the earth's magnetic poles are located north and south, the two magnetic poles are grossly referred to as *north* and *south*

Properties of Magnets

There are numerous characteristics that are important in understanding the usefulness of magnets, and a complete overview of these properties is beyond the scope of this text. Nonetheless, three of these parameters are crucial in evaluating the medical usefulness of a magnet. They are *energy product, coercivity*, and the *Curie constant.*

Energy Product

The energy product is a composite parameter determined by the strength of the magnet and the coercivity. This is the most frequently used and important parameter in evaluating the usefulness of a magnet [7]. The strength of a magnet depends on its constituent elements. As previously described, each atom in a magnetic substance has its own magnetic dipole moment, and the ultimate macroscopic magnetic strength is the resultant sum of the individual atomic moments. The energy product is measured in Gauss Oersted (GOe), or Joules/meter^3 (SI). One megaGOe (MGOe) is one million Gauss Oersted. For industrial use, the "strength" of a magnet is graded from N35 to N52. A magnet with a grade of N40 has a maximum energy product of 45 MGOe. As

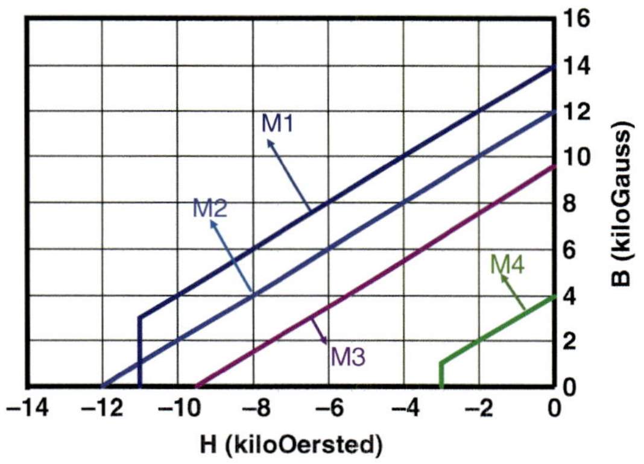

Fig. 2.2 Demagnetization curve (BH curve) of several hypothetical magnetic materials. The curve measures the strength of a given magnet and the force required to demagnetize it. The maximum energy product of a magnetic substance is the product of the B and H values along the curve (MGOe). Each magnetic substance has its unique demagnetization curve. *M* magnet. ("Magnetic field of an ideal cylindrical magnet with its axis of symmetry inside the image plane." by Geek3, Wikimedia Commons is licensed under CC BY-SA 3.0 and was partially modified)

the grade of the magnet increases, the strength of the magnet also increases.

The N grading system is based on the demagnetization curve (aka. BH Curve) (Fig. 2.2). This curve measures the strength of the magnet and the force required to demagnetize it. On the abscissa is the "H" value, which is measured in kilooersted, and on the ordinate is the "B" value, which is measured in kilogauss. The maximum energy product of a magnetic substance is the product of the B and H values along the curve; thus it bears the unit of MGOe [8]. Each magnetic substance has its unique demagnetization curve. While this grading system gives an overview of the strength of a particular magnetic substance, it is not a sufficient descriptor. A magnet's ultimate usefulness depends on a variety of other factors including the intended application, the shape, the cost, and the thickness of the final product.

Coercivity

Coercivity is the strength required of an external magnetic field in order to demagnetize a substance [7]. In essence, it measures how well a magnet stays a magnet. A material with a high coercivity means that it will require a higher external magnetic field for the substance to lose its magnetism. Recall that the macroscopic magnetic strength of a substance is the sum total of the individual atomic dipole moments, properly aligned. A high coercivity requires a crystal structure where the individual constituent dipole moments are oriented in such a way that its stability requires a high amount of external force to disrupt. Magnets resist demagnetization by imposing a high energy requirement to realign their atomic dipole moments. Accordingly, the coercivity of a magnetic product can be influence by the size, shape, as well as the orientation of its component molecules [9].

Curie Constant

Curie constant measures how the magnetic substance withstands heat. A magnet's ability to remain magnetic depends on the external energy required to disrupt the alignment of its dipole moments. In most ferromagnetic substance, the spontaneous alignment of these dipole moments is resisted by random external thermal forces. Thus, as these "disrupting forces" strengthen with rising temperature, the magnetic susceptibility of a ferromagnetic substance correspondingly decreases. In the late nineteenth century, the French physicist Pierre Curie (one half of the famous duo) first reported the observation that for many magnetic substance, their magnetic susceptibility is inversely related to the absolute temperature (T, Kelvin) [10]. His equation, $\chi = C/T$, where χ is the magnetic susceptibility, C is Curie constant, and T is absolute temperature. From this simple equation, it becomes apparent that the theoretical magnetic susceptibility of a ferromagnetic substance becomes infinite as the temperature approaches absolute zero. Today, the Curie constant is an important industrial parameter for magnet evaluation. How well a magnet can withstand heat significantly influences where and how it can be used.

Rare-Earth Magnets

By the nature of their chemical behavior, transition elements such as iron and cobalt have large magnetic dipole moments and are thus frequently used for their ferromagnetic properties. However, transition elements by their elemental nature often do not have high coercivity, and their industrial usefulness is significantly enhanced if their magnetocrystalline structure can be stabilized without diluting their magnetic dipole moments [7]. A handful of heavy elements on the periodic table have emerged as the ideal candidates for this task.

Rare-earth elements (REE) are a group of elements that includes the lanthanide series, lanthanum, scandium, and yttrium [11] (Fig. 2.3). Their misleading name notwithstanding, *rare-earth* elements are in reality not particularly rare. The REE's reserves in the earth's crust are 1600 times more abundant than silver and 3200 times more abundant than gold [11]. REE exist in a variety of minerals (e.g., haides, carbonates, oxides, phosphates, silicates, etc.) and are frequently used for industrial purposes. For example, the dominant REE, cerium, is used in catalytic converters, allowing them to run at higher temperatures. Lanthanum is used in telescope lenses, and gadolinium is a familiar contrast material in magnetic resonance imaging [12, 13].

Prior to the widespread use of REE in industrial magnets, transition metal (e.g., samarium and cobalt)-based magnets were the best available magnets. The original SmCo5 was discovered in the 1960s and play an important role in the postwar industrial economy [7]. Early iterations of REE-based magnets used a binary structure of REE-iron, and the common REE candidates were terbium, dysprosium, and samarium. Incorporation of these REEs gave the magnet much higher coercivity. Subsequent work led to the development of more complex structures, and ultimately the REE-iron-boron structure was developed.

Today, the most important industrial magnets, especially in medical use, are neodymium-based. Several attributes of neodymium-iron-boron (Nd-Fe-B) magnets make them particularly attractive for medical and industrial use. Neodymium magnets are significantly stronger than many of the other commonly encountered magnets. Nd-Fe-B can produce a maximum energy product of 474 kJ/M^3 [9]. At its surface, neodymium magnets can generate magnetic

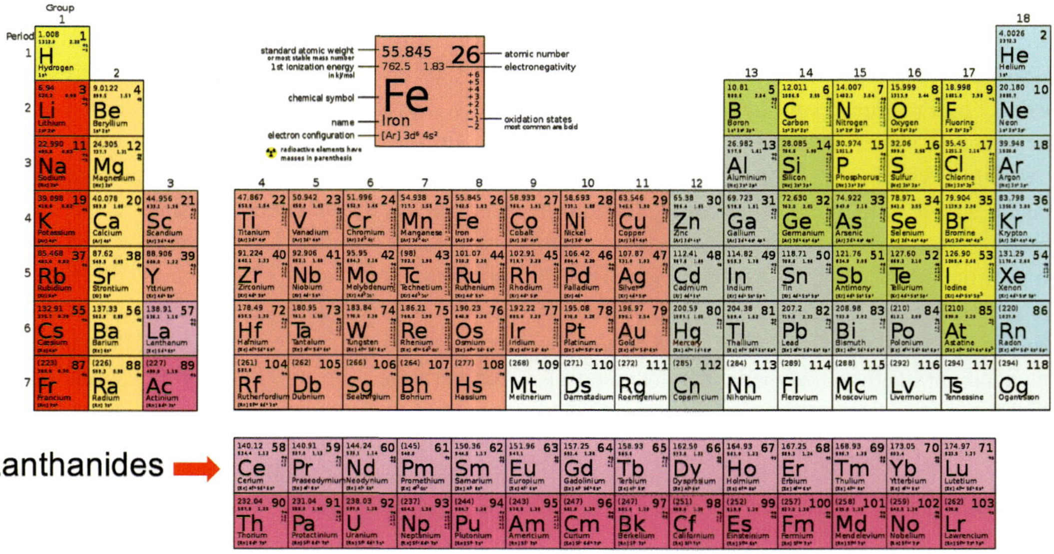

Fig. 2.3 Periodic table of elements. Rare-earth elements (REE) include the lanthanide series, lanthanum, scandium, and yttrium. ("Periodic table of the elements" by 2012rc, Wikimedia Commons is licensed under CC BY 3.0 and was partially modified)

fields up to 10,000 Gauss. This is roughly 100 times stronger than the household refrigerator magnet and about 10,000 stronger than the earth's magnetic field. It is comparable to a 1T MRI (1 Tesla = 10,000 Gauss). It also has a relatively high coercivity. The addition of the boron atom helps to stabilize the new compound. The resultant crystal structure is tetragonal, which is an anisotropic structure that is quite stable and thus contributing to the high coercivity [7]. The main limitation of the Nd-Fe-B magnet is its relatively low Curie constant of around 600 K, compared to samarium-cobalt magnet which has Curie constants >1000 K. However, in the realm of medical usage, this relatively low Curie constant is more than adequate to be compatible with physiologic processes.

Magnetic Field Strengths of Common Objects

Earth	0.5G
Household magnet	50–100G
Nd-Fe-B magnet	2000–12,500G
MRI	15,000–40,000G

Because of its overall magnetic strength and its relatively low cost of manufacture, Nd-Fe-B magnets have rapidly permeated into many aspects of modern life. Today, Nd-Fe-B magnets can be found in nearly every sector of consumer electronics including computer hard drives, speakers, power steering in cars, and hybrid automobiles. It is also the primary type of magnets used in medical and surgical devices.

Not only is neodymium crucial for medical and industrial usage; it also has an important place in the global geopolitical landscape. As noted earlier, contrary to their name, rare-earth elements are not particularly rare. They are simply rare in the United States and the rest of the western hemisphere. More than 90% of the global production of rare-earth metals is in one country, China [14]. China has historically exercised tight production control over rare-earth metals and has used this command on supply as an important leverage in global trade and security negotiations [15]. Because of the indispensable role that neodymium and other rare-earth metals play in our modern economy, securing its supply source has become a major national security priority for the United States and other western nations.

Elemental Magnetic Toxicity

Table 2.1 lists several important potential toxicities related to magnets. In its elemental form, neodymium is toxic to cells. At the cellular level, oxidative stress is believed to the main source of toxicity [16]. Neodymium is readily oxidized and, in the process, produces reactive oxygen species (ROS) which are cytotoxic. Donohue and colleagues reported results of in vitro testing of elemental magnetic toxicity [17]. They tested uncoated magnetized, uncoated demagnetized, coated magnetized, and uncoated demagnetized versions of the magnets to determine whether they were cytotoxic to either L929 mouse fibroblasts and/or human mucosal fibroblasts. They found that the coated magnetized, uncoated magnetized, and uncoated demagnetized versions of the magnet were cytotoxic to both cell lines. The coated demagnetized version of neodymium was also cytotoxic to the human mucosal fibroblast. They concluded that because these magnets were demagnetized, the observed cytotoxicity can only be attributed to the leaching of the metallic particles rather than the magnetic field itself.

Elemental neodymium can also have other physiologic toxicities. Dusts of the element, when inhaled, can cause lung embolisms. Accumulated elemental exposure can cause liver damage. Neodymium dusts are also irritating to the eye and other mucosal surfaces [12]. Other

Table 2.1 List of possible toxicities related to magnets

Elemental toxicities	Device toxicities
Oxidative stress to cells	Tissue injury (magnet shatter)
Pulmonary embolism (inhaled magnet dust)	Gastrointestinal complications following ingestion
Toxicity to alveolar macrophages (inhaled magnet dust)	Possible carcinogenicity

in vitro testing also demonstrated significant cytotoxicity to rat pulmonary alveolar macrophages, prompting investigators to consider these compounds to be cytotoxic to lung tissues as well [18].

Coating

In addition to their toxicity in pure elemental form, neodymium is also extremely susceptible to environmental corrosion, much more so than many of its REE counterparts. If left untreated, neodymium oxidizes rapidly when in contact with the air and moisture of the surrounding environment leading to rust and breakage. They are also very brittle and can break easily [19]. Therefore, for neodymium magnets to be useful, they must be coated with other more stable materials. Common industrial coating materials include nickel, which is the most commonly used nonmedical coating material. It has the advantage of being durable, low cost, and can withstand moderate abrasion and humidity [20]. Zinc is another commonly used coating material. It has the advantage of being highly resistant to environmental corrosion but not to salt water. Other common industrial coating materials include gold, epoxy, chrome, and Teflon.

Unlike coating for industrial use, coating of medical use has significantly more stringent prerequisites. In order for these otherwise brittle and toxic substance to be used safely in patients, coating must be durable, must not leach, and must be biocompatible. The two most commonly used medical-grade coating materials are parylene and titanium.

Parylene is a synthetic carbon polymer that is commonly used to coat a variety of medical and surgical materials, such as electrical surgical instruments used in laparoscopy [21]. It has the significant advantage of being chemically inert and biocompatible and has a long history of FDA approval for its usage in medical and surgical devices. It is often used as the initial coating, which is applied shortly after the neodymium magnet is produced in order to prevent any potential environmental corrosion.

Titanium coating provides the magnet with good chemical stability and corrosion resistance. Because of these characteristics, it has been used frequently in dental and surgical applications [22]. Some devices, especially those intended for long-term implantation into patients, are coated with more than one layer of coating in order to ensure safety. For example, the LINX device used in anti-reflux surgery, which has a Nd-Fe-B core, is coated with a parylene inner coating and then encased in a laser welded titanium outer coating. Other less frequently used material also includes RGD peptides, fibronectin, and dextran [16].

Physiologic Effects of Magnets

In addition to its elemental toxicities, neodymium magnets can also have many physical barriers to their safe use. As noted earlier, unlike the typical household magnets, these neodymium magnets exert a significantly stronger magnetic force. When brought sufficiently close, these magnets can snap together with such force and speed that they shatter. Moreover, any bodily tissue that is unfortunate enough to be in the trajectory of this uncontrolled force of attraction can sustain significant injury [12].

Once a Nd-Fe-B magnet is hermetically sealed with the proper coating material, there remains another category of potential physiologic toxicity that must be addressed: the magnetic field exerted by the device itself. The strength of electromagnetic forces exerted between any two objects diminishes exponentially as the distance between them increases. Therefore, the external force exerted by any magnetic hardware that a patient has will dissipate rapidly as the distance from the hardware grows.

Several areas of concern come to mind with respect to the potential physiologic toxicities that a magnetic device can exert. First is implanted cardiac defibrillators and pacemakers. Most of these devices are designed to turn off in the presence of a magnetic field. For example, many surgical patients with either implanted defibrillators or pacemakers will have a magnet placed over their chest to turn these devices off in order to prevent potential hazardous inference with electrical surgical instruments [23]. The safe threshold for most implanted defibrillators and pacemakers is to keep the magnetic field strength <5 Gauss. Studies have found that patients with implanted pacemakers can undergo MRI examination with systems that produce a static field strength of up to 1.5 T without any clinically significant adverse events [24]. Another theoretical concern is the potential of the implanted magnetic device to disrupt inherent cardiac electrical activity. However, this level of disruption will require a magnetic force significantly larger than anything possessed by the devices in use today.

Furthermore, an important consideration of any potential cardiac interference is the distance of the implanted device from the chest. For most intra-abdominal procedures involving magnets, this is a much smaller concern. As previously described, the force exerted by a magnet decreases exponentially as the distance from it increases. Most intra-abdominal devices are implanted sufficiently far from the chest to have any clinically meaningful cardiac effect. One potential exception is for devices that are placed sufficiently close to the chest where the magnetic strength becomes less negligible. For example, the LINX device used in anti-reflux procedures is placed just inferior to the diaphragm. The LINX device partially mitigates this concern with its geometry. Because the ultimate force and strength of a magnetic substance is determined by many factors including its shape, the implanted geometry is an important consideration. When the LINX device is opened, up, and straight, it exerts a magnetic field extending out to 7 cm. However, when the device is deployed and implanted in its final circular configuration, its magnetic field only extends to 2 cm [25]. Moreover, the LINX geometry also affects its MRI compatibility. When the device is implanted in a closed circular fashion, beads do not fly off toward the powerful magnetic force generated by the MRI. Instead, the entire circular device contorts its shape from an "O" configuration to a "D" configuration in the presence of a strong magnetic field. A more realistic concern is how a powerful MRI may demagnetize some of the LINX beads, which would affect its overall function and performance.

Another potential concern for these devices is whether the magnetic field generated by the device itself poses a danger to another person in the vicinity using a device that is magnetically sensitive. Once again, because the strength of the potential magnetic attraction drops exponentially with distance, this is often not a major source of concern. Nonetheless, some magnetic devices have a ferromagnetic shield on the outside in order to further decrease any potential unintended ambient magnetic field [26].

A more worrisome concern is accidental ingestion. When more than one piece of these magnets is ingested, they can be lodged in different portions of the gastrointestinal tract. The magnets can then be attracted toward one another, and they exert a sufficiently strong magnetic force to cause bowel obstruction, bowel wall necrosis, fistulae, and bowel perforation [27].

As the use of magnetic devices in medicine and surgery increases, one additional area of potential concern is the physiologic tolerance of long-term exposure to these devices. In particular, the specter of potential carcinogenic effects from long-term exposure to magnetic fields has been raised. The carcinogenic effects of several members of the electromagnetic spectrum (e.g., X-ray, gamma-ray) are well-known. However, most data on the cancer-causing effects of the electromagnetic spectrum have been on ionizing radiations such as X-rays and gamma-rays. Magnetic fields are nonionizing. For example, when patients undergo MRI scans, they can be exposed to radiofrequency in the 1 MHz to 100 MHz range, and there is no known adverse immediate or long-term effect [28].

What about long-term baseline exposure, such as to an implanted device or to a household appliance? Several epidemiological studies have been done examining potential links between exposure to nonionizing electromagnetic radiation and childhood leukemias. Most recent studies have not demonstrated a definitive link between nonionizing electromagnetic radiation and childhood leukemia [29]. An earlier study from the 1970s did suggest a possible link [30].

With regard to adult exposure, the data is similarly inconclusive. Vast majorities of epidemiological studies do not find a definitive linkage between nonionizing electromagnetic radiation and adult malignancies [31]. A few studies suggested a possible association [32]. The International Agency for Research on Cancer (IARC) empaneled a group of experts to evaluate the evidence linking nonionizing electromagnetic radiation to cancer in 2002. The group concluded that extremely low frequency electric and magnetic fields are "possibly carcinogenic to humans." They also classified static electric and magnetic fields as "not classifiable as to their carcinogenicity to humans" [33]. More recently, the European Commission's Scientific Committee on Emerging and Newly Identified Health Risks examined the available data concerning the link between nonionizing electromagnetic radiation and cancer. They concluded that extremely low frequency electric and magnetic fields harbored "an increased risk of childhood leukemias" with daily exposure greater than 0.3–0.4 μT [34]. Finally, studies examining potential risks to offspring with maternal exposure during pregnancy have similarly yielded inconclusive findings [35, 36].

While definitive long-term exposure data in humans is still accumulating, one of the greatest existing bodies of knowledge involving permanently implanted magnetic devices can be found in the veterinary literature. The "cow magnet" is a "a stack of cylindrical permanent magnets having intermediate disk-like spacers of a soft magnet material forming a tubular sleeve" [37] (Fig. 2.4). Because ruminants are not particularly discriminating when it comes to diet, they are at an increased risk of inadvertently ingesting loose hardware, which could result in obstruction or perforation. The cow magnet is administered to ruminants; following its ingestion, it is lodged in one of their four stomachs [38]. It resides there and attracts, thereby sequesters, all the loose nails, wires, and other metallic debris the animal consumes. The cow magnet in essence acts as the nucleus of a pseudobezoar. By sequestering these metallic debris in the rumen stomach, the cow magnet helps to prevent downstream migration of these debris and any potential obstruction or perforation. Within the available veterinary literature, there is no evidence of any long-term adverse health effects that these animals experience despite the widespread use of cow magnets.

With respect to human usage of magnetic devices, the regulatory safeguards are quite stringent. The Food and Drug Administration (FDA)

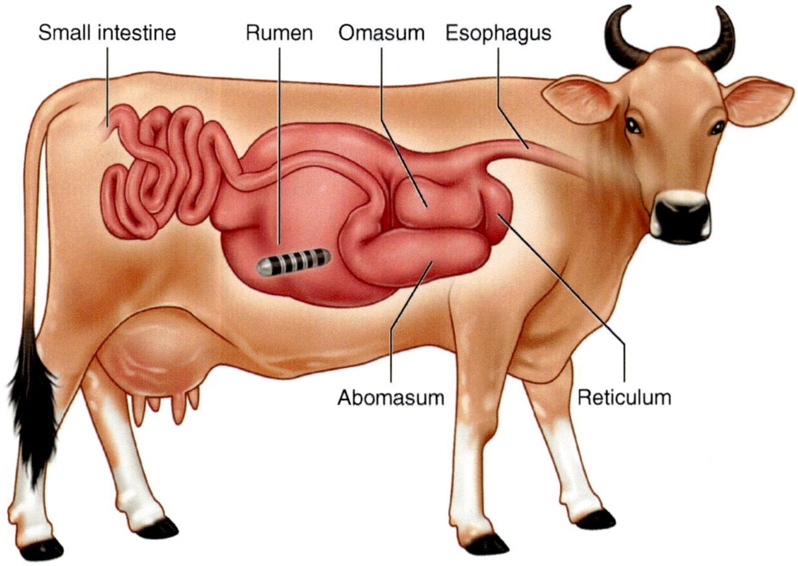

Fig. 2.4 Cow magnet. The cow magnet is ingested by the animal and then resides in one of its four stomachs. It then attracts the loose metallic debris that the cow consumes during grazing, sequestering them in the stomach, preventing the downstream migration of these debris and any potential obstruction or perforation

sets out an extensive list of biocompatibility and toxicology tests that potential devices are required to undergo. "An assessment of potential biocompatibility risk should include not only chemical toxicity, but also physical characteristics that might contribute to an unwanted tissue response. These characteristics can include surface properties, forces on surrounding tissues (e.g., electromagnetic), geometry, and presence of particulates" [39]. The exact level of scrutiny a potential device must undergo depends on the location and duration of the intended implant. The FDA divides implantation duration into three groups. Group A is for "limited" duration of up to 24 hours. Group B is for "prolonged" implantation between 24 hours and 30 days. Group C is for "permanent" implantation, which is >30 days. If the device is intended for implant <24 hours, and it only contacts tissue or bone, there are five categories of testing required: cytotoxicity, sensitization, irritation or intracutaneous reactivity, acute systemic toxicity, and material-mediated pyrogenicity. However, for any permanent implants (>30 days), in addition to these five categories, the potential devices must also undergo testing in subacute/subchronic toxicity, genotoxicity, implantation, and chronic toxicity.

Examples of Medical Usage of Nd-Fe-B Magnets

A detailed description of each of the following examples is beyond the scope of this introductory chapter, and a more detailed review of these devices will be provided in subsequent chapters. Nonetheless, it is worth briefly mentioning several examples to help highlight some of the principles covered earlier in the chapter as well as the importance of Nd-Fe-B magnets in the medical and surgical world.

Magnetic Mini-Mover

This is a device used in pediatric patients with pectus excavatum ("sunken chest"). It uses magnetic force to gradually remodel the chest deformity. A magnet is implanted on the sternum and is paired with an external magnetic brace [40]. This allows the device to apply a sustained outward force on the sternum. With time and force adjustment, the depressed chest gradually remodels until it assumes the correct anatomic position. An important factor to consider is the potential magnetic interference that the device could have on the nearby mediastinal organs. At a distance of 1 cm, which is the minimal distance from the sternum to the heart, the magnetic field strength is ~0.04 T, which is below the accepted safety limit [26, 41]. This once again invokes the principle that the force exerted by a magnetic substance diminishes exponentially with increased distance.

Magnamosis

This is a device that uses magnetic force to construct gastrointestinal anastomoses. It employs two convex-concave radially symmetric halves that, when brought together, will magnetically self-align [42]. Each half is made of a ring-shaped Nd-Fe-B magnet encased in a specially engineered polycarbonate coating. The two halves are inserted into the respective gastrointestinal segments to be anastomosed, they are then brought to close proximity, and the magnetic force attracts and aligns them. As described earlier, Nd-Fe-B is among the strongest magnetic substance available. Their magnetic force between the two halves will compress the bowel wall, and after the anastomosis is matured, the two halves are passed into the bowel lumen and excreted [43].

LINX

This device is implanted around the distal esophagus in patients with significant gastroesophageal reflux disease. The constriction provided by the deployed device helps to reinforce the lower esophageal sphincter. The potential magnetic interference with mediastinal organs was described above [25]. The LINX devices employ the principles of distance and geometry in its design to take advantage of the Nd-Fe-B magnet while mitigating its potential adverse effects. One challenge with this device is that ferromagnetic objects such as surgical and laparoscopic instruments or other metallic implants can be attracted to it if brought sufficiently close. This can be mitigated as more ferromagnetically insulated instruments are developed.

Conclusion

Since their discovery in antiquity, magnets and magnetic properties have played a major role in our scientific and technologic evolution. Today, magnets play an indispensable role in medical technology. Understanding the basic properties of magnets has enabled us to discover increasing numbers of diagnostic and therapeutic niches for these elements. This chapter provided an introductory overview of these properties and their consequences for medical use. In the coming chapters, you will explore, in depth, the various medical uses of magnetic derivatives.

References

1. Mills A. The lodestone: history, physics, formation. Ann Sci. 2004;61(3):273–319.
2. Chen C-W. Magnetism and metallurgy of soft materials. Elsevier; 1977.
3. Campbell WH. Chapter 1 – Nature's magnetism. In: Campbell WH, editor. Earth magnetism. San Diego: Academic Press; 2001. p. 1–23.
4. Cullity BD, Graham CD. Diamagnetism and paramagnetism. In: Introduction to magnetic materials. 2nd ed. Wiley-IEEE Press; 2008.
5. Miyazaki T, Jin H. The physics of ferromagnetism. 1st ed. Berlin Heidelberg: Springer; 2012.
6. Courtillot V, Le Mouël J-L. The study of Earth's magnetism (1269–1950): a foundation by Peregrinus and subsequent development of geomagnetism and paleomagnetism. Rev Geophys. 2007;45(3):1–31.
7. Robinson A. Powerful new magnet material found. Science. 1984;223(4639):920–2.
8. Zhou P, Lin D, Xiao Y, Lambert N, Rahman MA. Temperature-dependent demagnetization model of permanent magnets for finite element analysis. IEEE Trans Magn. 2012;48(2):1031–4.
9. Castle E, Sheridan R, Zhou W, Grasso S, Walton A, Reece MJ. High coercivity, anisotropic, heavy rare earth-free Nd-Fe-B by Flash Spark Plasma Sintering. Sci Rep. 2017;7(1):11134.
10. Kimura TGT, Shintani K, Ischizaka K, Arima T, Tokura Y. Magnetic control of ferroelectric polarization. Nature. 2003;426:55–8.
11. Panichev AM. Rare earth elements: review of medical and biological properties and their abundance in the rock materials and mineralized spring waters in the context of animal and human geophagia reasons evaluation. Achiev Life Sci. 2015;9(2):95–103.
12. Rim KT, Koo KH, Park JS. Toxicological evaluations of rare earths and their health impacts to workers: a literature review. Saf Health Work. 2013;4(1):12–26.
13. Charlton JR, Pearl VM, Denotti AR, Lee JB, Swaminathan S, Scindia YM, et al. Biocompatibility of ferritin-based nanoparticles as targeted MRI contrast agents. Nanomedicine. 2016;12(6):1735–45.
14. Binnemans K, Jones PT, Blanpain B, Van Gerven T, Yang Y, Walton A, et al. Recycling of rare earths: a critical review. J Clean Prod. 2013;51:1–22.
15. Bradsher K. China acts to tighten grasp on Rare Earth production. New York Times. 2011; Published on 2/16/2011. Retrieved on 1/13/2019.
16. Markides H, Rotherham M, El Haj AJ. Biocompatibility and toxicity of magnetic nanoparticles in regenerative medicine. J Nanomater. 2012;2012:1–11.
17. Donohue VEMF, Evans R. In vitro cytotoxicity testing of neodymium-Iron-boron magnets. J Appl Biomater. 1995;6(6):69–74.
18. Palmer RJ, Butenhoff JL, Stevens JB. Cytotoxicity of the rare earth metals cerium, lanthanum, and neodymium in vitro: comparisons with cadmium in a pulmonary macrophage primary culture system. Environ Res. 1987;43(1):142–56.
19. Croat JJ. Current status and future outlook for bonded neodymium permanent magnets (invited). J Appl Phys. 1997;81(8):4804–9.
20. Minowa T, Yoshikawa M, Honshima M. Improvement of the corrosion resistance on Nd-Fe-B magnet with nickel plating. IEEE Trans Magn. 1989;25(5):3776–8.
21. Noar JH, Wahab A, Evans RD, Wojcik AG. The durability of parylene coatings on neodymium-iron-boron magnets. Eur J Orthod. 1999;21:685–93.
22. Noar JH, Evans R. Rare earth magnets in orthodontics: an overview. Br J Orthod. 1999;26(1):29–37.
23. Mangar D, Atlas GM, Kane P. Electrocautery-induced pacemaker malfunction during surgery. Can J Anaesth. 1991;38(5):616–8.
24. Martin ET, Coman JA, Shellock FG, Pulling CC, Fair R, Jenkins K. Magnetic resonance imaging and cardiac pacemaker safety at 1.5-Tesla. J Am Coll Cardiol. 2004;43(7):1315–24.
25. Inc TM. Memo re: patients with previous metallic or electrical implants LINX Reflux Management System 2012.
26. Harrison MR, Estefan-Ventura D, Fechter R, Moran AM Jr, Christensen D. Magnetic Mini-Mover

Procedure for pectus excavatum: I. Development, design, and simulations for feasibility and safety. J Pediatr Surg. 2007;42(1):81–5; discussion 5–6.
27. Cauchi JA, Shawis RN. Multiple magnet ingestion and gastrointestinal morbidity. Arch Dis Child. 2002;87:539–40.
28. Zamanian A, Hardiman C. Electromagnetic radiation and human health: a review of sources and effects. High Frequency Electronics. 2005;4(3):16–26.
29. Kheifets L, Ahlbom A, Crespi CM, Draper G, Hagihara J, Lowenthal RM, et al. Pooled analysis of recent studies on magnetic fields and childhood leukaemia. Br J Cancer. 2010;103(7):1128–35.
30. Wertheimer N, Leeper E. Electrical wiring configurations and childhood cancer. Am J Epidemiol. 1979;109(3):273–84.
31. Schoenfeld EROLE, Henderson K, Grimson R, Kabat GC, Ahnn S, Kaune WT, Gammon MD, Leske MC, EBCLIS Group. Electromagnetic fields and breast cancer on Long Island: a case-control study. Am J Epidemiol. 2003;158(1):47–58.
32. Kluiukiene JTT, Andersen A. Residential and occupational exposures to 50-Hz magnetic fields and breast cancer in women: a population-based study. Am J Epidemiol. 2004;159(9):852–61.
33. Cancer WIAfRo. Non-ionizing radiation, part I: static and extremely low-frequency (ELF) electric and magnetic fields IRARC monographs on the evaluation of carcinogenic risks to humans. IARC Monogr Eval Carcinog Risks Hum. 2002;80:1.
34. Risks SCoEaNIH. Opinion on: Potential health effects of exposure to electromagnetic fields (EMF). SCENIHR. 2015.
35. Hug K, Grize L, Seidler A, Kaatsch P, Schuz J. Parental occupational exposure to extremely low frequency magnetic fields and childhood cancer: a German case-control study. Am J Epidemiol. 2010;171(1):27–35.
36. Infante-Rivard C, Deadman J. Maternal occupational exposure to extremely low frequency magnetic fields during pregnancy and childhood leukemia. Epidemiology. 2003;14(4):437–41.
37. Mozis, et al. Cow Magnet United States Patent. 1991; Patient No. 4,992,768.
38. Partington BP, Biller D. Radiography of the bovine cranioventral abdomen veterinary radiology and ultrasound. Vet Radiol Ultrasound. 1991;32(4):155–68.
39. Administration FaD. Use of International Standard ISO 10993-1, “Biological evaluation of medical devices - Part 1: Evaluation and testing within a risk management process”. Guidance for Industry and Food and Drug Administration Staff. 2016.
40. Harrison MR, Gonzales KD, Bratton BJ, Christensen D, Curran PF, Fechter R, et al. Magnetic mini-mover procedure for pectus excavatum III: safety and efficacy in a Food and Drug Administration-sponsored clinical trial. J Pediatr Surg. 2012;47(1):154–9.
41. Jamshidi R, Harrison M. Magnet-mediated thoracic remodeling: a new approach to the sunken chest. Expert Rev Med Devices. 2007;4(3):283–6.
42. Pichakron KO, Jelin EB, Hirose S, Curran PF, Jamshidi R, Stephenson JT, et al. Magnamosis II: magnetic compression anastomosis for minimally invasive gastrojejunostomy and jejunojejunostomy. J Am Coll Surg. 2011;212(1):42–9.
43. Jamshidi R, Stephenson JT, Clay JG, Pichakron KO, Harrison MR. Magnamosis: magnetic compression anastomosis with comparison to suture and staple techniques. J Pediatr Surg. 2009;44(1):222–8.

History of Magnets Used in Surgery

3

Michel Gagner

Introduction

This chapter deals with limited magnetic interventional applications for the abdomen and thorax, mainly gastrointestinal, biliary, colorectal, urological, and vascular applications. The time period studied was also taken into consideration, more specifically for the last 50 years, as very little was accomplished with the use of magnets in medicine before this time.

Colorectal Applications

Feustel and Hennig published an interesting article in German in 1975, entitled "Continent colostomy through magnetic closure in animal experiments on dogs" [1]. Canine experiments of a continent colostomy using magnetic occlusion were performed, with a silicon-coated ring magnet placed between muscular fascia and subcutaneous fascia (Fig. 3.1). Afterward, an end colon was pulled through the lumen of the ring and sutured to the skin. They demonstrated no leakage of gas and feces beneath the magnetic cap, and when the cap was removed, spontaneous defecation took place with expulsion of feces and gas. Hence, they moved to humans and published the same year in a different journal, also in German, the article entitled "Kontinente Kolostomie durch MagnetverschluB" [2], where continent colostomies were achieved by using a similar implanted circular magnet positioned subcutaneously and using a magnetic cover to provide sealing on top. Used in 17 patients after proctectomy where a permanent colostomy is inevitable, this device was proven to be highly successful. However, no long-term follow-up paper has been published by this team, and one wonders if long-term problems of erosion and skin breakthrough over time have relegated this to the past.

A Mount Sinai School of Medicine colorectal team was inspired by the German experience and published a small series of 12 dogs in 1977 [3]. They had one extrusion after a period of 8 months and two strictures that were easily dilated. Fortunately, no sinuses, fistulas, or infections were demonstrated. Their concerns were about the toxicity of the Erlangen magnet ring implanted, since it consisted of a samarium-cobalt magnetic ring encased in methyl methacrylate. No cobalt toxicity was ever demonstrated. It provided a force of 4–5 newtons over a distance of 10–30 mm (Fig. 3.2). This ring (Fig. 3.3) was implanted subcutaneously in the anterior abdominal wall around the stoma, and 4–6 weeks later, the cap obturated the colostomy. Germans followed with a paper published 3 years later [4], now called the "Erlangen magnetic stoma seal", and proposed it for ileostomies, not just colostomies. They stated it to be a simple technique but requiring proper

M. Gagner (✉)
Hôpital du Sacré-Cœur de Montréal, Montréal, QC, Canada

Chief of Surgery, Westmount Square Surgical Center, Westmount, QC, Canada

M. Gagner (ed.), *Magnetic Surgery*, https://doi.org/10.1007/978-3-030-73947-8_3

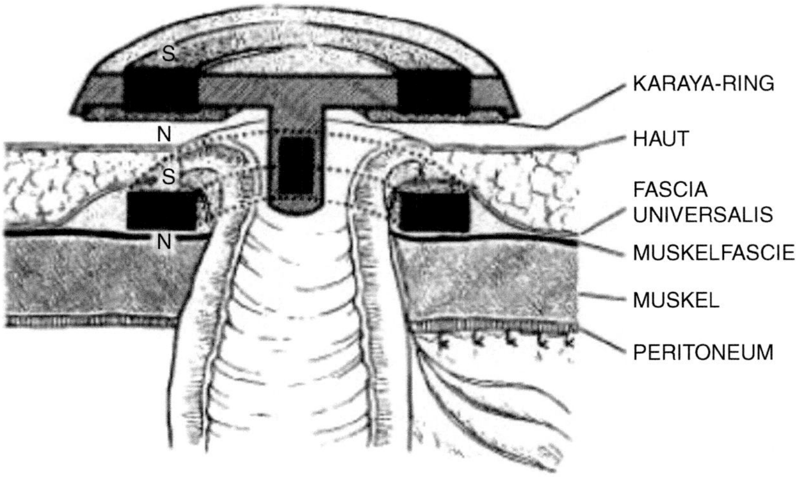

Fig. 3.1 The Erlangen magnet ring for stoma closure. The deeper ring is placed on the fascia, allowing fat and skin underneath, and the colon is sutured to the skin, passed through the ring. The cap is also magnetic but has a center rod, the karaya ring being on the skin itself between the two magnetic structures. (From Feustel et al. [1]. Reprinted with permission from Springer Nature)

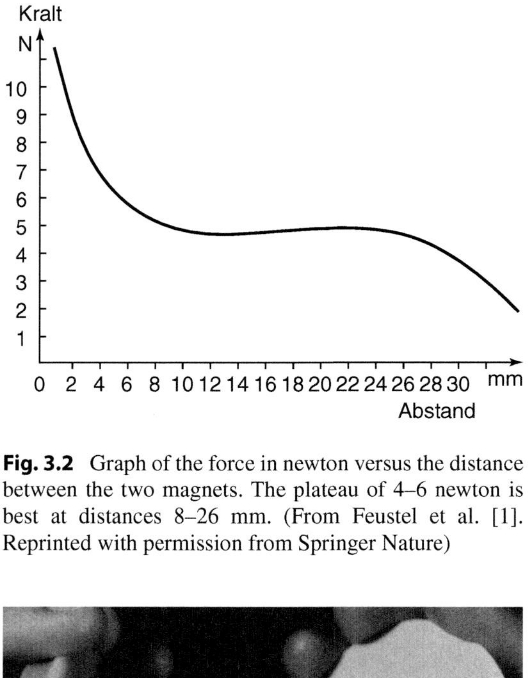

Fig. 3.2 Graph of the force in newton versus the distance between the two magnets. The plateau of 4–6 newton is best at distances 8–26 mm. (From Feustel et al. [1]. Reprinted with permission from Springer Nature)

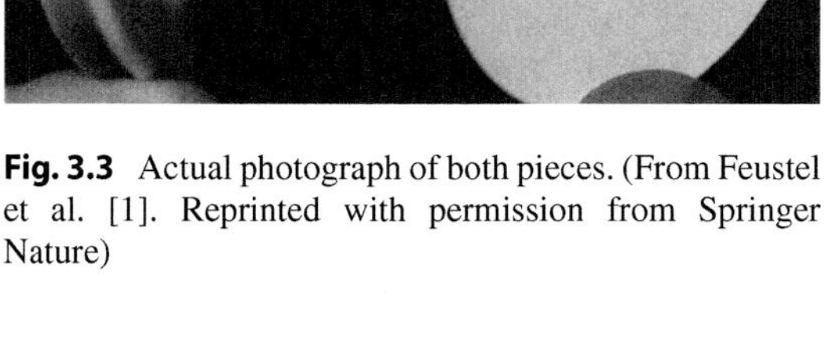

Fig. 3.3 Actual photograph of both pieces. (From Feustel et al. [1]. Reprinted with permission from Springer Nature)

patient selection and best performed in a colorectal unit where stoma therapists can follow carefully the patients, because approximately 15% of patients have adverse events requiring magnet explantation. Furthermore, continence is not always achieved. They tempered their enthusiasm in 1978, by stating that magnetic stoma seal requires further developments.

A much larger experience was gathered and published in 1984 by a different team [5]. The Erlangen magnetic ring colostomy closure was used in 240 patients, and close to 20% had to be explanted because of infection, pressure necrosis, parastomal hernia, invagination, prolapse, and stenosis. Continence was achieved in 68% of patients. By the mid-1980s, it was slowly being abandoned by patients. Only 43% of patients were still using the system, and many complained about the pain and weight. Improved techniques of coloanal anastomosis, sphincter preserving, and better stoma bags technology have relegated the Erlangen ring progressively.

Colorectal anastomoses using magnetic rings were tackled later in 1981 by Jansen et al. [6]. A device like the Erlangen magnetic ring was inserted in the bowel lumen to create a circular apposition. Progressive compression led to necrosis of the mucosal, submucosal, and serosa layers. The magnetic force was progressively increased with diminishing distances (especially below 6 mm), while intestinal healing took place.

The series of 21 patients included 11 sigmoidectomies and 9 low anterior resections. These magnets were obviously positioned by an open technique, as laparoscopic bowel surgery really started around 1990. After 7 to 12 days, the magnets cut through and migrated from the anastomotic space distally by intestinal peristalsis and eventually evacuated through the anus. Dehiscence of the connection was noted in two instances (10%). One patient required reoperation. Another patient had a small area of dehiscence at the anastomosis, noted after evacuation of an infected hematoma with a further uncomplicated course. So, one could say that imperfect healing took place in 15% of cases, a percentage too high to make it in the regular clinical arena at that time. One patient died on the third postoperative day of a recurrent myocardial infarct. Of the remaining 18 patients, primary bowel continuity was demonstrated radiographically and by endoscopy.

A Russian period of investigations followed with the study by Isakov et al. published in 1982 in Khirurgiia [7], concerning resection of the large intestine using permanent magnets. The translated title is misleading as it is the anastomosis and not the resection itself in which the magnets are used. In 1984, Stepanov et al. published an experience on the use of permanent magnets in digestive tract surgery in children [8].

Another team used permanent magnets in suture-free anastomoses in 1987 [9]. It includes an experimental design in 25 dogs, where creation of compressive intestinal anastomoses with the help of permanent magnets permitted "end-to-end" and "side-to-side" anastomoses in large and small intestines. The magnets were eliminated united, with necrotized walls, transanally on the 4–5th and 9–10th days after intervention. Further, the paper describes a small experience in six patients. In 1992 Stepanov et al. published (also in Russian) on the treatment of intestinal fistulae in children by applying a bypass anastomosis using magnetic devices [10]. Ten years had passed since the first paper in Russia, and this time they described a very specific application for the exclusion of intestinal fistulas by the formation of bypass anastomoses via a permanent magnet. The variants of the techniques of magnetic bypass anastomoses were discussed after the results of 46 children treated for external intestinal fistulas were elaborated. The mortality rate among children with intestinal fistulas operations decreased from 31% to 13%.

Vascular Applications

In 1978 Obora, Tamaki and Matsumoto published an avant-garde paper on using magnet rings to perform non-sutured microvascular anastomosis [11]. It took only 8.3 minutes for the anastomosis completion with a very high rate of patency. Obviously, these were inserted via an open vascular opening. According to histological studies, the vascular wall is continuous, and authors had declared this method to be simple, rapid, and reliable for the creation of microvascular anastomosis. Full data and the technique description were published in Japanese 2 years later in 1980, although unfortunately not very accessible [12]. The devices are well described in Figs. 3.4, 3.5, and 3.6. End-to-end anastomosis in animals was possible for very small vessels with diameters of up to 1 mm with an overall patency

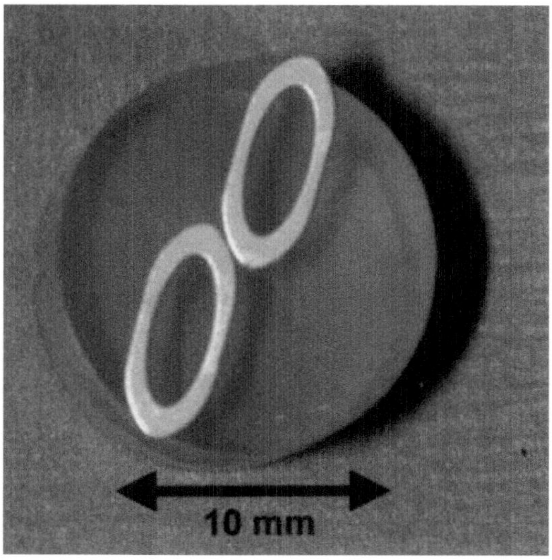

Fig. 3.4 Schematic representation of the small vessel magnet devices for microvascular anastomosis. (From Erdmann et al. [13]. Reprinted with permission from Elsevier)

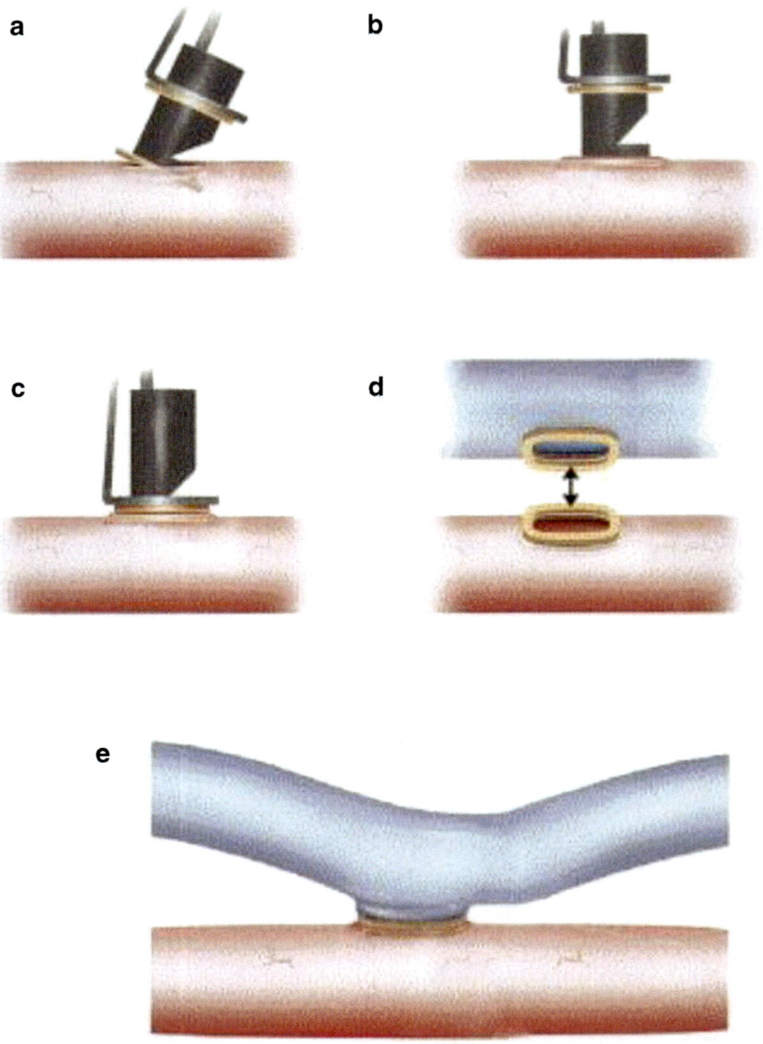

Fig. 3.5 Technical steps for a side-to-side vascular anastomosis. (**a**) Arteriotomy made, following with the insertion into the lumen of the inner magnet. (**b**) Inner magnet fully into the lumen and pulled against the wall. (**c**) External magnet descent against the inner magnet. (**d**) Same is created in a vein. (**e**) After full apposition. (From Erdmann et al. [13]. Reprinted with permission from Elsevier)

rate of 90%, requiring 8.0 minutes on average. In cases of end-to-side anastomosis, the patency rate was less at 84%, requiring 8.4 minutes on average [13]. Using electromagnetic flowmeter in end-to-end anastomosis, measurement showed no difference in blood flow between control and operated vessels. In end-to-side anastomosis, blood flow at the donor and recipient vessels were the same.

Histological examination in animals performed at 20 days after anastomosis revealed a continuity of the media and the intima, and after 180 days no abnormalities were defined. Finally, no disruption and flattening of longitudinal endothelial folds on the inner surface of the vessels were observed using electron microscopy. Further it showed that magnetic forces did not have any deleterious effect on vessel walls and surrounding tissues.

Urological Applications

Isakov et al., who had previously used bigger magnets for colo-intestinal anastomoses [7], used a smaller modified version for the treatment of urethral strictures in children in 1989 [14]. This article is in Russian and not easily accessible in

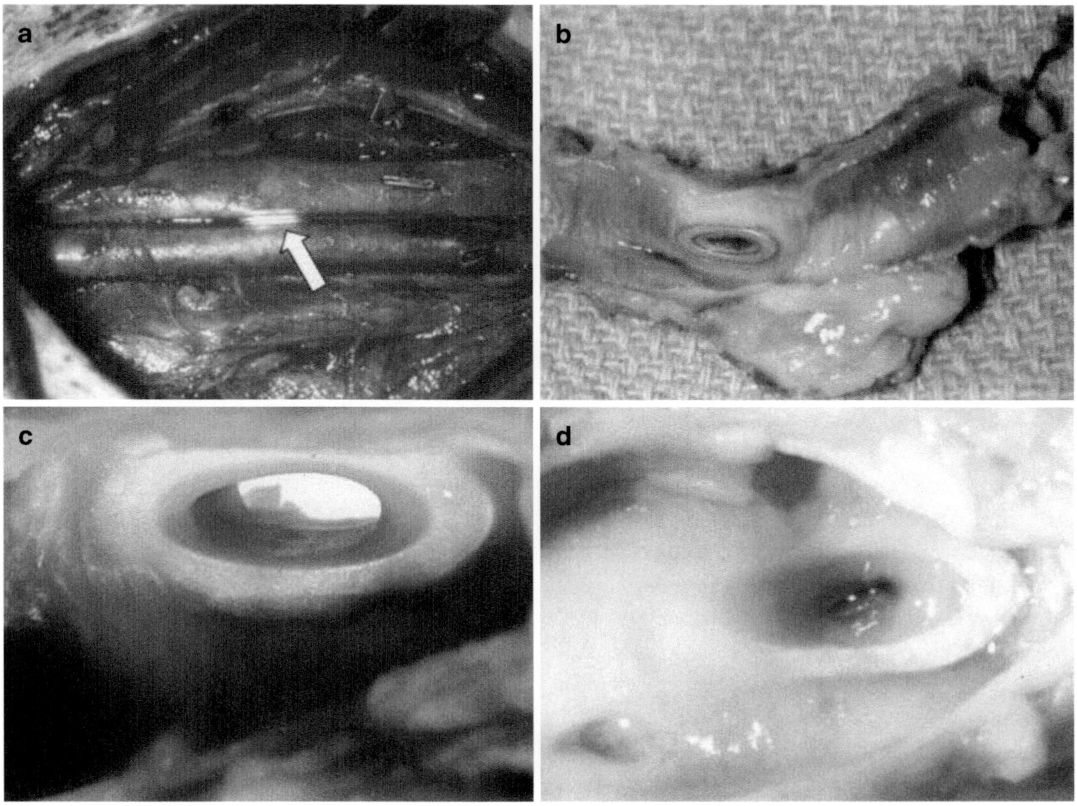

Fig. 3.6 Macroscopic aspects, after the anastomosis. (**a**) External view of the oval-shaped magnets, one being inside each vessel, and two external ones sticking to each other. (**b**) Internal view. (**c**) Tunnel created. (**d**) Vascular epithelialization. (From Erdmann et al. [13]. Reprinted with permission from Elsevier)

Western countries. Described are the results of treatment of posttraumatic strictures of the urethra in 34 children.

Permanent magnets were used to treat urethra strictures in dogs initially. Then children were treated. The results of a comparative group using the traditional surgical repair (19 patients) and by the proposed magnet method (15 patients) showed a twofold decrease in recurrences and complications during the follow-up period.

Biliary Applications

In 1993, a Russian team led by Savalev et al. published an experimental method of endoscopic biliodigestive anastomosis with the use of magnets (experimental and clinical study) [15]. Two variants of establishing postponed compression cholecystogastric anastomoses were developed in experiments on a model of obstructive jaundice in 50 inbred dogs, a variant of cholecystoenteric and enteroenteric anastomoses with the use of endoscopic techniques, which may be conducted in clinical practice.

Following this experimental protocol, procedures were performed in 16 patients, 4 cholecystogastrostomies, 1 cholecysto-duodenostomy, 10 choledocho-duodenostomies, and a single hepatico-duodenostomy. These operations were performed in patients with advanced nonresectable neoplasms, especially with distal obstruction of the common bile duct nonresectable and/or having a much higher operative risk with associated mortality. Technical details were published in English in the Journal of Laparoendoscopic surgery the same year [16]. The experiments carried out at the department of

Surgery at the Russian State Medical University in Moscow included a new type of combined endoscopic-laparoscopic surgery called magnetic cholecystodigestive anastomoses, as an alternative to conventional palliative treatment of mechanical neoplastic common bile duct obstruction. As the name indicates, this is achieved by endoscopic technique. Two methods of creating delayed magnetic cholecystogastric anastomoses and one modality of implanting cholecystoenteric and enteroenteric anastomosis have been worked out from series of experiment implemented on 50 mongrel dogs with obstructive jaundice, as stated before.

It requires a laparoscopic cholecystostomy to drop ring-shaped or rectangular magnets in the gallbladder, with simultaneous magnets transported into the stomach. Following the canine surgical research methodology, humans were treated. Specifically, four endoscopic cholecystogastric anastomoses and one cholecystoduodenal anastomosis were performed on patients suffering from malignant obstructions of the distal bile duct, mostly due to adenocarcinoma of the head of the pancreas. The preliminary results indicated that endoscopic magnetic cholecystodigestive anastomoses could serve as a form of palliative treatment of distal bile duct malignant obstructions. The Japanese took over after 2000 [17].

Gastric Applications

Cope described compression gastroenterostomy by means of the oral, percutaneous, or surgical introduction of magnets in a feasibility study in swine published in 1995 [18], in fact with two manuscripts back to back [19].

Of the nine surviving pigs, there were seven completely patent anastomoses and one partially patent anastomosis at 7–13 days. At 5 days, the anastomosis was not patent in the remaining animal. One anastomosis became occluded at 30 days. There was no anastomotic leakage, infection, or bleeding. This study revealed the difficulty of making magnetic anastomosis in thicker, more muscular tissue like stomach. These anastomoses had to be done with a minimal diameter; otherwise patency was limited. All anastomoses showed good apposition with no leakage and minimal inflammation. Anastomoses were fully patent in four CJs and one CG (mean, 12 days), partially patent in one CJ and one CG (mean, 15 days), and not patent in two CGs. Best results were noted with jacketed disc magnets with cutting rims and a 400–600-g pull. The rare-earth magnets were significantly weakened by gas sterilization in the first four CG experiments.

Two of four magnets used in CJ were retained despite a fully patent anastomosis. A repeat study published in 2001 with longer duration shower better patency at 6 months [20]. Magnets were introduced per orally with endoscopic and fluoroscopic guidance and were mated across the gastric and jejunal walls of five dogs. After a mean of 5.5 days a 12-mm diameter YO-YO stent was placed per orally in the resulting fistula.

The gastroenteric anastomosis (GEA) with stent was observed endoscopically and gastrographically at 1- to 2-month intervals. There was no morbidity and there were no significant weight changes. The GEA was widely patent at necropsy at 6 months ($n = 4$); partial membrane separation occurred at 5 months in the fifth dog. There was minor breakage of the stent prongs in two animals. More patients have been done by the same team and published in 2005 [21]. Fifteen patients (13 men, 2 women; mean age 64.5 years) with malignant obstruction underwent endoscopic gastroenteric anastomosis using magnets (EGAM) and had monthly follow-ups between December 2001 and May 2003. The procedure was successful in 13 patients (88.66%), with a mean survival of 5 months. There were four minor complications (30.76%) during the follow-up period. It was concluded that EGAM were feasible, safe, and efficacious to create a gastroenteric anastomosis. There was no mortality related to the procedure.

References

1. Feustel H, Hennig G, Filler D, Hübner E. [Continent colostomy through magnetic closure in animal experiments on dogs]. [Article in German] Langenbecks Arch Chir. 1975;Suppl:337–40.
2. Feustel H, Koning G. Kontinente Kolostomie durch MagnetverschluB. Dtsch. med, Wschr. 1975;100:1063–4.
3. Bauer JJ, Wertkin MG, Gelernt IM, Kreel I. A continent colostomy: the magnetic stoma cap. Am J Surg. 1977;134(3):334–7.
4. Filler D, Feustel H, Schwemmle K, Muhrer KH. [Continence of anus praeter -- a problem solved? Erlangen magnetic stoma seal (author's transl)]. [Article in German]. Zentralbl Chir. 1978;103(11):706–14.
5. Husemann B, Hager T. Experience with the Erlangen magnetic ring colostomy-closure system. Int Surg. 1984;69(4):297–300.
6. Jansen A, Brummelkamp WH, Davies GA, Klopper PJ, Keeman JN. Clinical applications of magnetic rings in colorectal anastomosis. Surg Gynecol Obstet. 1981;153(4):537–45.
7. Isakov IuF, Stepanov EA, Geraskin VI, Vasilev GS, Sharipov NA. [Resection of the large intestine using permanent magnets]. [Article in Russian] Khirurgiia (Mosk). 1982;(6):102–4.
8. Stepanov EA, Vasil'ev GS, Sharipov NA, Rudakov SS, Romakhin IuA. Use of permanent magnets in digestive tract surgery in children. [Article in Russian] V.estn Akad Med Nauk SSSR. 1984;(9):6–11.
9. Myshkin KI, Dolgushin NE, Zavalёv VI. [Use of permanent magnets in suture-free anastomoses]. [Article in Russian] Vestn Khir Im I I Grek. 1987;139(7):47–51.
10. Stepanov EA, Vasil'ev GS, Nikolaev VV. [The treatment of intestinal fistulae in children by applying a by-pass anastomosis using magnetic devices]. [Article in Russian] Khirurgiia (Mosk). 1992;(11–12):93–5.
11. Obora Y, Tamaki N, Matsumoto S. Nonsuture microvascular anastomosis using magnet rings: preliminary report. Surg Neurol. 1978;9(2):117–20.
12. Obora Y, Tamaki N, Matsumoto S. [Nonsuture microvascular anastomosis using magnet rings (author's transl)]. [Article in Japanese]. Neurol Med Chir (Tokyo). 1980;20(5):497–505.
13. Erdmann D, Sweis R, Heitmann C, Yasui K, Olbrich KC, Levin LS, Sharkawy AA, Klitzman B. Side-to-side sutureless vascular anastomosis with magnets. J Vasc Surg. 2004;40:505–11.
14. Isakov IuF, Stepanov EA, Erokhin AP, Nikolaev VV, Vasi'lev GS. [Surgical treatment of urethral strictures in children]. [Article in Russian]. Vestn Khir Im I I Grek. 1989;142(4):61–6.
15. Savelév VS, Avaliani MV, Kapranov SA, Bashirov AD, Boldina TB. [Endoscopic biliodigestive anastomosis with the use of magnets (experimental and clinical study)]. [Article in Russian] Khirurgiia (Mosk). 1993;(3):10–18.
16. Saveliev VS, Avaliani MV, Bashirov AD. Endoscopic magnetic cholecystodigestive anastomoses: personal technique for palliative treatment of distal bile duct obstruction. J Laparoendosc Surg. 1993;3(2):99–112.
17. Takao S, Matsuo Y, Shinchi H, Nakajima S, Aikou T, Iseji T, Yamanouchi E. Magnetic compression anastomosis for benign obstruction of the common bile duct. Endoscopy. 2001;33(11):988–90.
18. Cope C. Creation of compression gastroenterostomy by means of the oral, percutaneous, or surgical introduction of magnets: feasibility study in swine. J Vasc Interv Radiol. 1995;6(4):539–45.
19. Cope C. Evaluation of compression cholecystogastric and cholecystojejunal anastomoses in swine after peroral and surgical introduction of magnets. J Vasc Interv Radiol. 1995;6(4):546–52.
20. Cope C, Ginsberg GG. Long-term patency of experimental magnetic compression gastroenteric anastomoses achieved with covered stents. Gastrointest Endosc. 2001;53(7):780–4.
21. Chopita N, Vaillaverde A, Cope C, Bernedo A, Martinez H, Landoni N, Jmelnitzky A, Burgos H. Endoscopic gastroenteric anastomosis using magnets. Endoscopy. 2005;37(4):313–7.

Magnetic Interventions for Gastroesophageal Reflux

4

Luigi Bonavina

Current therapy for gastroesophageal reflux disease (GERD) is generally reported to be overall unsatisfactory by gastroenterologists, surgeons, and patients. About 40% of patients are resistant or only partial responders to proton-pump inhibitors (PPI) therapy [1, 2], and even doubling the dose may be inadequate to relieve regurgitation and improve quality of life. In addition, there are growing concerns over the long-term consequences of chronic acid suppression (reduced vitamin B12 and magnesium absorption, interaction with clopidogrel, risk of *Clostridium difficile* infection, hypergastrinemia, enterochromaffin-like cell hyperplasia, parietal cell hypertrophy leading to rebound acid hypersecretion, and risk of gastric cancer) [3–5]. Lastly, PPI therapy does not have any direct pharmacologic impact on the dynamics of the lower esophageal sphincter (LES) and the crural diaphragm. Persistent non-acid reflux and nocturnal acid breakthrough can still occur despite maximal PPI therapy and may lead to volume regurgitation with pulmonary aspiration and Barrett's metaplasia, the major risk factor for esophageal adenocarcinoma [6, 7].

Surgical therapy has the potential to cure GERD by reinforcing both the intrinsic (crural diaphragm) and the extrinsic sphincter (LES). Because of equivocal evidence and lack of robust and high-quality randomized trials, current guidelines suggest that the choice of an antireflux procedure should be left to the discretion of the individual surgeon and best suited to the individual patient [8–10]. The laparoscopic Nissen fundoplication remains the current gold standard and has been shown to be safe, effective, and durable when performed in specialized centers [11]. Systematic review and meta-analyses [12] and randomized clinical trials [13] suggest that the Toupet fundoplication provides equivalent results in terms of reflux control and a lower rate of side effects compared to the Nissen fundoplication, especially in patients with defective esophageal body motility and in those with increased esophageal hypersensitivity.

Despite the remarkably low incidence of morbidity and mortality rates, fundoplication is underused due to the perception of long-term side effects and fear of failure [14]. Also, variability in clinical outcomes related to inter-individual surgical expertise and/or unvalidated technical modifications [15] has limited the adoption of this procedure, especially in patients with early-stage GERD. Patients undergoing a Nissen fundoplication are especially at risk for potential side effects of the procedure such as bloating, the inability to belch and vomit, and the occurrence of persistent dysphagia that may occasionally require revisional surgery [16]. These are the main reasons why gastroenterolo-

L. Bonavina (✉)
Division of General and Foregut Surgery, Department of Biomedical Sciences for Health, University of Milano School of Medicine, IRCCS Policlinico San Donato, Milan, Italy
e-mail: luigi.bonavina@unimi.it

M. Gagner (ed.), *Magnetic Surgery*, https://doi.org/10.1007/978-3-030-73947-8_4

gists tend to refer for fundoplication only patients with long-lasting severe disease and large hiatal hernias.

A downward trend in the utilization of surgical fundoplication was noted in the USA over the past decade [17–19]. The decline in surgical volume has been attributed to the perceived risk of fundoplication failure, to the availability of over-the-counter PPI and endoscopic therapies, and to the rise of bariatric surgery. Paradoxically, underutilization of antireflux procedures is in contrast with the increasing recognition of GERD as a progressive disease leading to carditis, cardiac metaplasia, intestinal metaplasia, and eventually adenocarcinoma of the distal esophagus [20, 21]. The limitations of both PPI therapy and fundoplication have led many patients and clinicians either to tolerate a lifetime drug dependence with incomplete symptom relief or to undertake the risk of a surgical procedure that alters gastric anatomy, may have side effects, and may deteriorate over time. The Linx™ Reflux Management System is an FDA-approved device designed to provide a permanent solution to gastroesophageal reflux disease by augmenting the LES barrier with a standardized laparoscopic procedure. The Linx can be used with the intent to prevent progression of early-stage GERD or to treat established and more advanced disease associated to hiatus hernia.

Magnetic Sphincter Augmentation

The Linx is a mechanical device designed to augment the physiologic barrier to reflux by magnetic force. The device is manufactured in different sizes and consists of a series of biocompatible titanium beads with magnetic cores hermetically sealed inside. The beads are interlinked with independent titanium wires to form a flexible and expandable ring with a Roman arch configuration (Fig. 4.1). At rest, each bead is in contact with adjacent beads. The beads can move independently of the adjacent beads, creating a dynamic implant that does not compress the esophagus and does not limit its range of motion upon swallowing, belching, and vomiting (Fig. 4.2). Rather, the Linx device prevents reflux by limiting distension of the esophagogastric junction in response to challenges of intragastric pressure. Separation of the beads occurs when intragastric pressure overcomes the magnetic attraction force and is independent of the number of beads contained in the device. The Linx, while augmenting the LES, allows for expansion to accommodate a swallowed bolus or the escape of elevated gastric pressure associated with belching or vomiting. During the healing process after implantation, the device is encapsulated in fibrous tissue but is not incorporated in the esophageal wall [22]; this makes possible to remove the device without damaging the esophagus. The

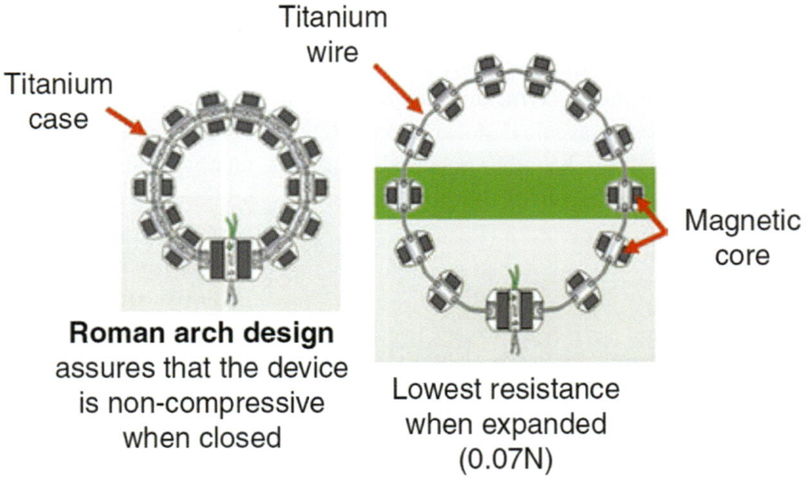

Fig. 4.1 Design of the Linx device. (From Mihura and Louie [48]. Reprinted with permission)

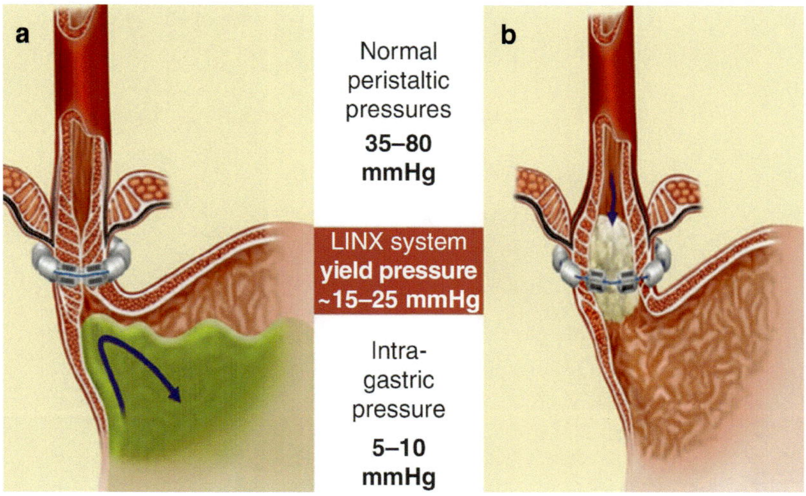

Fig. 4.2 Mechanism of action of the Linx device in the closed (**a**) and in the open (**b**) position. (From Mihura and Louie [48]. Reprinted with permission)

Linx has recently received magnetic resonance imaging (MRI) approval for scanning in systems up 1.5 Tesla.

Preoperative Work-Up

The preoperative assessment of patients who are candidates for a Linx procedure is essentially similar to any other antireflux intervention. Routine testing includes a barium swallow study, upper gastrointestinal endoscopy with biopsies, esophageal manometry, and esophageal pH monitoring. In selected patients, gastric emptying scintigraphy may be performed.

Surgical Technique

Compared to the current surgical standard, the Linx procedure in patients without hiatus hernia requires minimal dissection and preservation of the phrenoesophageal ligament [23]. The device is implanted with a standard laparoscopic approach under general anesthesia. There is no available data supporting the use of single-port access, three-dimensional camera, or robotics for performance of the Linx procedure. The steps of the procedure are illustrated in Fig. 4.3. Surgical dissection begins by dividing the peritoneum on the anterior surface of the gastroesophageal junction below the insertion of the inferior leaf of the phrenoesophageal ligament and above the junction of the hepatic branch to the anterior vagus nerve. The lateral surface of the left crus is dissected from the posterior fundic wall without dividing the short gastric vessels. The gastro-hepatic ligament is opened above and below the hepatic branch of the anterior vagus nerve to facilitate preparation of the retro-esophageal window. Gentle dissection from the right side is made toward the left crus just above the crural decussation to identify the posterior vagus nerve. A tunnel is created between the vagus and the posterior esophageal wall, and the esophagus is encircled with a Penrose drain. The circumference of the esophagus is measured to determine the proper size of the Linx device to be implanted. The sizing tool is a laparoscopic instrument with a soft, circular curved tip actuated by coaxial tubes through a handset. The handset contains a numerical indicator that corresponds to the size range of the Linx device. The sizing tool is placed around the esophagus in the tunnel dissected between the esophageal wall and the posterior vagus nerve bundle. The Linx device of appropriate size is introduced through the tunnel, and the opposing ends are brought to the anterior surface of the esophagus and simply connected together by engaging the two clasps. The decision to proceed with a posterior hiatal repair depends on the severity of GERD as assessed preoperatively, and the size of the hernia that is confirmed intraoperatively. Occasionally, simple correction of crura diastasis with one to two nonabsorbable stitches may be indicated. However, in the presence of hiatal hernia greater than 2 cm, division of

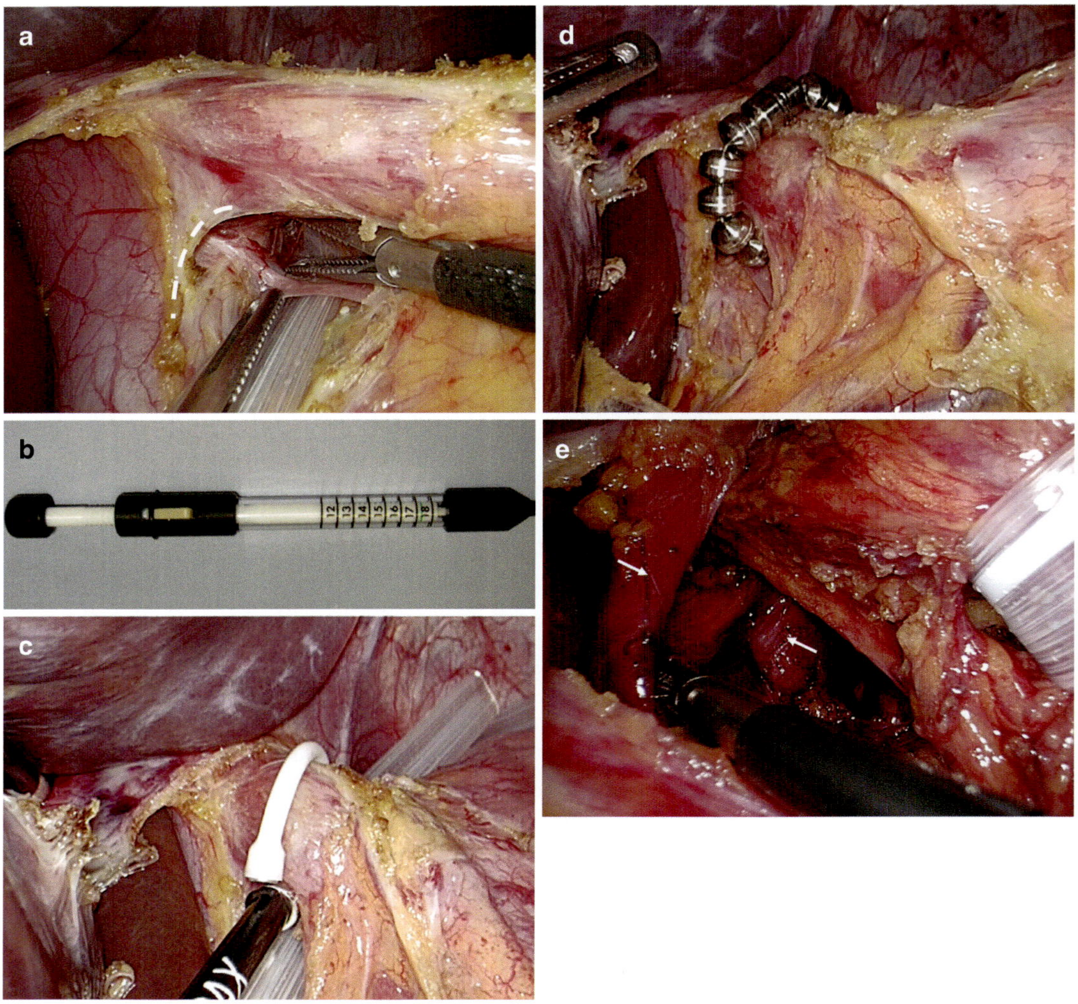

Fig. 4.3 Surgical steps of the Linx procedure. (**a**) The phrenoesophageal ligament is preserved and a tunnel is created between the posterior vagus nerve and the esophageal wall. (**b**) The circumference of the esophagus is measured using a special sizing tool. (**c**) Linx device locked in front of the esophagus after engagement of the two clasps. (**d**) No hiatus closure (minimal dissection). (**e**) Formal mediastinal dissection and posterior crura repair

the phrenoesophageal ligament and full mediastinal dissection is recommended to obtain an adequate length of intra-abdominal esophagus.

Postoperative Management

Patients are discharged the same day of surgery or on the first postoperative day after obtaining a chest film to control the position of the Linx (Fig. 4.4). Patients are encouraged to chew well, eat five small-volume meals during the day, and gradually discontinue PPI therapy. Dysphagia is considered normal during the first 3 months after surgery, with a peak generally occurring between the third and the sixth postoperative week. In such circumstances, a temporary switch to a semiliquid diet is recommended. Persistent dysphagia may occasionally require a short course of steroids and/or endoscopic pneumatic dilation.

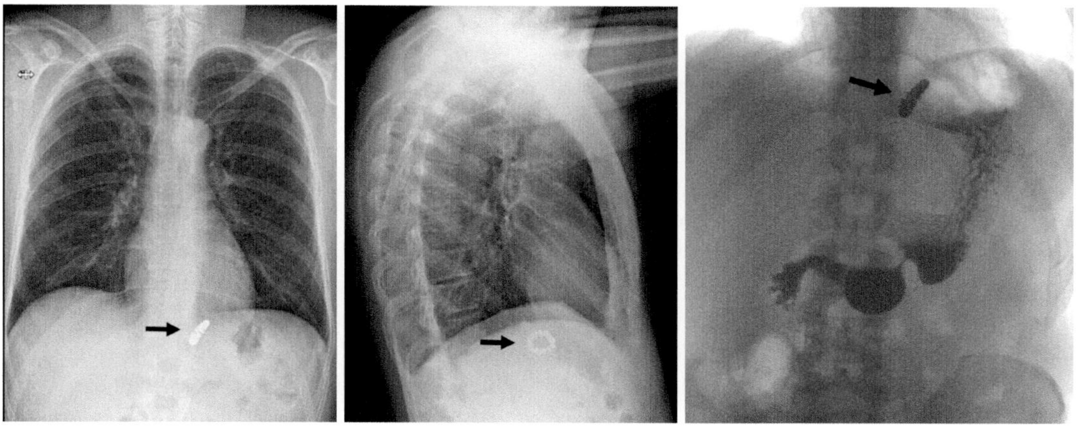

Fig. 4.4 Chest film and barium swallow study after Linx implant

Overview of Clinical Experience

Since the first human implantation in 2007, all reported studies investigating the long-term clinical outcomes of the Linx device have confirmed a high rate of symptom relief, discontinuation of PPI therapy, objective reduction of esophageal acid exposure, and improved quality of life. The feasibility study included 44 patients implanted with the Linx at 4 study centers in the USA and in Europe between February 2007 and October 2008; the short-term, midterm, 4-year, and final results of this study have been previously published [23–26]. Patients served as their own control to assess the effect of treatment on symptoms, use of PPI, and esophageal acid exposure. The primary criteria for inclusion in the feasibility trial were age >18 and <85 years, typical reflux symptoms at least partially responsive to PPI therapy, abnormal esophageal acid exposure, and normal contractile amplitude and wave form in the esophageal body. The primary criteria for exclusion from the trial were history of dysphagia, previous upper abdominal surgery, previous endoluminal antireflux procedures, sliding hiatal hernia >3 cm, esophagitis >grade A, and/or the presence of histologically documented Barrett's esophagus. Patients with abnormal manometric findings (distal esophageal contraction amplitude of less than 35 mmHg on wet swallows or <70% propulsive peristaltic sequences) were also excluded. All Linx devices were successfully implanted via a standard laparoscopic approach. The median operative time was 40 minutes. No intraoperative complications occurred. Patients were instructed to resume a regular diet after a chest film and radiological assessment of the esophageal transit were performed. Forty-three percent of patients complained of mild dysphagia during the postoperative period; in all individuals the symptom resolved by 90 days without treatment. Thirty-three patients (75%) were followed up to 5 years. The mean total GERD-HRQL score off PPI significantly decreased from 25.7 at baseline to 2.9, and 94% of patients had a greater than 50% reduction in the total score compared to baseline. Complete cessation of PPI or a reduction of 50% or more of the daily dose was achieved by 88% and 94% of patients, respectively, and 91% of patients declared to be satisfied with their current condition. Esophageal pH testing was completed in 20 patients at 5 years: 85% of patients either achieved normal esophageal acid exposure or had at least a 50% reduction from baseline, and 70% of patients achieved normalization of the pH profile. Three patients were explanted: one because of persistent dysphagia, one because of the need to undergo magnetic resonance imaging, and the last one elected to have a Nissen fundoplication for persisting GERD symptoms. All removals were safely performed via laparoscopy.

Similar rigorous inclusion criteria and perioperative subjective and objective assessment were used for a larger multi-institutional study involving 100 patients at 13 centers [27]. Significant improvements were seen in GERD-related quality of life, regurgitation, and esophageal acid exposure. Use of PPI dropped to 13% at 3 years and patient satisfaction with reflux control increased to 94% after implantation. Importantly, these positive results were stable showing no degradation over the study time period. Although 14% of patients reported bloating after implantation, no patients rated this symptom as severe. Patients retained their ability to belch and vomit. Dysphagia was present to some extent in 68% of patients but decreased to 4% by 3 years. Five percent of patients rated the dysphagia as severe, and the device was removed in three of them with complete symptom resolution.

Two single-center studies have further validated the efficacy of the Linx procedure. In Milan, Italy, 100 consecutive patients underwent Linx implantation between 2007 and 2012. The median implant duration was 3 years. There was a significant reduction of acid exposure time and improvement of GERD-HRQL score; freedom from daily dependence on PPI was achieved in 85% of the patients [28]. Another study from the USA, including 66 patients with an average follow-up of 5.8 months, showed similar satisfactory results [29].

Three recent case-control studies found comparable control of reflux symptoms after surgical fundoplication or Linx implant. However, in the Nissen fundoplication group, there was a higher rate of patients with inability to belch and vomit, along with more severe gas-bloat symptoms, whereas quality of life scores were similar in patients treated either by Linx or Toupet fundoplication [30–32]. A recent meta-analysis comparing Linx and fundoplication reported that the former was associated with less gas-bloat symptoms and an increased ability to vomit and belch, while PPI suspension rate, dysphagia requiring endoscopic dilatation, and GERD-HRQL were similar in the two patient groups [33].

It has been reported that the short-term results of the Linx procedure combined with systematic crural repair appear more favorable compared to Linx alone regardless of the size of hiatus hernia [34–38]. A multivariate logistic regression analysis confirmed that full mediastinal dissection with restoration of intra-abdominal esophageal length and crural repair was most likely to normalize esophageal acid exposure [39].

Regression of Barrett's has been observed in 72% of patients at 1 year after Linx implant; interestingly, patients with short-segment intestinal metaplasia in whom esophageal acid exposure reversed to normal were more likely to achieve regression [40]. It appears that early recognition of GERD is critical to prevent long-term complications, even in patients under continuous acid-suppressive medication [41]. A retrospective single-center review of 553 patients showed that the factors associated with a favorable outcome of the Linx procedure are age younger than 45 years, male sex, GERD-HRQL>15, and an abnormal DeMeester score [42].

Safety Profile

Concerns regarding the safety of this operation, especially the fear of erosions, stem from past adverse experience with the Angelchik device and, more recently, with the gastric banding device. An analysis of the safety profile of the first 1000 worldwide implants in 82 hospitals showed 1.3% hospital readmission rate, 5.6% need of postoperative endoscopic dilations, and 3.4% reoperation rate [43]. All reoperations were performed electively for device removal. The most commons symptoms were dysphagia and recurrence of reflux symptoms. In addition, 7% of patients enrolled in the US multicenter single-arm trial had the device removed due to persistent dysphagia in four, vomiting in one, chest pain in one, and reflux in one [44]. A study reported the results of reoperations for laparoscopic Linx removal in a series of 164 consecutive patients [45]. The reoperation rate was 6.7%, and a partial fundoplication was most commonly associated to Linx removal. The main presenting symptoms requiring device removal was recurrence of heartburn or regurgitation in 46%, dysphagia in 37%, and chest pain in 18%. In two patients

(1.2%), full-thickness erosion of the esophageal wall with partial endoluminal penetration of the device occurred (Fig. 4.5). The median implant duration was 20 months, with 82% of the patients being explanted between 12 and 24 months after the index operation. Operative time ranged from 25 to 150 minutes and postoperative course was uneventful. At the latest follow-up (12–58 months), the GERD-HRQL score was normalized in all patients.

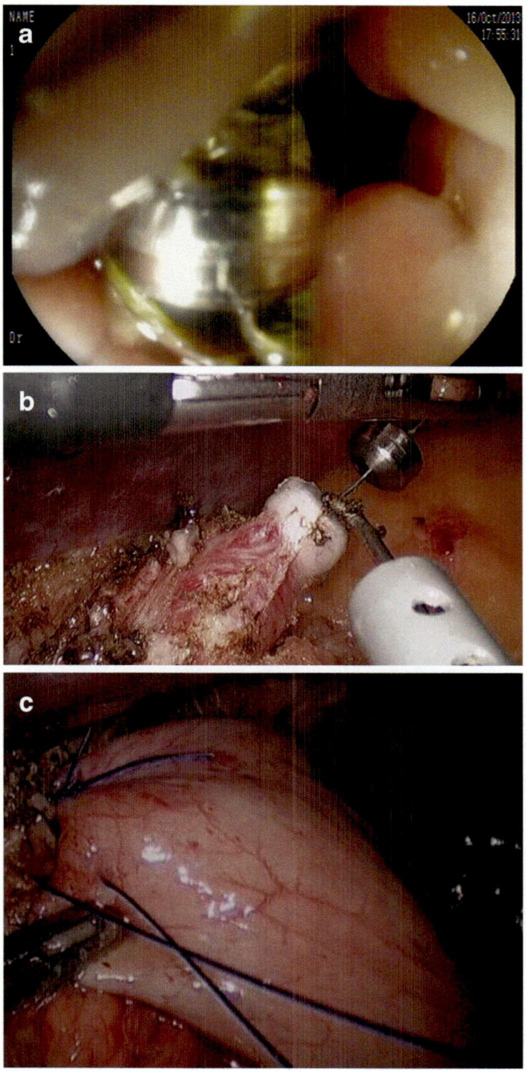

Fig. 4.5 Endoscopic view of erosion of Linx device (**a**) requiring laparoscopic removal (**b**) and Dor fundoplication (**c**)

Conclusion

The Linx procedure was developed to address the unmet needs of patients with unsatisfactory response to medical therapy and those with early-stage GERD who would not usually be considered ideal candidates for fundoplication [23, 46–49]. The Linx is highly effective in reducing typical symptoms with a favorable side-effect profile and therefore provides a standardized and physiological alternative to fundoplication. A randomized clinical trial has shown the superiority of Linx compared to daily PPI therapy in controlling moderate to severe regurgitation and reducing esophageal acid exposure [50]. Safety issues such as device erosions or migrations have been rare and not associated with mortality. The Linx can be easily removed if necessary, thereby preserving the option of fundoplication in the future. Among the potential limitations of this procedure are the current contraindication to undergo scanning in MRI systems >1.5 Tesla and the potential long-term consequences of a permanent foreign body implant. Randomized trials are needed to definitively assess the effectiveness of the procedure and to establish at which stage of disease severity magnetic sphincter augmentation may prove superior to fundoplication.

References

1. Toghanian S, Johnson DA, Stalhammar NO, Zerbib F. Burden of gastro-oesophageal reflux disease in patients with persistent and intense symptoms despite proton pump inhibitor therapy: a post-hoc analysis of the 2007 national health and wellness survey. Clin Drug Investig. 2011;31:703–15.
2. Kahrilas PJ, Howden CW, Hughes N. Response of regurgitation to proton pump inhibitor therapy in clinical trials of gastroesophageal reflux disease. Am J Gastroenterol. 2011;106:1419–25.
3. Heidelbaugh JJ, Kim AH, Chang R, et al. Overutilization of proton-pump inhibitors: what the clinician needs to know. Ther Adv Gastroenterol. 2012;5(4):219–32.
4. McColl K, Gillen D. Evidence that proton-pump inhibitor therapy induces the symptoms it is used to treat. Gastroenterology. 2009;137:20–2.
5. Poulsen AH, Christensen S, McLaughlin JK, et al. Proton pump inhibitors and risk of gastric cancer:

a population-based cohort study. Br J Cancer. 2009;100:1503–7.
6. Lord R, DeMeester S, Peters J, et al. Hiatal hernia, lower esophageal sphincter incompetence, and effectiveness of Nissen fundoplication in the spectrum of gastroesophageal reflux disease. J Gastrointest Surg. 2009;13:602–10.
7. Malfertheiner P, Nocon M, Vieth M, et al. Evolution of gastro-oesophageal reflux disease over 5 years under routine medical care – the ProGERD study. Aliment Pharmacol Ther. 2012;35:154–64.
8. Stefanidis D, Hope WW, Kohn GP, et al. Guidelines for surgical treatment of gastroesophageal reflux disease. Surg Endosc. 2010;24:2647–69.
9. Kohn GP, Price RR, DeMeester SR, et al. Guidelines for the management of hiatal hernia. Surg Endosc. 2013;27:4409–28.
10. Fuchs KH, Babic B, Breithaupt W, et al. EAES recommendations for the management of gastroesophageal reflux disease. Surg Endosc. 2014;28:1753–73.
11. Galmiche JP, Hatlebakk J, Attwood S, et al. Laparoscopic antireflux surgery vs esomeprazole treatment for chronic GERD: the LOTUS randomized clinical trial. JAMA. 2011;305(19):1969–77.
12. Broeders JA, Mauritz FA, Ahmed Ali U, et al. Systematic review and meta-analysis of laparoscopic Nissen (posterior total) versus Toupet (posterior partial) fundoplication for gastro-oesophageal reflux disease. Br J Surg. 2010;97:1318–30.
13. Hakanson BS, Lundell L, Bylund A, Thorell A. Comparison of laparoscopic 270° posterior partial fundoplication vs total fundoplication for the treatment of gastroesophageal reflux disease. A randomized clinical trial. JAMA Surg. https://doi.org/10.1001/jamasurg.2019.0047.
14. Niebisch S, Fleming FJ, Galey KM, et al. Perioperative risk of laparoscopic fundoplication: safer than previously reported – analysis of the American College of Surgeons National Surgical Quality Improvement Program 2005 to 2009. J Am Coll Surg. 2012;215:61–9.
15. Richter JE, Dempsey DT. Laparoscopic antireflux surgery: key to success in the community setting. Am J Gastroenterol. 2008;103:289–91.
16. Khajanchee YS, O'Rourke R, Cassera MA, et al. Laparoscopic reintervention for failed antireflux surgery: subjective and objective outcomes in 176 consecutive patients. Arch Surg. 2007;142:785–91.
17. Finks JF, Wei Y, Birkmeyer JD. The rise and fall of antireflux surgery in the United States. Surg Endosc. 2006;20:1698–701.
18. Colavita PD, Belyansky I, Walters AL, et al. Nationwide inpatient sample: have antireflux procedures undergone regionalization? J Gastrointest Surg. 2013;17:6–13.
19. Khan F, Maradey-Romero C, Ganocy S, Frazier R, Fass R. Utilisation of surgical fundoplication for patients with gastro-oesophageal reflux disease in the USA has declined rapidly between 2009 and 2013. Aliment Pharmacol Ther. 2016;43:1124–31.
20. Labenz J, Chandrasoma PJ, Knapp LJ, DeMeester TR. Proposed approach to the challenging management of progressive gastroesophageal reflux disease. World J Gastrointest Endosc. 2018;10:175–83.
21. Pinto D, Plieschnegger W, Schneider NI, et al. Carditis: a relevant marker of gastroesophageal reflux disease. Data from a prospective central European multicenter study on histological and endoscopic diagnosis of esophagitis (histoGERD trial). Dis Esophagus. 2019;32(1). https://doi.org/10.1093/dote/doy073.
22. Ganz R, Gostout C, Grudem J, et al. Use of a magnetic sphincter for the treatment of GERD: a feasibility study. Gastrointest Endosc. 2008;67:287–94.
23. Bonavina L, Saino G, Bona D, et al. Magnetic augmentation of the lower esophageal sphincter: results of a feasibility clinical trial. J Gastrointest Surg. 2008;12:2133–40.
24. Bonavina L, DeMeester TR, Fockens P, et al. Laparoscopic sphincter augmentation device eliminates reflux symptoms and normalizes esophageal acid exposure. Ann Surg. 2010;252:857–62.
25. Lipham JC, DeMeester TR, Ganz RA, et al. The Linx reflux management system: confirmed safety and efficacy now at 4 years. Surg Endosc. 2012;26:2944–9.
26. Saino G, Bonavina L, Lipham J, Dunn D, Ganz RA. Magnetic sphincter augmentation for gastroesophageal reflux at 5 years: final results of a pilot study show long-term acid reduction and symptom improvement. J Laparoendosc Adv Surg Tech A. 2015;25:787–92.
27. Ganz RA, Peters JH, Horgan S, et al. Esophageal sphincter device for gastroesophageal reflux disease. N Engl J Med. 2013;368:719–27.
28. Bonavina L, Saino G, Bona D, et al. One hundred consecutive patients treated with magnetic sphincter augmentation for gastroesophageal reflux disease: 6 years of clinical experience from a single center. J Am Coll Surg. 2013;217:577–85.
29. Smith CD, Devault KR, Buchanan M. Introduction of mechanical sphincter augmentation for gastroesophageal reflux disease into practice: early clinical outcomes and keys to successful adoption. J Am Coll Surg. 2014;218:776–81.
30. Louie BE, Farivar AS, Schultz D, et al. Short-term outcomes using magnetic sphincter augmentation versus Nissen fundoplication for medically resistant gastroesophageal reflux disease. Ann Thorac Surg. 2014;98:498–504.
31. Riegler M, Schoppman SF, Bonavina L, et al. Magnetic sphincter augmentation and fundoplication for GERD in clinical practice: one-year results of a multicenter, prospective observational study. Surg Endosc. 2015;29:1123–9.
32. Reynolds J, Zehetner J, Wu P, et al. Laparoscopic magnetic sphincter augmentation vs laparoscopic Nissen fundoplication; a matched-pair analysis of 100 patients. Ann Surg. 2015;221:123–8.
33. Aiolfi A, Asti E, Bernardi D, et al. Early results of magnetic sphincter augmentation versus

fundoplication for gastroesophageal reflux disease: systematic review and meta-analysis. Int J Surg. 2018;52:82–8.
34. Rona KA, Reynolds J, Schwameis K, et al. Efficacy of magnetic sphincter augmentation in patients with large hiatal hernias. Surg Endosc. 2017;31(5):2096–102.
35. Kuckelman JP, Phillips CJ, Hardin MO, et al. Standard vs expanded indications for esophageal magnetic sphincter augmentation for reflux disease. JAMA Surg. 2017;152(9):890–1.
36. Buckley FP, Bell RCW, Freeman K, et al. Favorable results from a prospective evaluation of 200 patients with large hiatal hernias undergoing LINX magnetic sphincter augmentation. Surg Endosc. 2018;32:1762–8.
37. Schwameis K, Nikolic M, Morales Castellano DG, et al. Crural closure improves outcomes of magnetic sphincter augmentation in GERD patients with hiatal hernia. Sci Rep. 2018;8:7319.
38. Tatum JM, Alicuben E, Bildzukewicz N, et al. Minimal versus obligatory dissection of the diaphragmatic hiatus during magnetic sphincter augmentation surgery. Surg Endosc. 2019;33:782–8.
39. Irribarra MM, Blitz S, Wilshire CL, et al. Does treatment of the hiatus influence the outcomes of magnetic sphincter augmentation for chronic GERD? J Gastrointest Surg. 2019;23:1104–12.
40. Alicuben ET, Tatum JM, Bildzukewicz N, et al. Regression of intestinal metaplasia following magnetic sphincter augmentation device placement. Surg Endosc. 2019;33:576–9.
41. Bonavina L, Fisichella PM, Gavini S, Lee YY, Tatum RP. Clinical course of gastroesophageal reflux disease and impact of treatment in symptomatic young patients. Ann N Y Acad Sci. 2020. https://doi.org/10.1111/nyas.14350.
42. Ayazi S, Zheng P, Zaidi AH, et al. Clinical outcomes and predictors of favorable results after laparoscopic magnetic sphincter augmentation: single-institution experience with more than 500 patients. J Am Coll Surg. 2020. doi.org/10.1016. ISSN 1072-7515-20.
43. Lipham JC, Taiganides PA, Louie BE, et al. Safety analysis of first 1000 patients treated with magnetic sphincter augmentation for gastroesophageal reflux disease. Dis Esophagus. 2015;28:305–11.
44. Ganz RA, Edmundowicz SA, Taiganides PA, et al. Long-term outcomes of patients receiving a magnetic sphincter augmentation device for gastroesophageal reflux. Clin Gastroenterol Hepatol. 2016;14:671–7.
45. Asti E, Siboni S, Lazzari V, et al. Removal of the magnetic sphincter device. Surgical technique and results of a single-center cohort study. Ann Surg. 2017;265:941–5.
46. Bonavina L, DeMeester TR, Ganz R. LINX TM reflux management system: magnetic sphincter augmentation in the treatment of gastroesophageal reflux disease. Expert Rev Gastroenterol Hepatol. 2012;6(6):667–74.
47. Worrel SG, Greene CL, DeMeester TR. The state of surgical treatment of gastroesophageal reflux disease after five decades. J Am Coll Surg. 2014;219:819–30.
48. Mihura M, Louie BE. Laparoscopic antireflux surgery: magnetic GEJ augmentation. In: Grams J, Perry K, Tavakkoli A, editors. The SAGES manual of foregut surgery. Cham: Springer; 2019. p. 171–92.
49. Bonavina L, Boyle N, Schoppmann S. The role of magnetic sphincter augmentation in the treatment of gastroesophageal reflux disease. Curr Opin Gastroenterol. 2021. https://doi.org/10.1097/mog.0000000000000748.
50. Bell R, Lipham J, Louie BE, et al. Magnetic sphincter augmentation superior to proton pump inhibitors for regurgitation in a 1-year randomized trial. Clin Gastroenterol Hepatol. 2020;18(8):1736–1743.e2.

Use of Magnets for Double-J Ureteral Stents

5

Marie-Claire Rassweiler-Seyfried

Abbreviations

€	Euro
BMI	body mass index
DJ	ureteral stents
F	French = 1/3 millimeter
USSQ	ureteral stent symptom questionnaire
VAS	visual analogue scale

Introduction

The first ureteral double-J (DJ) stent implantation was described almost 40 years ago [1, 2]. Today, the placement of a ureteral stent is the most frequent urologic intervention if drainage of the upper urinary tract is required. New stent technologies to improve patient care and comfort are evolving lately [3]. Certain prophylactic and therapeutic indications exist to insert a ureteral stent, for example, after an ureterorenoscopy (URS) and heavy stone removal. Eighty percent of the patients complain of irritative voiding problems, sometimes accompanied by macrohematuria, after the placement of a ureteral stent [4]. The rate for a secondary urinary tract infection is 2–4% [5]. The DJ stents are removed after endoscopic stone removal, usually within 1–2 weeks [6]. The standard procedure to remove a DJ is a cystoscopy, which might be painful and requires local anesthesia or sedation. Especially for young male patients, the DJ removal is the most unpleasant part of the stone treatment [7, 8]. The idea to develop a magnet attached to the DJ to remove the stent without the need of a cystoscope was first reported by Macaluso et al. in 1989 [9]. Later, Taylor and McDougall used a magnetic retrieval catheter to catch the steel bead which was attached to the end of the DJ [10]. The idea of a DJ removal without cystoscopy using a magnet was implemented in real life, but the steel bead was not easy to find and catch in the bladder. Also, irritative symptoms occurred due to the heavy steel bead [10]. Other study groups developed new materials and shapes of ureteral stents to improve patients' comfort, but there is no ideal ureteric stent currently available [10–12]. To assess patient's quality of life regarding the side effects of ureteral stents, Joshi and colleagues developed a validated symptom questionnaire [13].

It still took more than 10 years to implement the idea of using the strength of two magnets to remove a DJ without using a cystoscope. The breakthrough point was the development of small magnets with enough power to stay together and not cause too much discomfort to the patient while staying in the bladder. Up to now, two stud-

M.-C. Rassweiler-Seyfried (✉)
Department of Urology and Urosurgery, University Medical Center Mannheim, Medical Faculty Mannheim, University of Heidelberg, Mannheim, Germany
e-mail: marie-claire.rassweiler@medma.uni-heidelberg.de

M. Gagner (ed.), *Magnetic Surgery*, https://doi.org/10.1007/978-3-030-73947-8_5

ies have been published using the new magnetic DJ and comparing it to a standard DJ [14, 15].

The Magnetic DJ

The magnetic DJ (Blackstar, Urotech [Achenmuehle, Germany]) is a standard 7F(French) ureteral polyurethane stent with a cylinder-shaped magnet fixed through a string on the distal loop of the stent. The size of the magnet varies depending on the length of the stent (Fig. 5.1):

- 9F: external diameter 3 mm, internal diameter 1.42 mm, length 4.5 mm, volume 31.8 mm^3
- 7F: external diameter 2.33 mm, internal diameter 1.14 mm, length 3.5 mm, volume 14.9mm^3

A specific catheter-shaped retrieval device made of soft polyurethane with a magnetic tip is used for the removal of the magnetic DJ (Fig. 5.2). The retrieval device has a Tiemann tip with a 30-degree curve. To remove the DJ, the retrieval device is inserted, the two magnets connect in the bladder and the retrieval device can be removed together with the DJ (Fig. 5.3). The patient is lying supine as for a catheter insertion. The standard position for a cystoscopic DJ removal is the lithotomy position. Therefore, the patient is more comfortable when using the retrieval device. The first case was performed under fluoroscopic control to see the two magnets connect (Fig. 5.4). Later, all magnetic DJ removals were performed by trained nurses.

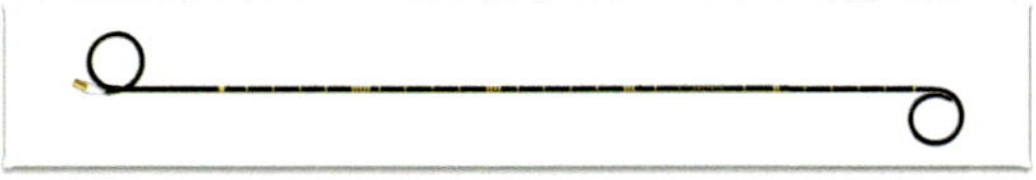

Fig. 5.1 Magnetic DJ with magnetic cube on a string on the distal part of the DJ

Fig. 5.2 Retrieval device with the magnet on the tip

Clinical Studies

Two studies have shown the advantages and disadvantages of the magnetic DJ so far (Table 5.1) [14, 15]. Consecutive patients for a ureterorenoscopic stone removal and the need for a DJ due to extensive stone burden with or without laser lithotripsy either got a standard DJ or the new magnetic DJ. In our study, we used a specific validated questionnaire (USSQ, Ureteral Stent Symptom Questionnaire) to determine the problems with the indwelling DJ [15]. Furthermore, the time of the DJ removal and the pain during the removal (questions P1-3) using a VAS (visual analogue scale) were examined. Sevcenco et al. just used the VAS to determine the discomfort with the indwelling DJ, but with a bigger patient population [14]. The DJ was removed within 2 weeks with cystoscope when the standard DJ was used or with the retrieval device. In the study by Sevcenco et al., 12 female patients who underwent a laparoscopic pyeloplasty with a magnetic DJ placement were followed. In this population, the DJ was removed after 4 weeks.

Results

A total of 170 magnetic DJ stents were placed combining the two studies together. No intra- or post-interventional complications or early stent removals or replacements were documented. The mean age of the first study group was around 50 years and more male patients were included. The detailed data are shown in Table 5.1.

Stent Irritation

Stent irritation was slightly higher in patients with an indwelling magnetic stent than in those with a regular stent, with a median VAS score of 3 versus 2, according to the study of Sevcenco [14].

In our study [15], no significant difference could be shown ($p = 0.156$). With the magnetic DJ, the median VAS was stated at 3, with the standard DJ at 5, respectively. No significant dif-

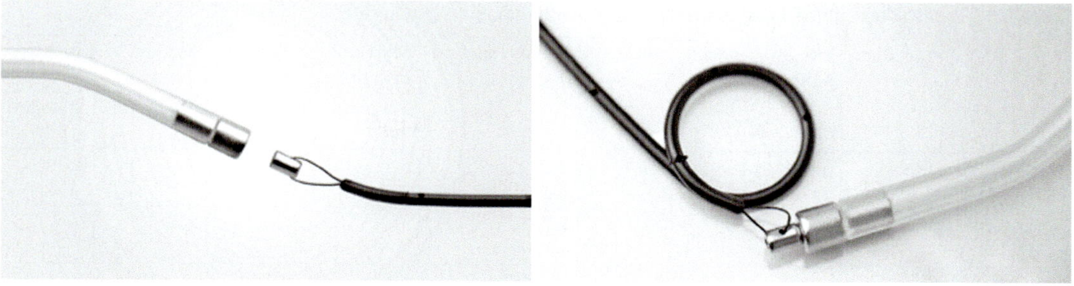

Fig. 5.3 Retrieval device with magnet and connecting magnet of the DJ

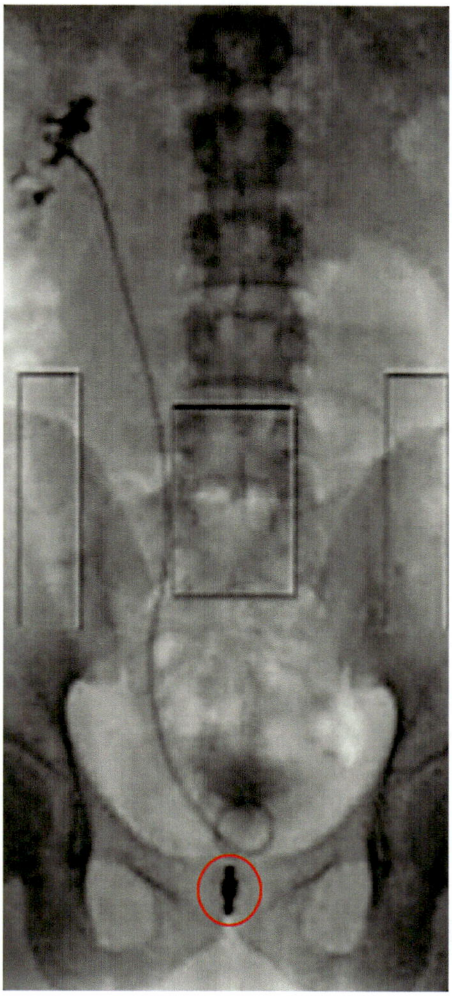

Fig. 5.4 First clinical case with magnetic DJ removal under fluoroscopy. The connecting magnets are circled in red

ferences in stent irritation were found in patients who carried a magnetic stent for 4 weeks after laparoscopic pyeloplasty (p = 0.20). The pain location differed significantly with the indwelling DJ. In our study, almost half of the patients with the magnetic DJ (48%) experienced pain in the lower abdomen or around the bladder, whereas most patients in the standard DJ group (54%) described pain around the flank. This difference could be related to the small magnet, which might cause discomfort in the bladder and abdomen. Just 18% of the patients with the magnetic DJ complained about flank pain. Other parts of the USSQ regarding sexual life, physical activity, sleep, micturition, etc., are shown in Fig. 5.5. Altogether no significant difference between the two groups could be shown.

Stent Removal

Both study groups experienced significantly less pain during the magnetic DJ removal compared to the standard cystoscopic removal, even when using a flexible cystoscope, especially in men. The median VAS was 2.5 and 3 compared to 6 and 4, respectively (Table 5.1). In contrast, Kuehhas et al. reported astonishing low mean VAS scores of 2.1 and 2.5 during cystoscopic stent removal in women and men, respectively, especially because the removal was performed using rigid cystoscopy. Patients with recurrent stone formation had a significantly lower VAS scores at stent removal

Table 5.1 Two studies comparing the magnetic to a standard double-J stent (DJ)

	Procedure	No. of patients	Mean age	w/m	Magnet/standard DJ stent	Median VAS stent irritation		Median VAS stent removal	
						Magnetic DJ	Standard DJ	Magnetic DJ	Standard DJ
Rassweiler et al. [15]	URS	60	48	13/47	40/20	3	5	3	4
Sevcenco et al. [14]	URS	163	50	12/151	130/33	3	2	2.5	6

VAS visual analogue scale

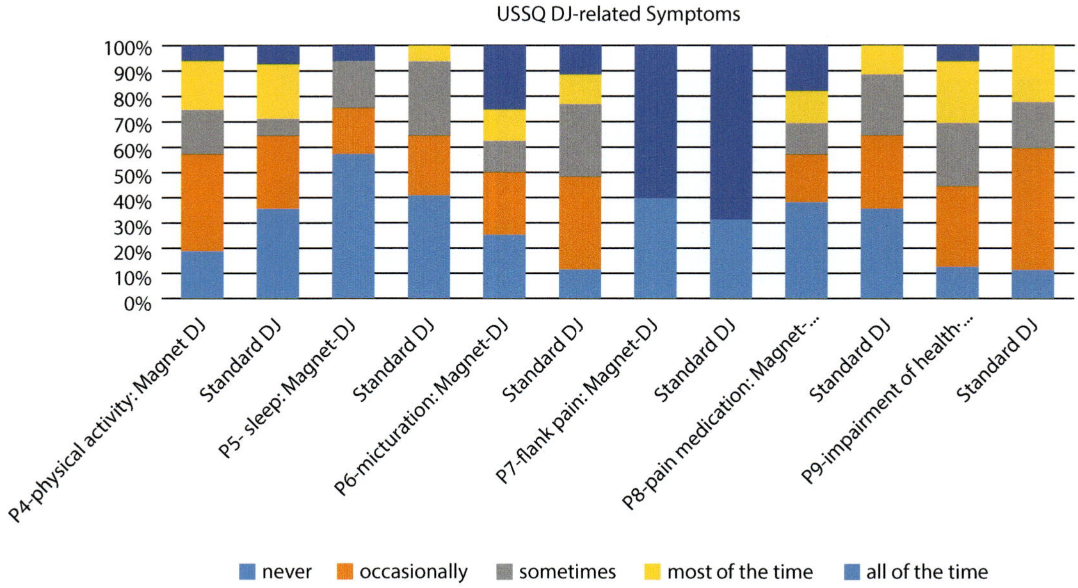

Fig. 5.5 Detailed data of the USSQ different pain questions comparing the standard and magnetic DJ. The results are listed in percentage of each study group. P1-3 (pain scale) with the DJ is described separately. USSQ = ureteral stent symptom questionnaire

[16]. Due to a big median lobe of the prostate, the retrieval instrument could not be inserted in the bladder and a cystoscopy was need. Furthermore, one female patient needed a cystoscopy because after 4 weeks, an encrustation around the magnet made it impossible to remove the DJ with the retrieval instrument. Every other removal was without complication and could be done by a trained nurse.

Economic Assessment

A cost analysis at our institution calculated a reduction of around € 100 using the magnetic DJ (Table 5.2). The main reason for the reduction is that trained urologists or residents and operating rooms are not needed. The time of the staff is one of the most expensive elements of the procedure. Furthermore, no cystoscope and sterilization procedures are needed.

Other Magnetic Stents and New Interventions

Two different study groups have been working with the idea of a magnetic DJ and removal without cystoscopy. A Chinese group uses a spiral elastic wire at the distal part of the DJ and a retrieval device with a magnetic tip and several small hooks to catch the elastic spiral wire for the

Table 5.2 Comparison of the cystoscopic and magnetic DJ removal in regard of costs, time, and staff

	Cystoscopic removal	Magnetic removal
Mean procedure time (min)	7	1
No. of physicians needed	1	1
Preparation time for the physician (min)	3	2
No. of nurses needed	1	0
Preparation time for the nurse (min)	15	5
Costs of the double-J stent	20,- €	80,- €

min minutes, *No* number, € Euro

removal [17]. Currently, no in vivo studies have proven this kind of magnetic DJ suitable for every day clinical praxis. The stent was tested in a bench model for removal, and the biocompatibility was examined in a rat model.

Altarac et al. describe a similar stent with a magnet on the distal part of the DJ. The retrieval device is a Nelaton catheter with a magnetic tip, meaning that there is no curved tip as in the retrieval device in our study [18]. This results in poor mobility of the retrieval device in the bladder with problems in removing the stent. To date, just female patients were treated with this magnetic DJ and no comparative study was conducted.

Another idea to remove the DJ without any additional procedure includes the use of a string attached on the distal part of the DJ, which hangs out of the urethra. Just by pulling the string, the DJ can be easily removed by the patient him/herself. This method is convenient and is used in daily clinical praxis when the DJ should stay in place for a few days. The risk of urinary tract infection or accidental loss of the DJ increases if the DJ needed to stay longer. Althaus et al. found, in a three-center study with 512 cases, that 5.3% of men and 24.4% of women accidently dislodged the string. According to their study, 15% of all patients with strings will have inadvertent stent dislodgement, whereas women have a fourfold higher risk. This could be crucial if the patient has an infection, perforation, or a ureteral stricture [19].

Other inventions to overcome a cystoscopic procedure to removal the ureteral stent include biodegradable stents that dissolve in urine after a period of 2 weeks. These stents are made of polysaccharides and were proven to dissolve in artificial urine in an in vitro study [20, 21]. There are no clinical studies so far. Other study groups cover the ureteral stent with pain medication (ketoprofen) or anticancer drugs, such as paclitaxel and doxorubicin, to treat a renal colic or urothelial tumors of the upper urinary tract, respectively [21, 22]. One in vivo animal study (pigs) has been conducted to date [23]. Biodegradable drug eluting stents are also a promising future development.

Conclusion

The magnetic DJ causes comparable stent irritation, mostly due to the attached magnet on the distal end of the ureteral stent, which can cause bladder irritation and lower urinary tract symptoms. The DJ removal is less painful and much faster than the standard cystoscopic removal, whether a flexible or rigid cystoscope.

References

1. Finney RP. Experience with new double J ureteral catheter stent. 1978. J Urol. 2002;167:1135–8; discussion 1139.
2. Hepperlen TW, Mardis HK, Kammandel H. Self-retained internal ureteral stents: a new approach. J Urol. 1978;119:731–3.
3. Chew BH, Knudsen BE, Denstedt JD. The use of stents in contemporary urology. Curr Opin Urol. 2004;14:111–5.
4. Chew BH, Knudsen BE, Nott L, Pautler SE, Razvi H, Amann J, et al. Pilot study of ureteral movement in stented patients: first step in understanding dynamic ureteral anatomy to improve stent comfort. J Endourol. 2007;21:1069–75.
5. Moltzahn F, Haeni K, Birkhäuser FD, Roth B, Thalmann GN, Zehnder P. Peri-interventional antibiotic prophylaxis only vs continuous low-dose antibiotic treatment in patients with JJ stents: a prospective randomised trial analysing the effect on urinary tract infections and stent-related symptoms. BJU Int. 2013;111:289–95.

6. Haleblian G, Kijvikai K, De La Rosette J, Preminger G. Ureteral stenting and urinary stone management: a systematic review. J Urol. 2008;179:424–30.
7. Türk C, Neisius A, Petřík A, Seitz C, Thomas K, Skolarikos A. EAU guidelines on urolithiasis 2018. Eur Assoc Urol Guidel 2018 Ed. Arnhem: The European Association of Urology Guidelines Office; 2018.
8. Jeong YB, Doo AR, Park HS, Shin YS. Clinical significance of ureteral stent removal by flexible cystoscopy on pain and satisfaction in young males: a prospective randomised control trial. Urolithiasis. 2016;44:367–70.
9. Macaluso JN, Deutsch JS, Goodman JR, Appell RA, Prats LJ, Wahl P. The use of the magnetip double-J ureteral stent in urological practice. J Urol. 1989;142:701–3.
10. Taylor WN, McDougall IT. Minimally invasive ureteral stent retrieval. J Urol. 2002;168:2020–3.
11. Chew BH, Lange D. Advances in ureteral stent development. Curr Opin Urol. 2016;26:277–82.
12. Forbes C, Scotland KB, Lange D, Chew BH. Innovations in ureteral stent technology. Urol Clin North Am. 2019;46:245–55.
13. Joshi HB, Newns N, Stainthorpe A, MacDonagh RP, Keeley FX, Timoney AG. Ureteral stent symptom questionnaire: development and validation of a multidimensional quality of life measure. J Urol. 2003;169:1060–4.
14. Sevcenco S, Eredics K, Lusuardi L, Klingler HC. Evaluation of pain perception associated with use of the magnetic-end ureteric double-J stent for short-term ureteric stenting. World J Urol. 2018;36:475–9.
15. Rassweiler MC, Michel MS, Ritter M, Honeck P. Magnetic ureteral stent removal without cystoscopy: a randomized controlled trial. J Endourol. 2017;31:762–6.
16. Kuehhas FE, Miernik A, Sharma V, Sevcenco S, Javadli E, Herwig R, et al. A prospective evaluation of pain associated with stone passage, stents, and stent removal using a visual analog scale. Urology. 2013;82:521–5.
17. Wang J, Feng J, Hu W, Song Y, Xu X, Fan M, et al. Preclinical evaluation of a newly designed ureteral stent and magnetic retrieval catheter for minimally invasive stent removal. Urology. 2014;84:960–6.
18. Altarac S, Vražić M. A new type of ureteral stent will facilitate stent removal. Eur. Urol. 2012;61:225–6.
19. Althaus AB, Li K, Pattison E, Eisner B, Pais V, Steinberg P. Rate of dislodgment of ureteral stents when using an extraction string after endoscopic urological surgery. J Urol. 2015;193:2011–4.
20. Barros AA, Rita A, Duarte ARC, Pires RA, Sampaio-Marques B, Ludovico P, et al. Bioresorbable ureteral stents from natural origin polymers. J Biomed Mater Res Part B Appl Biomater. 2015;103:608–17.
21. Barros AA, Oliveira C, Reis RL, Lima E, Duarte ARC. Ketoprofen-eluting biodegradable ureteral stents by CO2 impregnation: in vitro study. Int J Pharm. 2015;495:651–9.
22. Barros AA, Oliveira C, Reis RL, Lima E, Duarte ARC. In vitro and ex vivo permeability studies of paclitaxel and doxorubicin from drug-eluting biodegradable ureteral stents. J Pharm Sci. 2017;106:1466–74.
23. Barros AA, Oliveira C, Ribeiro AJ, Autorino R, Reis RL, Duarte ARC, et al. In vivo assessment of a novel biodegradable ureteral stent. World J Urol. 2018;36:277–83.

6 Magnets for Colorectal Anastomosis

Zhongfa Xu and Ya'nan Zhen

Physiological Processes of Anastomotic Healing

Physiologically, the healing process of intestinal anastomosis can be divided into an acute inflammatory phase, proliferative phase, and tissue remodeling phase or mature phase. Collagen plays an important role in the tensile strength of the intestinal wall. After anastomosis, collagen begins to degrade within 24 hours, and the degradation lasts for approximate 4 days. Seven days after surgery, collagen synthesis begins, especially in the site near the anastomosis [1]. Five to six weeks after surgery, the degradation and synthesis of collagen are balanced, and there is no longer a significant increase in the amount of collagen at the anastomotic site. The tensile strength of the scar gradually increases to the optimal level over time.

The bursting pressure of the anastomosis was used as a parameter for evaluation. After completion of anastomosis, the bursting pressure increased rapidly in the early stage, reaching 60% of the tensile strength of the surrounding intestinal canal in 3–4 days and completely recovering within a week [2]. Halsted [3] found that the tensile strength of the gastrointestinal tract is mainly derived from the submucosa, which includes a large amount of collagen, the vasculature, the lymphatic system, and nerve fibers. At the early stage after anastomosis, the tensile strength of the anastomosis is very weak. Before the synthesis of a large amount of new collagen, the tensile strength of an anastomosis mainly depends on suture, staples, and existing collagen. The risk of anastomotic leakage is very high 1 or 2 days after anastomosis.

In addition to the regeneration function of the tissue cells, anastomotic healing is closely related to alignment of the tissue layers, blood supply, and tension of anastomosis. The accurate alignment of the layers of the digestive tract wounds, especially the complete alignment of the mucosa and submucosa, is an important condition for the good healing of the anastomosis. The serosa is a thin layer of connective tissue covering the muscularis propria. A good alignment of the serosa layer during anastomosis can greatly reduce the risk of anastomotic leakage [2]. Adequate blood circulation provides a nutrient supply for tissue regeneration during anastomotic healing and ensures rapid tissue regeneration and reconstruction. Poor local blood circulation will lead to

Z. Xu (✉)· Y. Zhen
Department of Gastrointestinal Surgery, The Third Affiliated Hospital of Shandong First Medical University (Affiliated Hospital of Shandong Academy of Medical Sciences), Jinan, Shandong, People's Republic of China

M. Gagner (ed.), *Magnetic Surgery*, https://doi.org/10.1007/978-3-030-73947-8_6

excessive formation of granulation tissue, difficulty of anastomosis healing, or cicatricial stenosis after healing.

History of Intestinal Anastomosis

Hand-Sewn Anastomosis

In 1826, Lembert proposed and established the principle of serosal alignment in intestinal anastomosis, that is, "Lembert-type vertical mattress suture." This represents the modern origin of intestinal anastomosis. This suture technique was well-accepted by many surgeons in the early nineteenth century [4]. In 1880, Czerny et al. proposed the technique of a mucosa suture based on the Lembert method, namely, the Czerny-Lembert method. Compared with the Lembert method, the Czerny-Lembert method is a double-layer inverting suture method [5]. Since then, various improved double suture techniques have been reported, including double-layer intermittent everting suture, intermittent full-layer suture for the inner layer, and continuous serosa suture for the outer layer.

Based on the theory that collagen is abundant in the submucosa, Halsted first proposed the single-layer anastomosis technique [3], which was popularized as the "single-layer horizontal mattress suture method." The advantage of this method lies in the reduced incidence of anastomotic stenosis. However, this method of anastomosis was not widely used at that time due to the concern of whether the anastomosis method is more likely to cause anastomotic leakage. There was a dispute about advantages between single-layer anastomosis and double-layer anastomosis. In 1951, Gambee invented the "intermittent full-layer vertical inverting mattress suture," which was successfully used in the clinical practice and then gradually promoted [6]. Taken together, single-layer anastomosis is associated with shorter time, less impact on tissue blood supply, faster healing, and milder stenosis, but the sutures in the lumen side may increase inflammation and affect healing. Double-layer anastomosis can cause compression of the inner layer of tissue to affect blood supply and result in poor healing and stenosis. Thus, it was used less and less in clinical practice. However, it is still an option for anastomosis of fragile, edematous, and vascular-rich tissues because it can increase the tensile strength of the anastomosis.

The suture material also has an important effect on anastomosis. In addition to inert substances, most foreign bodies can cause inflammatory reactions in the human body. It is well known that the silk sutures that are now widely used can cause an inflammatory reaction in the human body for several weeks. Polypropylene suture, catgut suture, and polyglycolic acid sutures caused relatively mild reactions. The tensile strength of the anastomosis is almost the same between uses of the absorbable and nonabsorbable threads.

Stapled Anastomosis

In 1908, Hultl [7] first invented the modern stapler and successfully applied it in gastrectomy. Its design concept is widely used even today, including two rows of staples on each side, stapler-type anastomosis using metal staples, and tissue stapled by "B"-shaped staples. Since 1950, the researchers in the Institute for Experimental Surgical Instruments of the former Soviet Union had systematically studied the stapler and had been leading this field. In 1958, American researcher Ravitch introduced the stapler technique to the United States. At this time, the stapler can be used to complete the cutting and stapling of the intestine and can perform the end-to-end inverting anastomosis of the intestine [8]. The first single-use stapler in the United States was manufactured by Ethicon in 1979. This enabled the mass production and wide application of staplers to reach a new level.

The widely used stapler for anastomosis works in a similar way to a regular stapler, that is, two rows (three rows) of intertwined staples are implanted into the tissue to cross-stitch the tissue to form tight approximation and to prevent leakage. The "B-shaped" staples allow small blood vessels to pass through it to maintain the blood supply to the anastomosis and its distal end. The cutter on the top of the stapler can be used to remove the excess inverted tissue from the intestine in order to keep the intestine lumen patent.

The advantages of using a stapler for anastomosis include the following: (1). The staples are generally made of titanium, which causes milder tissue reactions than those caused by regular sutures. (2). Because the staples are arranged neatly with equal space and the tightness of the stitch is controlled by a scale, this method can avoid the over-tightening and over-loosening commonly seen in the hand-sewn suture to ensure good healing of the tissue. (3). It can simplify the operation of the procedure with quicker anastomosis and lower operative time. (4). A stapler can be easily used for low anastomosis, which is difficult to complete by hand-sewing, to improve the chance of sphincter preservation.

The disadvantages of using a stapler for anastomosis include the following: (1). Metal staples are still foreign bodies for the human body and can cause local inflammatory reaction in anastomosis, which is associated with risk of anastomotic bleeding and anastomotic leakage. (2). Anastomotic stenosis is more likely to occur if (a) the size of the stapler selected is too small; (b) the adipose tissue or the loose connective tissue around the anastomosis or the folded intestinal wall that were embedded in the anastomosis were stitched by mistake (this can result in overgrowth of granulation tissue later); and c) inappropriate suture of the seromuscular layer in the anastomosis causes excessive tissue inversion and widened scars during healing. (3). Retained staples in the body will affect the postoperative computed tomography (CT) and magnetic resonance imaging (MRI) examinations, radiation therapy, and thermal therapy. (4). Higher cost of a stapler limits the application in clinical practice. (5). The detached staples may lead to pain, hematochezia, and discomfort. (6). The occurrence of segmental motility-disturbance syndrome (named by the authors).

The concept of segmental motility-disturbance syndrome: The retained staples cause anastomotic inflammation and formation of scar tissue or excessive granulation tissue, which reduce intestinal wall elasticity and compliance and cause stiff anastomosis, stiff adjacent intestinal wall tissue, and loss of the function of relaxing and contracting. The intestinal peristalsis is resisted when it reaches the anastomosis, causing interrupted propulsive and peristaltic waves or even antiperistalsis. The intestinal contents accumulated above the anastomosis produce a certain pressure. When the pressure reaches the nerve stimulation threshold, the bowel peristalsis can be triggered to push the stool out, and multiple episodes of bowel peristalsis are required for defecation. Therefore, diarrhea and constipation occur alternatively. Clinically, patients often have a sensation of abdominal emptiness after multiple diarrhea episodes and then become constipated for several days. In severe cases, symptoms similar to intestinal obstruction may occur.

Comprehensive evaluation: In terms of tissue alignment and blood supply in the anastomosis, stapled anastomosis can achieve outcomes between those achieved by the single-layer and the double-layer hand-sewn anastomosis, and it has better mechanical healing. The current literature has not confirmed that stapled anastomosis has more advantages than simple hand-sewn anastomosis. Selection of a method often depends on the surgeon's experience and the clinical conditions (Fig. 6.1).

Compression Anastomosis

Compression anastomosis was first reported by Denan in 1826 [9]. The main idea was to compress the two segments of the intestinal wall together to produce tissue necrosis and then healing, resulting in recanalization of the two segments of the intestine. The principle is to use two opposite anastomosis rings to create patent anastomosis through ischemic necrosis and shedding of the excess tissue, and the shed tissue and the rings, together with the intestinal content, are expelled from the body. No foreign material is retained in the body. Therefore, this anastomotic

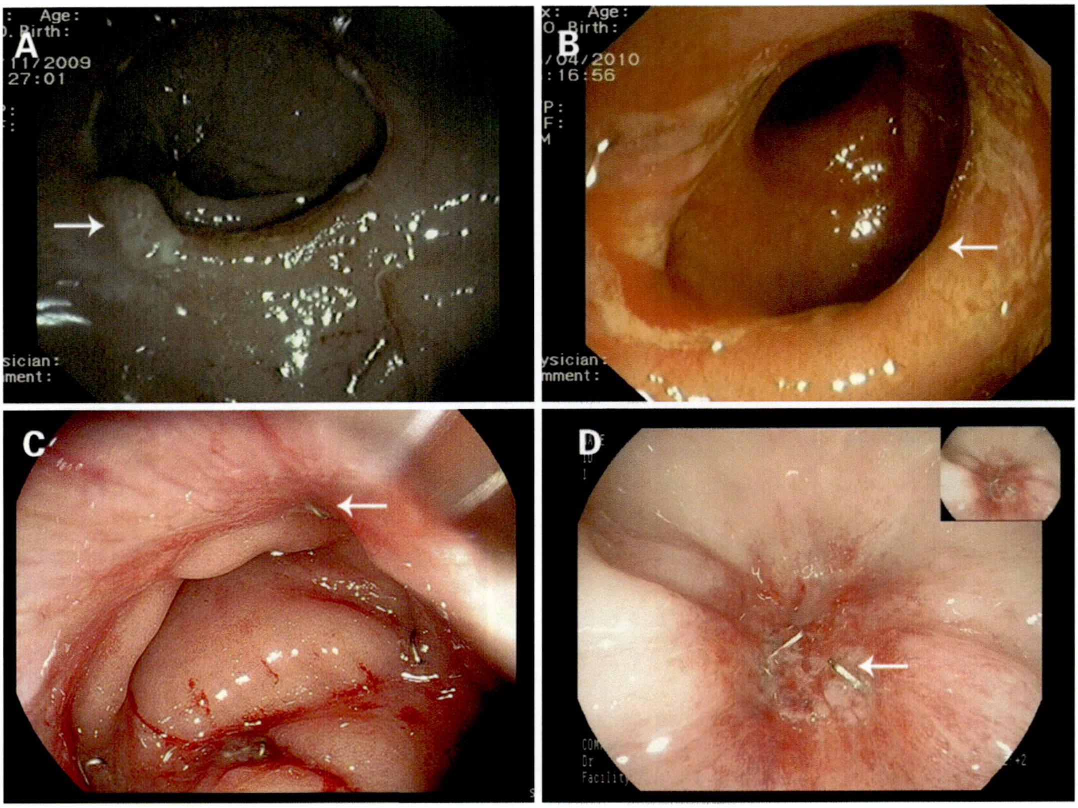

Fig. 6.1 Common endoscopic inflammatory manifestations after stapled anastomosis. (**a**) Granuloma at the anastomosis (*arrow*). (**b**) Stiff and narrow anastomosis with obvious inflammation (*arrow*). (**c**) Mucosal hemorrhage, visible staples (*arrow*), and obvious stenosis at the anastomosis. (**d**) Visible staples (*arrow*) and completely occluded anastomosis

technique does not cause an inflammatory reaction, stenosis, and foreign body reactions and is expected to solve the problem of anastomotic stenosis and leakage.

Murphy's Button

In 1892, the famous American surgeon Murphy invented a device called the Murphy button [10]. This device consists of two hollow, mushroom-shaped metal pieces. The tissues of the intestinal wall at both ends are fixed on the device by a purse-string suture. The built-in spring causes the mushroom-shaped metal pieces to compress the intestinal wall together. The device is expelled with necrotic intestinal wall tissue from the body. This device is simpler than Denan's metal ring and has been used ever since.

Biofragmentable Anastomosis Ring (BAR)

In 1985, Hardy et al. [11] invented the BAR. The BAR consists of two rings made of biomaterial containing absorbable polyglycolic acid (87.5%) and absorbable barium sulfate suspension (12.5%). The two segments with scalloped rims are attached together on a central frame. There is a gap of 1.5 mm, 2 mm, or 2.5 mm in its closed position to accommodate different thicknesses of the intestinal wall. This design prevents compressed necrosis to a certain extent. The two rings of the BAR are placed at each end of the intestine and then are locked after placement of a pursue-string suture to complete the anastomosis. The retained BAR will be passed out in the stool within 2–3 weeks after the operation. BAR has been widely used in gastrointestinal anastomosis.

There is no significant difference in the incidence of complications in the use of BAR compared with stapled anastomosis and hand-sewn anastomosis. The procedure for BAR is simpler and less time-consuming than the other two methods, and microscopy shows that it causes a minimal degree of anastomotic tissue necrosis [12, 13]. However, the anastomosis with BAR may fail if the surgeon failed in the placement of a purse-string suture or selected the wrong device size.

Slesser et al. [14] performed a meta-analysis of postoperative conditions in 1969 patients undergoing hand-sewn, stapled, and compression anastomosis (mostly using BAR) from 10 randomized controlled trials. There was no statistically significant difference in the incidence of anastomotic stenosis between compression anastomosis and hand-sewn or stapler anastomosis. The compression anastomosis was associated with early postoperative intestinal function recovery [weighted mean difference (WMD): −1.02; 95% confidence interval (CI): −1.37, −0.66; $p < 0.001$] and shorter length of postoperative hospital stay (WMD: −1.13; 95% CI: −1.52, −0.74; $p < 0.001$). However, it was more prone to postoperative intestinal obstruction [odds ratio (OR) 1.87; 95% CI: 1.07, 3.26; $p = 0.03$].

AKA-2

In 1984, Kanshin et al. [15] developed the AKA-2 device, which can be used for transanal compression anastomosis. The working principle of the device is similar to that of the stapler. It consists of two plastic anastomosis rings, one of which is a base ring including metal staples and metal springs. After completion of the compression anastomosis, the two anastomosis rings and the necrotic tissue within the rings are expelled from the body in stools within 4–6 days. The advantage of this device is that the anastomosis can form a good lumen to ensure the smooth passage of intestinal contents. However, early expulsion of the anastomosis ring increases the risk of anastomotic leakage. Although there are few reports on the use of AKA-2, they have shown its feasibility and safety in intestinal anastomosis [16].

Compression Anastomotic Clip (CAC)

CAC is made of nonbiologically active Nitinol alloy [17]. After heating, it is made into a high-toughness Nitinol ring. The double-ring device with a diameter of 30 mm can produce a compressive force of 400 g/cm^2. This material is featured by changing its shape with external temperature and having a memory function. In ice water at 0 °C, the anastomosis ring opens at an angle of 30° to 40° due to loss of toughness, and when the device is placed in the human body, the angle is restored to the closed state by the action of the human body temperature. The elliptical design of the device facilitates the expulsion of the anastomosis ring. This device has been used clinically and is considered simple, safe, and effective in both laparotomy and laparoscopic surgery [18].

Compared with stapled anastomosis, the CAC anastomosis has the following advantages. (1) After CAC anastomosis, the intestinal wall is relatively intact and smooth without retained staples, and the incidence of anastomotic stenosis is low. (2) The strength required for CAC closure is small. Thus, both ends of the intestinal wall can be continually compressed, and the risk of damage to the intestinal wall of the anastomosis is greatly reduced. However, because of the expensive CAC material and complicated manufacturing process, the price of CAC is relatively high.

Endoluminal Compression Anastomosis Ring (EndoCAR)

The principle of EndoCAR anastomosis is similar to that of CAC, and its application is similar to that of the stapled anastomosis. It can not only complete the side-to-side anastomosis but also complete the end-to-side anastomosis and end-to-end anastomosis, especially for low rectal anastomosis. When the two EndoCARs are closed, tissue necrosis and healing occur under a constant continuous pressure (approximately 7.7 N) produced by titanium alloy compression. The device is expelled from the body in 7–10 days [17].

Compared with stapled anastomosis, it has the following advantages. (1) The tensile strength of the anastomosis is greater during the period with risk of anastomotic leakage, and this indicates that it can reduce the incidence of anastomotic leakage. (2) There is no foreign body retained in the intestinal wall after anastomosis, and the internal diameter of the anastomosis is relatively large. These can reduce the incidence of postoperative anastomotic stenosis. (3) Postoperative pathology shows mild anastomotic inflammatory reaction and unobvious scar growth [19].

Tabola et al. [20] analyzed the postoperative data of 565 patients who underwent EndoCAR anastomosis and traditional colorectal anastomosis (including hand-sewn and stapled anastomosis). They found that EndoCAR anastomoses were not significantly different from traditional anastomoses in terms of anastomotic leakage, exhaust time, time for returning to normal diet, and the length of hospital stay.

Magnetic Anastomosis Device

If the compression anastomosis only mechanically aligns the tissue without long-lasting pressure, when anastomotic leakage occurs before the anastomosis device has been expelled from the body, there will be very serious consequences. Magnetic anastomosis has the above-described advantages of EndoCAR and can produce a long-lasting and gradually increasing pressure on the intestinal wall. When ischemic necrosis occurs in the intestinal wall that is clamped into the anastomosis ring, the intestinal wall becomes thinner, and the distance between the two magnetic rings reduces, but the compression force increases to thereby accelerate tissue necrosis and shedding. Moreover, the cost of the magnetic anastomosis device is lower than that of EndoCAR. Magnetic anastomosis has been widely used in bile duct and vascular anastomosis [21, 22]. However, due to issues in patent anastomosis and stent fixation, the application in intestinal anastomosis is limited.

The Work We Have Done

Spherical Magnetic Compression Colorectal Anastomosis Device

Using the magnetic compression anastomosis technique, we designed a new type of spherical magnetic compression colorectal anastomosis device and carried out experimental research in a pig model of colorectal anastomosis. The purpose of the experiment was to determine the magnetic force of the magnetic anastomosis rings in vitro and in vivo and the bursting pressure at the anastomosis at different time points after operation. The gross anatomical observation and histopathological examination of the anastomotic specimen were performed to detect the healing process of the anastomosis to evaluate the feasibility, safety, advantages, and disadvantages of the device.

Device Design

The spherical magnetic compression anastomosis device is composed of two structurally mated hemispheres, each of which is equipped with a magnetic anastomosis ring. At the intestinal anastomosis, the intestinal stumps are respectively fixed on the hemisphere parts, which are brought together to form a complete spherical device in the intestinal lumen. The cylindrical channel can maintain the patency of the intestinal lumen. The magnetic force between the magnetic rings exerts a continuous pressure on the intestinal wall, thereby completing the anastomosis to restore the continuity of the intestinal tract. The sphere device and necrotic tissue are expelled by bowel movement.

Related parameters: The spherical device is made of nontoxic polyethylene material, with 3 different specifications (outer/inner diameter of 32/15 mm, 28/13 mm, and 26/11 mm, respectively). The magnetic anastomosis ring is made of neodymium-iron-boron magnetic materials with a surface magnetic force of 2000 G/2000 G and outer diameters of 29 mm, 26 mm, and

24 mm, which correspond to inner diameters of 25 mm, 22 mm, and 20 mm, respectively. The weight of the ball is 10 g. The surface of the spherical body and the internal passage channel is smooth and will not cause damage to the intestinal mucosa. The intestinal contents can pass smoothly. It can be applied to colorectal or small intestine anastomosis (Fig. 6.2).

Experimental Procedure

We selected 15 female pigs with an average weight of 40 kg and divided them into five groups of three pigs. In each group, two pigs were assigned to the experimental group. The magnetic compression anastomosis device with a magnetic ring (outer diameter of 29 mm) was used for end-to-end anastomosis in the rectum 15 cm away from the anus. The other pig was

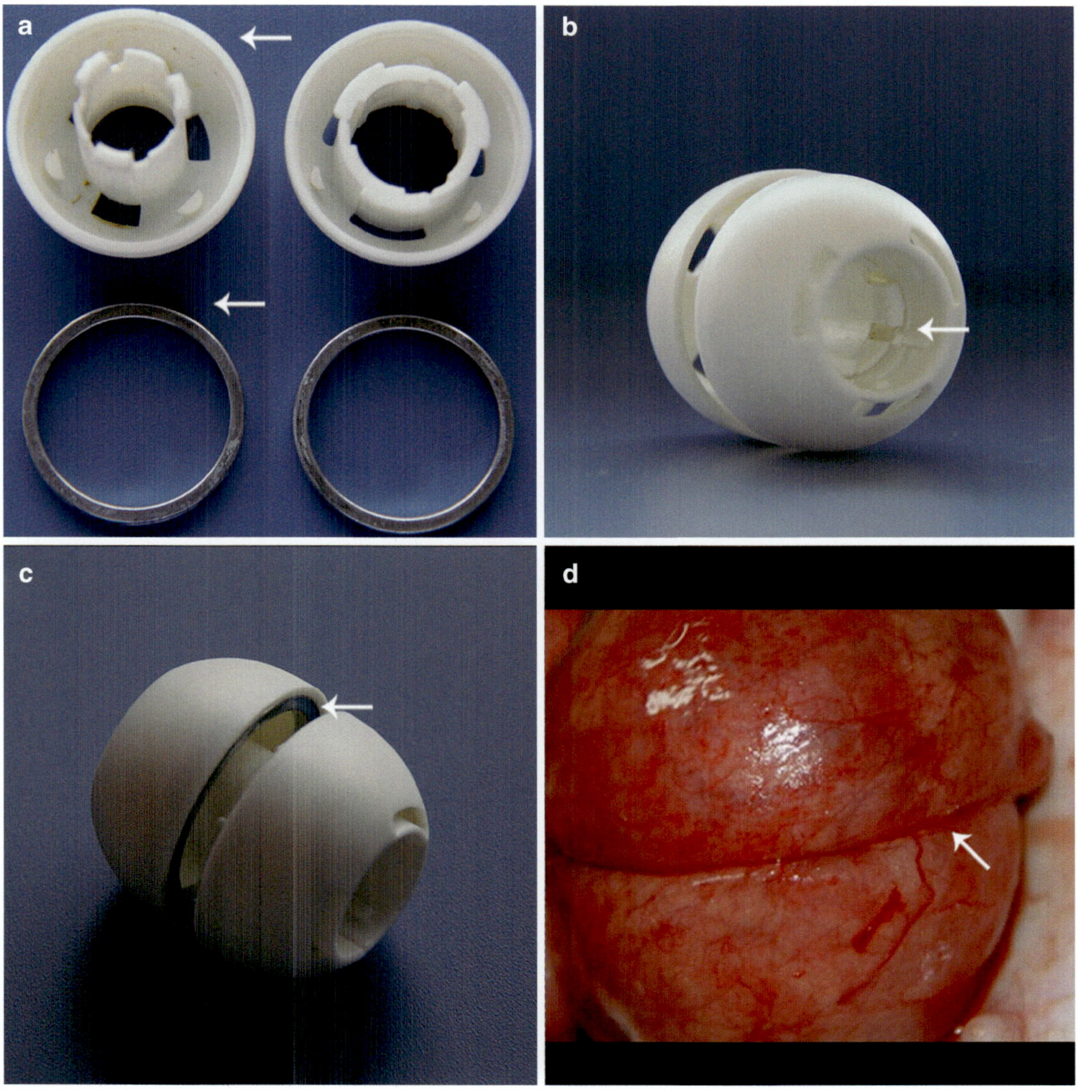

Fig. 6.2 Spherical magnetic compression anastomosis device. (**a**) The mated hemisphere body is indicated by the arrow in the top, the bottom arrow points to the magnetic ring. (**b**) The arrow indicates the internal passage channel. (**c**) A spherical magnetic compression colorectal anastomosis device. (**d**) A complete spherical structure after the completion of an anastomosis. The arrow points to the anastomotic site

assigned to the control group. The Johnson & Johnson 29-mm circular stapler was used to complete the end-to-end anastomosis at the same position. The anastomosis was not enforced with silk suture in either the experimental or control groups. After the operation, the animals were housed individually. The technician recorded the feeding status, general condition, defecation, and expulsion time of the anastomosis device. The pigs were sacrificed on the 3rd, 5th, 7th, 9th, and 14th postoperative days. The anastomosis specimens were harvested for determination of bursting pressure, gross anatomical observation, and pathological examination. The specific experimental procedure was described in previous literature [23].

Experimental Results

Intraoperative and Postoperative Recovery

The anastomosis in the experimental group and the control group was completed in approximately 10 minutes.

Both groups of animals were fed with fluid food on the second day, and the average defecation time was 4 days. The average expulsion time of the magnetic anastomosis device in the experimental group was 7.5 days, and the anastomosis rings were intact. In the control group, anastomotic leakage occurred in one case (1/5), adhesions around the small intestine were seen in two cases (2/5), and no anastomotic stenosis was reported. There was no anastomotic leakage or anastomotic stenosis in the experimental group, but there were two cases of abdominal adhesion.

Intraoperative magnetic force measurement: the largest magnetic force was detected at the anastomosis. The average magnetic force was 132.67 G. The magnetic force was attenuated to 9.75 G at 1.5 cm from the anastomosis and was negligible at more than 3 cm from the anastomosis. No magnetic force was detected on the body surface of the abdomen, back, chest, and hip. As the distance from the anastomosis increased, the magnetic force decayed rapidly and did not affect the surrounding tissue.

Determination of anastomotic bursting pressure: The lowest bursting pressure of the two anastomoses was detected on the 5th day, with an average of 117.5 mmHg and 72.5 mmHg for the experimental and control groups, respectively. The experiment showed that the bursting pressure of the experimental group reached 280 mmHg at the 7th day, and there was no air leakage at the anastomotic site, but the surrounding normal intestinal wall tissues were ruptured under this pressure. The bursting pressure in the control group was 200 mmHg, at which the air leak of the anastomosis was present. After 7 days, the bursting pressure of the anastomosis increased slightly and remained stable, at 300 mmHg in the experimental group and 280 mmHg in the control group.

Gross and Histopathological Results

On the third day after operation, the gross anatomical examination showed inflammatory hyperemia of the intestinal wall around the anastomosis, well-healed anastomosis and no leakage, nonexpanded proximal bowel, and patent anastomosis in the experimental group. The gross anatomical examination showed a large amount of inflammatory exudation of the intestinal wall around the anastomosis without leakage or stenosis in the control group. The histopathological examination showed obvious anastomotic inflammatory exudation, a few fibroblasts and blood vessels, and no obvious collagen deposition in the experimental group. The histopathological examination showed obvious inflammatory exudation and no obvious fibroblasts and blood vessels in the control group.

On the 5th day after operation, the gross anatomical examination in the experimental group showed that the inflammatory exudation of the intestinal wall around the anastomosis was significantly reduced and the serosa surface was smooth, without leakage and stenosis. In the control group, inflammatory exudate was in the intestinal wall tissue around the anastomosis, granuloma formation was observed, and the serosa surface was rough.

The histopathological examination in the experimental group showed fibroblast proliferation, capillary proliferation, decreased inflammatory exudation, and a small amount of collagen fibers. The histopathological examination in the control group showed fibroblast and capillary proliferation, decreased inflammatory exudation, and a small number of collagen fibers.

On the 7th day after surgery, the gross anatomical examination in the experimental group showed the healed serosa, disappeared anastomotic gap, slightly rough serosa surface, and significantly reduced inflammatory exudation. The gross anatomical examination in the control group showed visible inflammatory exudation in the anastomosis, vague anastomotic gap, and rough serosa surface.

The histopathological examination in the experimental group showed proliferative granulation tissue accompanied by inflammatory exudation and partial collagen formation. In the control group, fibroblasts, vascular endothelial cells, fibroblasts, and collagen fibers were observed with a small number of inflammatory cells.

On the 9th day after surgery, the gross anatomical examination in the experimental group showed healed anastomosis with scar and no obvious inflammatory exudation. The gross anatomical examination in the control group showed anastomotic scar, retained staples, rough surface, and local tissue necrosis.

The histopathological examination in the experimental group showed increased fibroblasts and collagen fibers, decreased blood vessels, and scar formation. Most inflammatory exudation was absorbed. The histopathological examination in the control group showed increased fibroblasts and collagen fibers and decreased blood vessels. Inflammatory exudation was partially absorbed.

On the 14th day after surgery, the gross anatomical examination in the experimental group showed "serosalized" anastomosis. The morphology of the anastomosis was difficult to distinguish. Anastomotic scar healing was observed by dissection. The gross anatomical examination result in the control group was basically consistent with that in the experimental group. After the dissection of the anastomosis, healed anastomosis with scar and retained staple were observed. The scar was wide, and the inner diameter of the intestine was slightly narrow.

The histopathological examination in the experimental group showed obviously proliferated fibroblasts and collagen fibers, scar formation, and disappearance of inflammatory exudation. Grown mucosa mostly covered the wound that was almost healed. The histopathological examination in the control group showed obviously proliferated fibroblasts and collagen fibers, scar formation, disappearance of inflammatory exudation, mucosal hyperplasia, and a nearly healed wound.

Please refer to [23] for the specific data and pictures.

Magnetic Compression Colorectal Stapler

The results of the first phase of animal experiments suggest that the new spherical magnetic compression colorectal anastomosis device has potential advantages compared with traditional stapler anastomosis in terms of anastomotic results, anastomotic bursting pressure determination, anastomotic healing, and complication rate.

To facilitate the anastomosis operation and be more conducive to clinical application, we modified the magnetic compression anastomosis device and assembled it with the auxiliary components to form a complete magnetic compression colorectal stapler. The release of the magnetic compression anastomosis device can be performed after the anastomosis is completed. With the aid of the auxiliary components, the operation (such as low anal sphincter preservation) in the deeper surgical sites can be completed.

Device Design

Magnetic Compression Anastomosis Device

The magnetic compression anastomosis device comprises two mated "primary magnet" and "secondary magnet." The surfaces of the two magnets are smooth with curved sides. Each magnet consists of a shell and a magnetic ring. There are adjustable gaps in the vertical direction between the shell and the ring to accommodate the intestinal wall tissue with different thicknesses and to ensure that the intestinal wall tissue is firmly compressed. The center of the device is a passage channel. When the magnets were brought together, the passage channels of the two magnets connected to maintain the patency of the intestinal lumen. After completion of the anastomosis, the device is generally a "sphere-like structure" and can eventually be passed in the stool.

Related parameters: The shell is composed of nontoxic polyethylene material. The magnetic ring is made of neodymium-iron-boron magnetic material. The surface of the magnetic ring is coated with an epoxy resin that is harmless to biological tissues. The magnetic force and external diameter are kept the same. Because the magnet has a connection structure to the auxiliary component, the total weight of the anastomosis device is increased to approximately 15 g.

Auxiliary Component Assembly

Similar to a conventional round staple stapler, the component includes an anvil for mounting the primary magnet and a stapler for mounting the second magnet. The first magnet is connected to the anvil by an elastic latching structure, and the inner diameter of the passage channel is equal to the outer diameter of the anvil. After completion of the anastomosis, the anvil can be separated from the magnetic compression anastomosis device through the passage channel. The second magnet is coupled to the stapler main body by an annular elastic latching structure, and the top end of the stapler main body includes an annular cutter at a position within the channel of the magnetic ring to cut the compressed intestinal wall tissue. To increase safety, we also tried to install the staple cartridge between the cutter and the magnetic ring and to complete the "double anastomosis," that is, the stapled anastomosis and the magnetic compression anastomosis. This procedure was carried out as another experimental group.

Releasing the magnetic compression anastomosis device from the auxiliary component into the intestinal lumen after anastomosis depends on the assembly method of the second magnet and the main stapler components. To this end, we designed a variety of assembly tools and release methods, including push-up assembly tools, pull-down assembly tools, drawstring assembly tools, and rotary assembly tools. Through repeated verification, the push-up assembly tool was finally selected. In this design, the second magnet and the operating rod are connected by an elastic latching structure. After completion of the anastomosis, the latching part is disengaged from the card slot by the push-up operation, and the two magnets that are mated are released. The "push up" is an action along the vertical axis of the magnetic ring and is operated in the homeward direction, and thus it has the highest stability (Fig. 6.3).

Experimental Process

We selected 15 male Bama miniature pigs with an average weight of 40 kg and divided them into five groups of three animals. In each group, an animal was assigned to the experimental group A. In group A, the magnetic compression anastomosis device with a magnetic ring outer diameter of 29 mm was used for end-to-end anastomosis in the rectum 15 cm away from the anus. The top of the main component of the stapler was equipped with a staple cartridge within the magnetic ring. "Double anastomosis," that is, stapler anastomosis and magnetic compression anastomosis, was performed. An animal was assigned to the experimental group B, and magnetic compression anastomosis was performed at the same site as for group A. The other animal was assigned to the control group C. A Johnson & Johnson 29-mm circular stapler was used to complete the end-to-end anastomosis at the same site. The anastomosis was not enforced with silk suture in either the experimental or control groups. As in the previous experiment, after the surgery, the pigs were housed individually. The technician recorded the feeding status, general condition, defecation, and expulsion time of the anastomosis device.

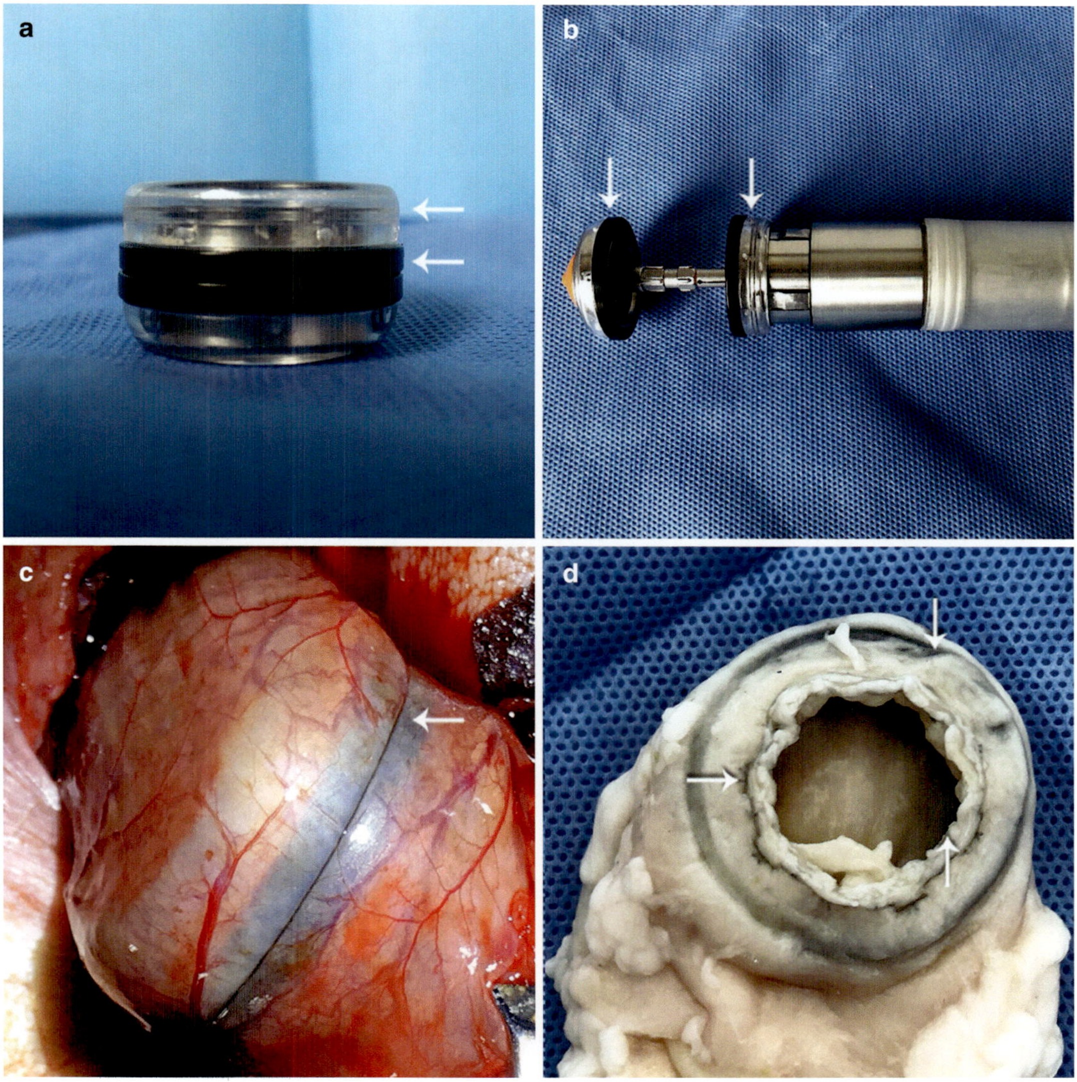

Fig. 6.3 Magnetic compression stapler. (**a**) Magnetic compression anastomosis device: the state of the primary magnet and the secondary magnet is mated. The upper arrow indicates the shell of the primary magnet; the lower arrow indicates the magnetic ring of the primary magnet. (**b**) The arrow left of the magnetic compression stapler indicates the primary magnet mounted on the anvil; the right arrow indicates the secondary magnet that is mounted on the stapler main component. (**c**) The magnetic compression anastomosis device after the completion of anastomosis. The arrow points to the anastomotic site. (**d**) The cross-sectional structure of the tissue after completion of the anastomosis: the top arrow indicates the track of the magnetic ring, the left arrow indicates the closed staple, and the lower arrow indicates the wound edge after the circular cutting

The timepoints of postoperative observation were different than in the previous experiment. The anastomotic specimen was harvested 1 day before expulsion of the anastomosis device (approximately 6 days after surgery), 1 day after expulsion of the anastomosis device (approximately 8 days after surgery), and at sacrifice at 2 weeks, 4 weeks, or 12 weeks after surgery for the determination of the magnetic force and bursting pressure, and the gross anatomical observation and histopathological examination of the anastomosis site. Enteroscopy was performed for 2 weeks, 4 weeks, and 12 weeks to provide a more intuitive understanding of mucosal healing in the intestinal lumen.

Experimental Results

Intraoperative and Postoperative Recovery

The anastomosis of the experimental groups A and B and the control group C was completed in approximately 10 minutes. There was no significant difference from the previous experimental results.

Both groups of animals were fed fluid food on the second day, and the average defecation time was 3.5 days. The average expulsion time of the magnetic anastomosis device in the experimental group was 7 days, and the anastomosis rings were intact. In the control group, anastomotic leakage occurred in one case (1/5), adhesions around the small intestine were seen in one case (1/5), and no anastomotic stenosis was reported. No anastomotic leakage or anastomotic stenosis was observed in the experimental group. There was no significant difference from the previous experimental data.

The magnetic force measurement results were basically consistent with the previous experimental results.

Determination of anastomotic bursting pressure: The lowest bursting pressure of the two anastomoses was observed on the 6th day, with an average of 180 mmHg and 135 mmHg for the experimental group and the control group, respectively. The experiment showed that the bursting pressure of the experimental group reached 280 mmHg on the 8th postoperative day. Under this pressure, rupture of the surrounding normal intestinal wall tissue of the anastomosis site occurred. The bursting pressure in the control group was 200 mmHg, at which air leak of the anastomosis was observed. After 8 days, the bursting pressure in the experimental group was stable at approximately 300 mmHg, and the bursting pressure of the control group was stable at approximately 280 mmHg. Good tensile strength was observed in the anastomosis in both groups. Because the selected magnetic ring has consistent magnetic force, the magnetic force measurement and the anastomotic bursting pressure measurement are basically consistent with the previous experimental data.

Over time, the anastomotic healing of the experimental group and the control group improved. At 2 weeks (W), 4 W and 12 W after surgery, the anastomotic scar was becoming smaller and the anastomosis was more patent in the experimental group; in the control group, more visible staples and more obvious inflammatory reaction were noted in the anastomosis. As shown in Fig.6.4e, the track of the anastomosis was almost invisible in the experimental group at 12 W, while the anastomosis shown in Fig.6.4f was easier to identify.

Gross and Histopathological Results (Fig. 6.5)

The results on the 6th and 8th postoperative days and 2nd postoperative week were consistent with the previous results and are not shown here.

Four weeks after operation, the gross anatomical observation in the experimental group showed well-healed anastomosis with complete coverage of the mucosa, smooth serosa surface, and a thin-line scar difficult to recognize with the naked eye. The gross anatomical observation in the control group showed well-healed anastomosis with complete coverage of the mucosa, mild adhesion to the surrounding tissue on the serosa surface, and a more obvious scar than that in the experimental group.

The histopathological examination in the experimental group showed fibrous scar formation, no inflammatory exudation, mucosal growth completely covering the wound surface, and basically healed mucosal surface. The morphology of the new mucosa was close to the normal one. The tissue layer was relatively clear. The histopathological examination in the control group showed fibrous scar formation, inflammatory exudation, and basically healed mucosa. The morphology and structure of the new mucosa were disordered.

Twelve weeks after operation, the gross anatomical observation in the experimental group showed well-healed anastomosis with complete coverage of the mucosa, smooth serosa surface, and a scar difficult to recognize with naked eyes. The gross anatomical observation in the control group showed well-healed anastomosis with

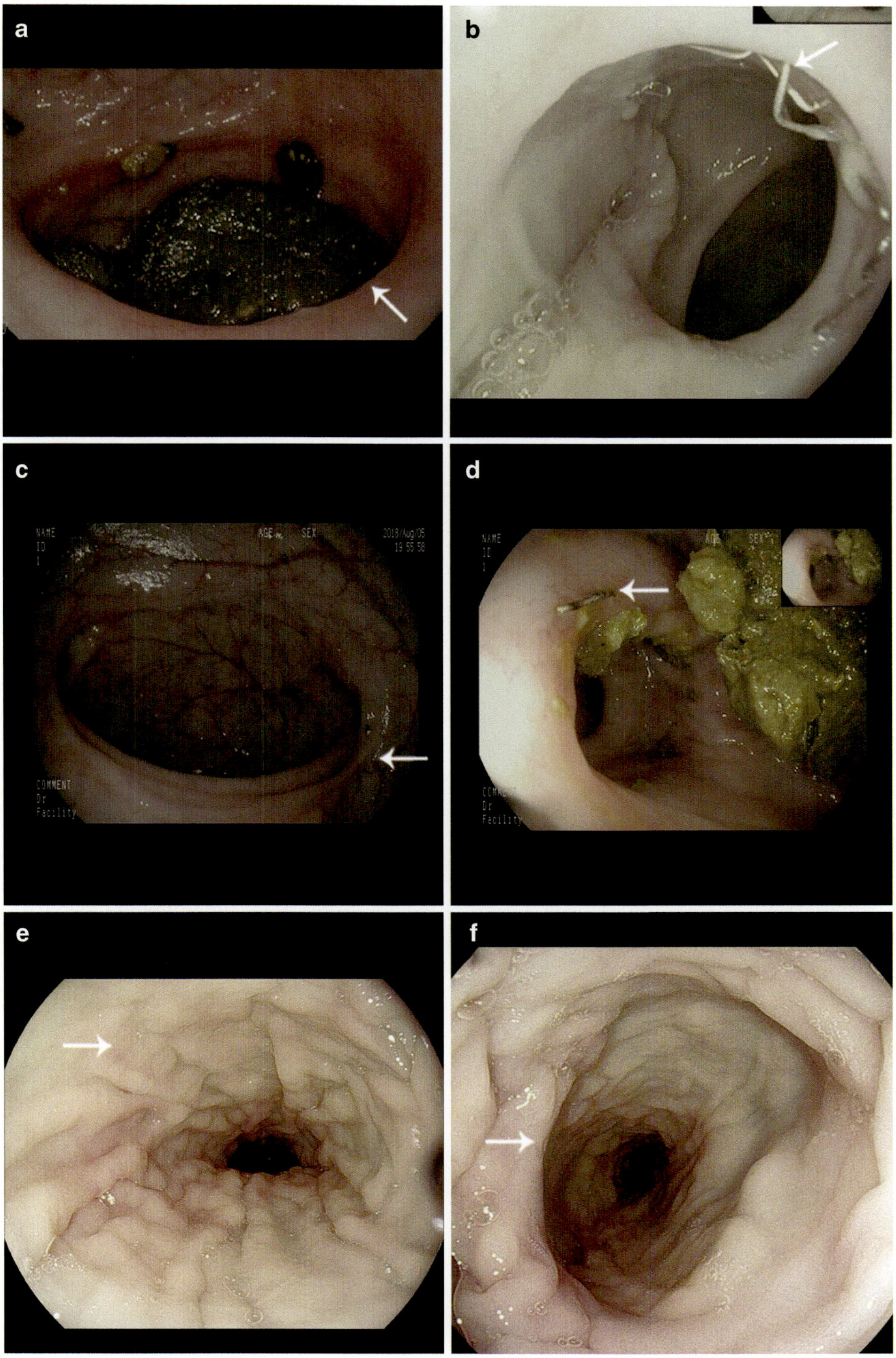

Fig. 6.4 Photograph of anastomosis under colonoscopy. (**a**) At 2 weeks after surgery in the experimental group. (**b**) At 2 weeks after surgery in the control group. (**c**) At 4 weeks after surgery in the experimental group. (**d**) At 4 weeks after surgery in the control group. (**e**) At 12 weeks after surgery in the experimental group. (**f**) At 12 weeks after surgery in the control group. The arrows indicate the anastomosis, where the exposed staples are visible in panels B and D

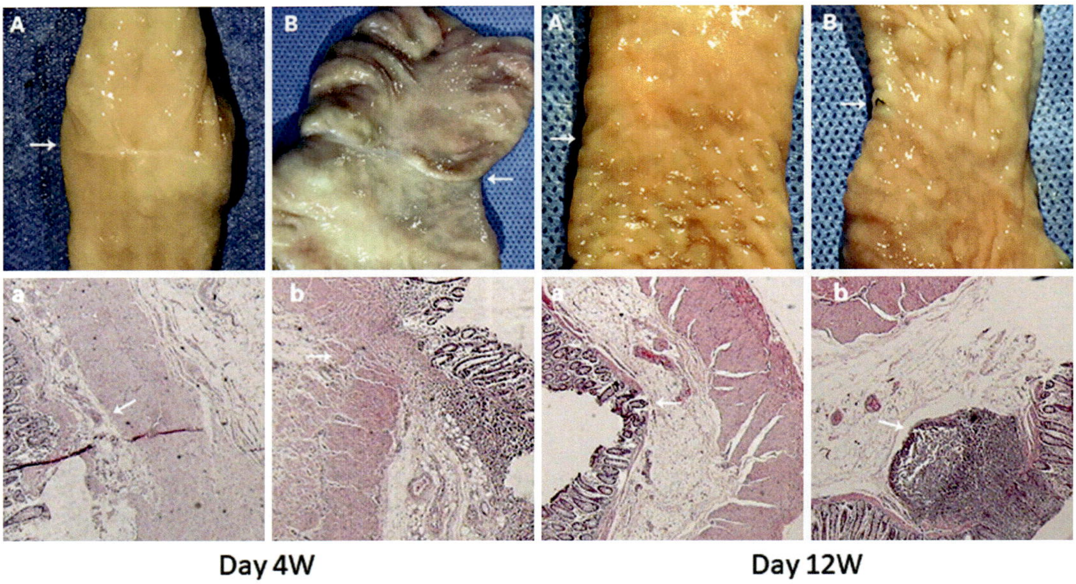

Fig. 6.5 Gross anatomical and histological examinations on day 4 W and day 12 W. A gross anatomical examination of (**a**) the pigs in the experimental group and (**b**) the pigs in the control group, and a histological examination of (**a**) the pigs in the experimental group and (**b**) the pigs in the control group. The arrow points to the anastomotic site

complete coverage of the mucosa, mild adhesion to the surrounding tissue on the serosa surface, exposed staples, and obvious scar compared with that in the experimental group.

The histopathological examination in the experimental group showed fibrous scar formation, no obvious inflammatory exudation, mucosal growth completely covering the wound surface, and well-healed mucosal surface. The morphology of the new mucosa was close to the normal one. The tissue layer was clearer. The histopathological examination in the control group showed fibrous scar formation, a small amount of inflammatory exudation, and basically healed mucosa. The morphology and structure of the new mucosa were disordered.

Discussion

Based on the principle of continuous magnetic compression, we designed the original "concept version" of the spherical magnetic compression colorectal anastomosis device. The magnetic anastomosis rings bring the two ends of the anastomosis intimately close together by magnetic force. The pressure causes the intervened tissue to gradually become ischemic and necrotic. The site of the anastomotic intestine is gradually healed through the inflammatory repair process, and the continuity of the intestinal tract is restored. As the tissue gradually becomes necrotic, the two magnetic rings gradually approach to produce further enhanced pressure. Therefore, the persistent tight anastomosis accelerates the necrosis of the intervening tissue. Meanwhile, after completion of the anastomosis, the inner space of the spherical device forms a sufficiently large passage channel so that the contents in the intestinal tract are easily passed. This can lower the pressure on the anastomosis. Finally, the anastomosis is completely healed approximately 7 days after surgery, and the anastomosis device falls off with the necrotic tissue and is passed in the stool. The results of the first-phase animal experiments have demonstrated the safety and superiority of a spherical magnetic compression colorectal anastomosis device.

Furthermore, to facilitate the anastomosis operation and clinical application, we reduced the volume of the anastomosis device with unchanged magnetic force and outer diameter of the magnetic ring and assembled it onto the auxiliary component to form a complete colorectal magnetic compression anastomosis device. The stapler can easily release the anastomosis device into the intestinal lumen when the anastomosis is completed. From the actual operation point of view, the use of the spherical magnetic compression anastomosis device or the magnetic compression colorectal stapler did not increase the operative time compared with the use of a circular stapler.

Previous studies have shown that the greater magnetic force of the anastomosis ring is associated with greater compression strength, shorter time to complete necrosis and healing, earlier falling off of the magnetic ring, and greater impact on the surrounding tissue. If a magnetic force of 3000–6000 G is applied, the intestinal wall tissue in the anastomosis falls off due to necrosis 48 hours after surgery. As a consequence, an anastomotic leakage occurs [24]. Therefore, we used a magnetic force of 2000 G, which not only ensures the firmness and tightness of the anastomosis but also makes the rings fall off smoothly after the anastomosis is healed. Moreover, the appropriate magnetic force avoids magnetic interference on the surrounding tissue.

In this study, we designed magnetic rings with different outer diameters and inner diameters, which matched with the shell, including passage channels. We selected the 29 mm magnetic ring for the experiment because it is matched to the pig's colorectal diameter. Based on the current technique, more clinically applicable devices can be produced. These devices can ensure the smoothness of the anastomosis and passage of intestinal contents through the passage channel without resistance. The total weight of the anastomosis device is approximately 15 g, which is roughly equivalent to the weight of the stool with similar volume. Thus, it does not cause compression on the anastomosis and should not cause discomfort.

In both experiments, no anastomotic leakage occurred in the experimental group, but an anastomotic leakage occurred in the control group (1/5). The early stage is a period having high possibility of anastomotic leakage because of the lack of collagen and the weak tensile strength of the anastomosis. Compared with stapler anastomosis, magnetic compression anastomosis can provide greater tensile strength. The tensile system is mainly present in the submucosa layer, and the magnetic compression anastomosis can directly bring the submucosa layers together. Meanwhile, it can maintain blood flow of the serosal layer, which provides good support for healing and reduces the occurrence of anastomotic leakage. The histopathological examination of the anastomosis has provided proof. There was no anastomotic leakage in the experimental groups A and B. This indicated that magnetic compression anastomosis is very safe, and there is no need for the aid of stapled anastomosis.

In this study, significant advantages in colonoscopy and gross and histopathological examination were noted in the experimental group. In the early stage after anastomosis, the anastomosis in the experimental group was superior to that of the control group in terms of mucosal smoothness, inflammatory reaction, and scar formation. In the later stage, the magnetic compression anastomosis was superior to the stapled anastomosis in terms of retained foreign body and scar healing.

Prospective

There are many different types of magnetic compression bowel anastomosis devices that have achieved promising results in animal experiments. Jamshidi et al. [24] designed two self-orienting magnetic devices of uniform compression and gradient compression for intestinal side-to-side anastomosis in experimental pigs and compared this with hand-sewn anastomosis and stapled anastomosis. Their results demonstrate the safety and effectiveness of the magnetic compression anastomosis and that the gradient compression device has higher strength and earlier patency than the uniform compression device. The magnetic compression anastomosis device designed by Pichakron et al. [25] has a concavo-convex surface and specially engineered radial topography of the mating surfaces to promote gradual remodeling. Gastrointestinal anastomosis and jejunostomy were performed in experimental pigs. The results showed that the strength of magnetic compression anastomosis was equal to or greater than the strength of hand-sewn or stapled anastomosis. Thus, the magnetic compression anastomosis technique may be a safe, effective, and minimally invasive method to replace the current anastomotic techniques. Wall et al. [26] demonstrated in the porcine animal model that MAGNAMOSIS was feasible in performing a hybrid natural orifice transluminal endoscopic surgery (NOTES) colorectal anastomosis, and it has the advantage over circular staplers of precise endoscopic delivery throughout the entire colon.

Our initial spherical magnetic compression colorectal anastomosis device experiment yielded a promising result similar to the above-depicted experiments, demonstrating the feasibility, safety, effectiveness, and superiority of magnetic compression anastomosis. Further improvement of magnetic compress devices can move the device closer to clinical application. The application of magnetic compression anastomosis techniques is expected to overcome the many disadvantages of stapled anastomosis, reduce the incidence of anastomotic leakage, eliminate the reaction caused by retained foreign body in the intestinal tract, and ultimately improve the quality of life of patients. Unquestionably, there are still some problems that need to be fixed, for instance, the magnetic interference of the magnetic ring on the metal surgical instrument during operation.

References

1. Syk I, Agren MS, Adawi D, et al. Inhibition of matrix metalloproteinases enhances breaking strength of colonic anastomoses in an experimental model[J]. Br J Surg. 2001;88(2):228–34. https://doi.org/10.1046/j.1365-2168.2001.01649.x.
2. de Hingh IH, de Man BM, Lomme RM, et al. Colonic anastomotic strength and matrix metalloproteinase activity in an experimental model of bacterial peritonitis[J]. Br J Surg. 2003;90(8):981–8. https://doi.org/10.1002/bjs.4146.
3. Halsted WS. Circular suture of the intestine-an experimental study[J]. Am J Med Sci. 1970;94(3):436–60. https://doi.org/10.2307/852864.
4. Fraser I. An historical perspective on mechanical aids in intestinal anastomosis[J]. Surg Gynecol Obstet. 1982;155(4):566–74. https://doi.org/10.1002/pd.1970020414.
5. Senagore A, Milsom JW, Walshaw RK, et al. Direct comparison between Czerny-Lembert and circular-stapled anastomotic techniques in colorectal anastomosis: a similar pattern of healing for both[J]. Dis Colon Rectum. 1992;35(9):862–9. https://doi.org/10.1007/BF02047874.
6. Gambee LP, Garnjobst W, Hardwick CE. Ten years' experience with a single layer anastomosis in colon surgery[J]. Am J Surg. 1956;92(2):222–7. https://doi.org/10.1016/S0002-9610(56)80063-9.
7. Hultl H. Zweite Kongress der Gesellschaft fur Chirurgie. Budapest. 1908[J]. Pester Med-Chir Presse. 1909;45:108–10.
8. Moran BJ. Stapling instruments for intestinal anastomosis in colorectal surgery[J]. Br J Surg. 1996;83(7):902–9. https://doi.org/10.1002/bjs.1800830707.
9. Steichen FM, Ravitch MM. History of mechanical devices and instruments for suturing[J]. Curr Probl Surg. 1982;19(1):1–52. https://doi.org/10.1016/0011-3840(82)90004-1.
10. Musana K, Yale SH. John Benjamin Murphy (1857-1916)[J]. Clin Med Res. 2005;3(2):110–2. https://doi.org/10.3121/cmr.3.2.110.
11. Hardy TG Jr, Pace WG, Maney JW, et al. A biofragmentable ring for sutureless bowel anastomosis. An experimental study[J]. Dis Colon Rectum. 1985;28(7):484–90. https://doi.org/10.1007/BF02554090.
12. Thiede A, Geiger D, Dietz UA, et al. Overview on compression anastomoses: biofragmentable anastomosis ring multicenter prospective trial of 1666 anastomoses[J]. World J Surg. 1998;22(1):78–87. https://doi.org/10.1007/s002689900353.
13. Forde KA, Goodell KH, DellaBadia M. A 10-year single-institutional study of the biofragmentable anastomosis ring[J]. Am J Surg. 2006;191(4):483–7. https://doi.org/10.1016/j.amjsurg.2006.01.005.
14. Slesser AA, Pellino G, Shariq O, et al. Compression versus hand-sewn and stapled anastomosis in colorectal surgery: a systematic review and meta-analysis of randomized controlled trials[J]. Tech Coloproctol. 2016;20(10):667–76. https://doi.org/10.1007/s10151-016-1521-8.
15. Kanshin NN, Lytkin MI, Knysh VI, et al. [First experience with application of compression anastomoses with the apparatus AKA-2 in operations on the large intestine][J]. Vestn Khir Im I Grek. 1984;132(1):52–7.

16. Wullstein C, Gross E. Compression anastomosis (AKA-2) in colorectal surgery: results in 442 consecutive patients[J]. Br J Surg. 2000;87(8):1071–5. https://doi.org/10.1046/j.1365-2168.2000.01489.x.
17. Szold A. New concepts for a compression anastomosis: superelastic clips and rings[J]. Minim Invasive Ther Allied Technol. 2008;17(3):168–71. https://doi.org/10.1080/13645700802103126.
18. Zhang D, Zheng C, Song C. A modified method of using laparoscopic compression anastomosis clip for gastrointestinal anastomosis[J]. Minim Invasive Ther Allied Technol. 2010;19(6):350–4. https://doi.org/10.3109/13645706.2010.527777.
19. Chun J, Parikh P, Lee D, et al. Safety of the NiTi EndoCAR following chemoradiation in a porcine model[J]. Surg Innov. 2011;18(4):394–9. https://doi.org/10.1177/1553350611398879.
20. Tabola R, Cirocchi R, Fingerhut A, et al. A systematic analysis of controlled clinical trials using the NiTi CAR™ compression ring in colorectal anastomoses[J]. Tech Coloproctol. 2017;21(3):177–84. https://doi.org/10.1007/s10151-017-1583-2.
21. Itoi T, Yamanouchi E, Ikeuchi N, et al. Magnetic compression duct-to-duct anastomosis for biliary obstruction in a patient with living donor liver transplantation[J]. Gut Liver. 2010;4(Suppl 1):S96–8. https://doi.org/10.5009/gnl.2010.4.S1.S96.
22. Liu SQ, Lei P, Cao ZP, et al. Nonsuture anastomosis of arteries and veins using the magnetic pinned-ring device: a histologic and scanning electron microscopic study[J]. Ann Vasc Surg. 2012;26(7):985–95. https://doi.org/10.1016/j.avsg.2012.04.003.
23. Xu ZF, Li ZJ, Sun YL, et al. A novel spherical magnetic compression device for colorectal anastomosis in a swine model[J]. J Laparoendosc Adv Surg Tech A. 2015;25(4):323–9. https://doi.org/10.1089/lap.2014.0404.
24. Jamshidi R, Stephenson JT, Clay JG, et al. Magnamosis: magnetic compression anastomosis with comparison to suture and staple techniques[J]. J Pediatr Surg. 2009;44(1):222–8. https://doi.org/10.1016/j.jpedsurg.2008.10.044.
25. Pichakron KO, Jelin EB, Hirose S, et al. Magnamosis II: magnetic compression anastomosis for minimally invasive gastrojejunostomy and jejunojejunostomy[J]. J Am Coll Surg. 2011;212(1):42–9. https://doi.org/10.1016/j.jamcollsurg.2010.09.031.
26. Wall J, Diana M, Leroy J, et al. MAGNAMOSIS IV: magnetic compression anastomosis for minimally invasive colorectal surgery[J]. Endoscopy. 2013;45(8):643–8. https://doi.org/10.1055/s-0033-1344119.

Magnets for Fecal Incontinence

7

Mauro Bortolotti

Abbreviations

ABS	Artificial bowel sphincter
CCIS	Cleveland Clinic Incontinence Severity
EAS	External anal sphincter
FI	Fecal incontinence
FIQoL and FIQL	FI Quality of Life
IAS	Internal anal sphincter
MAS	Magnetic anal sphincter
SNS	Sacral nerve stimulation

Introduction

Fecal incontinence (FI) is the involuntary loss of liquid and/or solid stools from the anus, varying from a simple soiling of underpants to complete discharge. It represents a most embarrassing and disabling social problem, causing a poor quality of life, sometimes with severe psychopathological consequences. The prevalence in the general population ranges from 0.8% to 6.2% [1] and from 2.2% to 15% [2], depending on different data collection methods, reaching highest values in women and in elderly people living in community dwellings [3], up to 47% in those confined to bed and/or mentally impaired [2]. Severe incontinence affects 1% of the general population increasing with age [4]. These values are likely underestimated, under-investigated, underdiagnosed, and, consequently, undertreated, because many patients do not seek medical help being ashamed of their condition.

Causes of Fecal Incontinence

The anal canal is surrounded from the interior to the exterior by mucosal and submucosal layers made of smooth, elastic, and expansible connective tissue with a fibrovascular cushion, and by circular bundles of smooth muscle (internal anal sphincter—IAS), adjacent to bundles of striated musculature (external anal sphincter, EAS). The tonic contraction of the sphincters maintains closure of the lumen, with a pressure of about 50–80 mmHg for a length of about 3–4.5 cm and is aided by the fibrovascular cushions to tightly seal the anal canal, the reduction of which is associated with idiopathic FI [5]. In addition, the tonic contraction of puborectalis muscle produces an angle between the axis of the rectum and anal canal forming a kink to the passage of stool contributing to maintain continence especially during the increase of abdominal pressure [6].

Fecal incontinence is chiefly due to a loss of the tonic contraction of anal sphincters, which does not retain the stools in the rectum. Damage of the IAS is responsible for passive inconti-

M. Bortolotti (✉)
Gut Motility Laboratory, Section of Pathophysiology of Digestion, Internal Medicine and Gastroenterology, S.Orsola-Malpighi Polyclinic, University of Bologna, Bologna, Italy

M. Gagner (ed.), *Magnetic Surgery*, https://doi.org/10.1007/978-3-030-73947-8_7

nence and post-defecatory leakage, whereas damage of the EAS is liable for urge incontinence. The causes of FI are numerous (Box 7.1): myopathies, local traumatic lesions, surgical interventions for anal fissure and fistula and hemorrhoids, including the disruption of fibrovascular cushions (Lord's and stretch methods), obstetric perineal injury, spinal cord lesions or peripheral nerves alterations such as impairment of pudendal nerves due to perineal descent caused by weakness of pelvic floor, and severe diarrhea, too. In patients with skeletal muscle diseases, the puborectalis muscle is weakened as well as the external anal sphincter, favoring incontinence, whereas smooth muscle diseases, such as progressive systemic sclerosis, can affect continence by altering rectal compliance and weakening the internal anal sphincter [7]. The "idiopathic" incontinence is commonly due to a traumatic neuropathy of pudendal nerve [8], resulting from an obstetric injury or a straining during defecation, sometimes occurred long before. In addition, there are spontaneous relaxations of the sphincter, not only during the night but also during the day, that facilitate the fecal loss [9]. These different causes can be ascertained with structural and functional specific tests, such as endoscopy, radiology, including defecography, dynamic MRI and MRI proctography, endo-anal ultrasonography (especially the three-dimensional one), anal manometry with balloons for compliance and sensations, as well as neurophysiologic tests, such as electrophysiology and electromyography, on single fiber too. The results of these tests may inform the best way of FI management.

Box 7.1 Causes of Fecal Incontinence

Anorectal Injury
- Childbirth
- Accidental
- Sexual
- Surgical
  - Hemorrhoidectomy
  - Sphincterotomy
  - Prostatectomy
  - Colectomy
  - Pouch procedure
  - Fistulectomy
- Radiation (pelvic)

Gut Diseases
- Rectal prolapse
- Severe diarrhea (any cause)
- Infections (anorectal)
- Crohn's disease
- Cancer (anorectal)

Muscle and Connective Diseases
- Myasthenia gravis
- Muscular dystrophy
- Other myopathies
- Progressive systemic sclerosis
- Degeneration IAS

Neurologic Diseases

Central Nervous System
- Dementia
- Stroke, brain tumors
- Spinal cord lesions
- Multiple sclerosis
- Tabes dorsalis

Peripheral Nervous System
- Cauda equina lesions
- Polyneuropathies
  - Diabetes mellitus
  - Sky-Drager syndrome
  - Toxic Neuropathy

Traumatic neuropathy
- "Idiopathic" incontinence
- Perineal descent

Decreased Rectal Sensation
- Fecal impaction
- "Delayed rectal sensation" syndrome

Treatment

This is a short excursus among the various FI therapeutic possibilities currently available despite the magnetic option.

Nonsurgical

Dietary and lifestyle modifications, together with the use of *disposable bodyworns and underpads,* are useful in cases of mild or occasional incontinence.

Drugs like valproate were used in patients with ileo-anal anastomosis to increase the strength of the anal sphincters with some improvement [10], whereas drugs such as loperamide, diphenoxylate + atropine (Lomotil), codeine, amitriptyline, alosetron, and cholestyramine (in cases of idiopathic bile acid diarrhea) are chosen to increase the fecal consistency and reduce the rectal filling.

In selected cases, one can try to activate the cortical centers that are implicated in voluntary contraction of the anal sphincter [11] with the *biofeedback technique* [12], using surface EMG or manometry of the external anal sphincter, obtaining a certain degree of improvement according to some authors [13], but not others [14]. Anal muscle weakness has been treated with *electrostimulation,* with electrodes applied to the anal canal in order to stimulate muscle contraction, but the results were disappointing [15, 16]. Conversely, the *posterior tibial nerve stimulation* performed both percutaneously and transcutaneously in some randomized clinical trials obtained significant improvements in the number of FI episodes and quality of life [17], comparable to that of SNS at 12 months [18]. Another technique is the application of *radiofrequency electrical energy (Stretta procedure)* to the anal canal [19], a safe, minimally invasive, and rather effective tool in treating patients with mild or moderate fecal incontinence [20]. This procedure should induce morphological changes in the IAS and EAS reminiscent of normal sphincter structure [21], but manometry testing did not show any increase in resting tone [22]. Therefore, prospective, sham-controlled, randomized clinical trials are awaited.

Lastly, there are harsh nonsurgical treatments such as the use of *anal plugs* or *balloons inflated* above the anal canal or in the vaginal lumen to keep the stools from passing into the anal canal.

Surgical

Surgical treatments are indicated when medical interventions have failed. They are numerous, not only due to the different causes of FI, but also because the definitive solution of FI has not yet been found, especially for the most severe cases.

Sphincteroplasty is appropriate when there is an organic interruption of the anal sphincter and offers substantial improvement in 75% of patients [23, 24], but long-term results are disappointing with a less than 50% success rate at 10 years [25]. In cases of neuropathic fecal incontinence due to perineal descent, a *total pelvic floor repair* may be performed with success reported in 41% and 67% of patients [26, 27]. *Narrowing of the anal canal lumen* may be done in patients with mild or moderate FI by means of anal encirclement with meshes (Thiersch procedure) [28, 29], anal slings [30], or, more recently, infiltrations of the sphincter complex with biocompatible materials (autologous fat, collagen, silicone, Durasphere or synthetic gel, PTQ, Coaptite, NASHA/Dx, etc.) [31–36]. The results of the latter treatment vary depending on the material and technique used, but in general are considered good with about a 50% reduction in number of incontinence episodes and quality of life. The technique is easy to perform and with rare adverse events, but the beneficial result is not long lasting. A "neosphincter," obtained with skeletal *muscles transplant,* such as gluteus maximus or gracilis muscle [37], may be attempted especially when there is a severe disruption of the anal sphincter. The results are satisfactory, especially associating muscle electrostimulation, but it is a very complex procedure with a high morbidity exposure [38]. Nerve impairment, and not only, was counteracted by *sacral nerve stimulation* (SNS), which is a scientifically validated solution in the absence of organic sphincter lesions and applied after a 14-day stimulation period test. In a study by Hull et al. [39], 76% of 120 patients were followed for a minimum of 5 years. Eighty-nine of them showed a $\geq$ 50% improvement with a reduction from 9.1 to 1.7 in the number of incontinence episodes/week and a significant improvement in all 4 scales of FI Quality of Life scores.

Similar results were obtained by Mellgreen in 120 patients [40] with a mean of 3.1 years of follow-up. In a report from Matzel on the clinical outcome of SNS [41], all studies demonstrated a statistically significant highly improved function across all outcome measures, which remained stable at long-term follow-up. However, 35.5% of patients in the study by Hull et al. [39] required device revision, replacement, or explants, whereas in the study of Mellgreen et al. [40] a 5% rate of explants were necessary, due to the occurrence of infections (10%) and implant site pain (28%). This treatment is expensive, invasive, and rather complicated with many adverse events, but considering the good results it is considered cost-effective [42].

The treatment with *artificial bowel sphincter* (ABS) may be performed in some selected and motivated patients with severe FI, especially if the latter is due to a traumatic disruption of the sphincter complex. This device is implanted in the abdominal cavity and is an inflatable ring surrounding the distal portion of the rectum that is distended by a semiautomatic pump up to a normal sphincter tone and deflated on request. In some patients, it gives good results, as in a study of Devesa et al. [43], where good continence was obtained in 63% of patients with an improvement of CCIS score from 17 to 4, sometimes with complete continence. However, the implantation procedure is difficult and subsequently the device may often give rise to more or less severe complications, requiring surgical revision in 46–50% of cases, the majority of which were due to infections (25–40%), and explantation in 37% of cases [44–46]. Diversion of the feces with *colostomy* or *ileostomy* is an extreme remedy in the most severe cases not responding to other treatments [47, 48], as well as *antegrade continence enemas* via cecostomy [49].

All these surgical FI treatment options relieve, but do not completely resolve, the problem in the large majority of patients, especially those with severe incontinence. Sometimes they are scarcely tolerated, burdened by more or less severe adverse events, whereas the long-term outcome is uncertain [50]. Therefore, there was a need for a new device in cases of severe fecal incontinence that should be simple, effective, devoid of severe adverse effects, and not too expensive.

The "Magnetic" Way for FI Treatment

Following is a history of the efforts to apply the magnetic force in the prevention of fecal incontinence, from the first failed attempt to one already realized that seemed the ultimate solution of the problem, up to a novel device in development.

The First Attempt

The use of magnets in the treatment of fecal incontinence started about 40 years ago. The first attempt was made in 1979 by Willital et al. [51] who conceived a magnetic device consisting of two hollow semicylindric sections with a height of 3.1 cm, thickness of 6.3 mm, and an inner diameter of about 3 cm when assembled. These sections are surgically assembled and fixed around the rectum just above the anus, which is then encircled by a magnetic cylinder. A tampon of polyvinyl formal foam, similar to a menstrual tampon, with the diameter of the anal canal and a central longitudinal metallic stick, was inserted through the anus into the anal canal, closing it to avoid the loss of feces. The tampon, with its metallic stick, was kept "in situ" by the magnetic ring attraction force and was detached three times a day, allowing the bowel to empty. This device was implanted in seven patients with fecal incontinence. The main problems were the risk of stenosis and dilatation of the intestine, irritation of the mucosa, and intolerance, especially when sitting down. The results were considered satisfactory by the authors [52], but the outcome is unknown and nobody to date published a reiteration of this experiment.

The "Two Plaques" Magnetic System

In 2003, I sent a bench study to the Journal of Biomechanics detailing the use of a magnetic valve for the esophagogastric junction to prevent gastro-esophageal reflux in patients with a weak lower esophageal sphincter, but the paper was published belatedly in 2006 [53]. This study showed that a device made of two magnetic plaques can operate as a valve pressure-control when applied to a tube simulating the esophagus. See Fig. 7.1 for the explanation of how it works. The idea of a mechanism based on magnets to reinforce the closure of a weak gut sphincter came to my mind from the observation that two magnetic disks positioned one in front of the other in two adjacent intestinal loops were used to obtain a bypass between them. In fact, the portions of the walls clinched by the magnets fall in necrosis, creating a communication between the lumens of the two loops, so bypassing an obstruction due to cancer or other causes [54, 55]. I surmised that a pair of magnets with less attraction force placed face to face outside the opposite walls of a sphincter would gently bring themselves closer, closing the lumen without damaging the tissues.

This system may be applied to any sphincter that has lost its tone, causing reflux or incontinence, located either at the cardias or the anus. In regard to the anal sphincter, a pair of magnets in the form of small plaques covered by a biocompatible material may be surgically positioned in two pouches in the distal 3–4 cm of the anal canal on the right and left sides of the incontinent anal sphincter, outside or between the sphincter muscle bundles. These two plaques, provided with suitable holes, may be properly fixed with sutures to the surrounding tissue, with the opposite polarities face to face, so that, attracting to each other, they gently but firmly compress the opposite walls of the anal canal, closing the anal lumen (Fig. 7.2). When the defecation muscles contract, the pressure of the rectal lumen with its fecal content increases, exceeding the attraction force of the magnets, which detach and open the lumen of the anal canal. Once the stools are passed, the endoanal pressure decreases and the magnetic

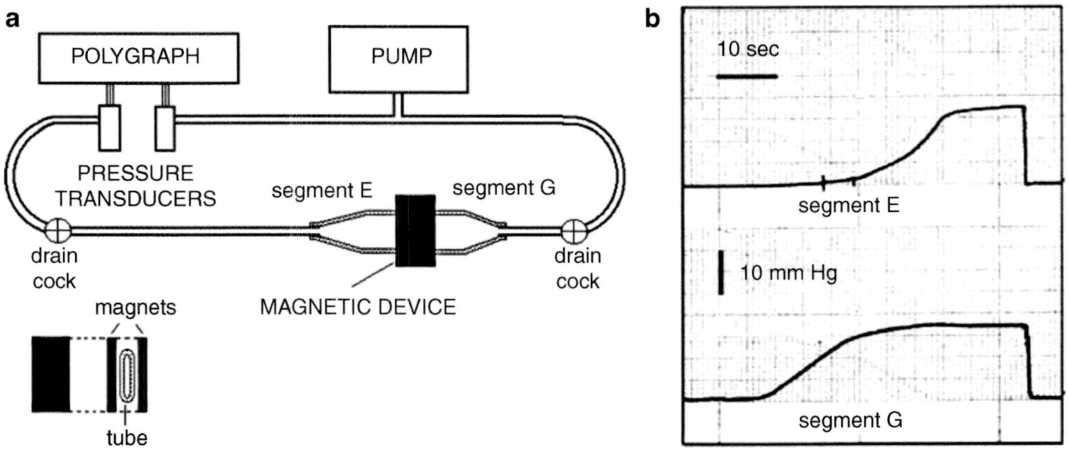

Fig. 7.1 (**a**) Schematic illustration of the bench model used to study the new anti-reflux device based on magnets. On the right is a flaccid polyethylene tube of 2.8 cm of diameter, mimicking the gastro-esophageal junction. It is squeezed perpendicularly by two rectangular magnets made of plastoferrite (Flexo) 2 × 4 × 0.5 cm with an attraction force of 0.36 N/cm^2 when put at contact and 0.16 N/cm^2 at 7 mm distance. It creates a high-pressure zone 2 cm wide, which divides the tube in the segment E (esophagus) and G (stomach). The tube is perfused with water by a pump, and the pressure variations of each segment are detected with two pressure transducers and recorded by a polygraph. (**b**) Intraluminal pressure variations in segment G (bottom) and E (top). The pressure of the segment G (stomach) was progressively increased by the pump, and when it reaches the value of about 11.5 mmHg, the magnets, simulating the sphincter, get detached, so that the pressure in the segment E (esophagus) starts to increase, mimicking a gastro-esophageal reflux and reaching the level of the segment G. Once the pump stops, the pressure falls and the magnets adhere again, closing the passage. Exchanging the letter E for G and G for E, this sequence of events may represent the passage of a bolus through the zone squeezed by the magnets. (From Bortolotti [53]. Reprinted with permission from Elsevier)

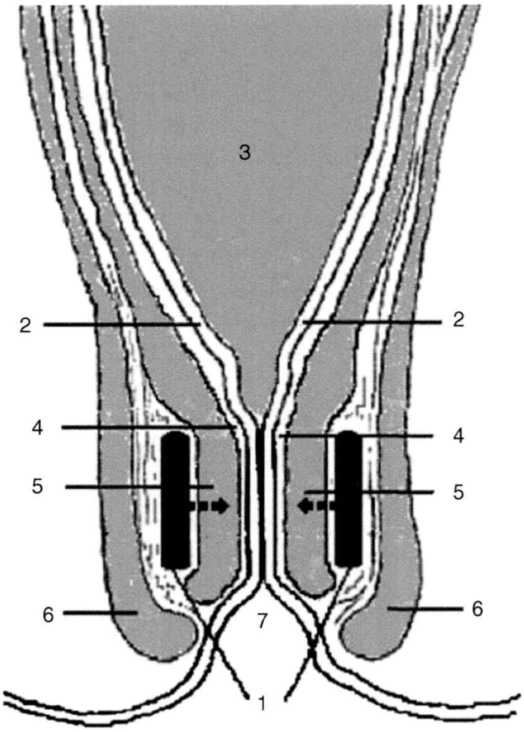

Fig. 7.2 Schematic section following a vertical frontal plane of the recto-anal region showing the pair of magnets in profile (1) inserted between the muscular bundles of the internal (5) and external (6) anal sphincters, with the opposite polarities attracting each other face to face. Note: 2 = mucosa; 3 = rectal ampulla; 4 = submucosa; 7 = anus. (From: Bortolotti et al. [56]. Reprinted with permission from Springer Nature)

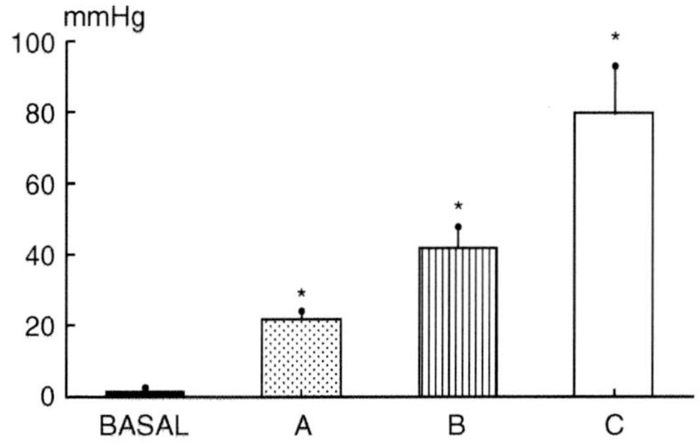

Fig. 7.3 Anal pressure measured manometrically in basal conditions and after the insertion of the magnets made of plastoferrite (**a**), those made of ferrite (**b**), and those made of neodymium (**c**) * = $p < 0.05$
The endoanal pressure after the insertion of neodymium magnets was 79.7 ± 13.1 mmHg (mean ± SD), after ferrite magnets it was 42.1 ± 5.6 mmHg, and after plastoferrite magnets it was 21.6 ± 4.6 mmHg, all of them significantly higher than the pressure recorded in basal conditions (1.72 ± 0.71 mmHg). (From: Bortolotti et al. [56]. Reprinted with permission from Springer Nature)

attraction prevails, allowing the magnets to close the lumen again.

The effectiveness of the magnetic closure was evaluated with a pilot study [56] in a series of porcine anatomical preparations obtained by sectioning the posterior half of swine weighing from 25 to 35 kg. Three pairs of magnets of ovoidal shape with a diameter of about 20–30 mm and a thickness of about 1.5–2.5 mm, made of materials with different magnetic force (neodymium> ferrite> plastoferrite), were examined. The two magnets of each pair were surgically inserted in two pouches on both sides of the anal canal, between the external and internal anal sphincters, taking care that their opposite polarities were positioned face to face. The effectiveness of the magnets in closing the anal lumen was tested in each anatomical preparation by measuring the endoanal pressure with three trans-anal pull-throughs of a thin side-hole manometric catheter perfused with a pneumo-hydraulic pump and connected to a Statham P23 Db pressure transducer and a Beckman R 612 polygraph. The measurements were done both before and after magnet implantation, and the mean endoanal pressures obtained in the two conditions were statistically compared with Student t test. The results are illustrated in Fig. 7.3. The endoanal pressure after the insertion of neodymium magnets was 79.7 ± 13.1 mmHg (mean ± SD), after ferrite magnets it was 42.1 ± 5.6 mmHg, and after plastoferrite magnets it was 21.6 ± 4.6 mmHg, all of them significantly ($p < 0.05$) higher than the pressure recorded in basal conditions (1.72 ± 0.71 mmHg). This experiment demonstrated that the implantation of a pair of magnets in the wall of the anal canal was able to create a high-pressure zone, with values that could increase to a level sufficient to prevent fecal incontinence.

The main advantage of this magnetic system is that the magnets create a "dynamic closure," the mechanism of which has been previously demonstrated [53] and illustrated in Fig. 7.1. When the magnets are detached by an endoluminal pressure increase above the pressure of closure, they leave a passage that allows an easy transit of contents, while other systems, such as the systems that narrow the anal lumen more or less consistently and continuously, create an obstacle to the passage of stool, not only under resting conditions, but also during defecation. Another advantage of this method lies in the fact that the characteristics of the high-pressure zone could be chosen by using magnets of various attraction force and dimensions. In this manner, we could tailor the force of anal sphincter closure. The value of the new high-pressure zone should be sufficiently high to prevent fecal incontinence, including fluid leakage, but low enough to be overcome by the endorectal pressure increase during defecation. As the basal pressure of the anal closure measured with manometry is important in preventing leakage, especially of liquid feces [57], the most suitable pair of magnets may be chosen on the basis of a manometric measurement of the incompetent sphincter pressure performed before intervention [58], or even during magnet implantation. In fact, the force of attraction between the magnets, and consequently the pressure obtained, depends not only on the type and size of the magnets but also on the distance between them, due to the thickness of the interposed tissues. Obviously, we must choose magnets with an attraction force that generates a value of endoanal pressure that does not damage the below tissues but is sufficient to prevent fecal incontinence. To avoid this drawback, the rigid magnetic plaque may be covered toward the lumen by some soft biocompatible material to reduce the trauma to the tissues compressed by the magnets.

This system may be applied to any other gut sphincter that has lost its tone and function. In fact, we also employed a similar magnetic device to reinforce the incompetent *lower esophageal sphincter* with the aim of preventing gastroesophageal reflux [59].

The "Magnetic Collar" System

More recently the idea of using magnets to reinforce weak sphincters was exploited with the creation of a "magnetic collar" to be placed around the sphincter. In 2010, Lehur et al. [60] applied the FENIX magnetic device augmentation (TORAX Medical, Inc. Share View, Minnesota, USA) to the anal canal of patients with fecal incontinence. This device is similar to another magnetic device, the LINX reflux management system of the same TORAX Medical Inc., that is applied around a weak gastro-esophageal sphincter to prevent gastro-esophageal reflux, the first results of which were published in the Annals of Surgery in 2010 by Bonavina et al. [61].

This magnetic anal sphincter (MAS) [62] resembles a collar and consists of an annular series of 5 mm wide titanium beads with magnetic cores interlinked along an independent flexible titanium wire. The beads slide against one another along the wire, self-attracting by magnetic force (Fig. 7.4). The number of beads varies from 14 to 20, adapting the "collar" to different circumferences of the anal canal measured with a sizing tool [63]. This string of beads is introduced into a channel surgically created around the external muscle of the anal canal and the sutures at each end of string tied, so that the sphincter remains encircled by a "collar" of magnetic beads attached to one another. During evacuation, the increase in pressure into the anal canal separates the beads, which slide along the wire, so that the collar and the anal lumen widen.

The patients selected for this kind of implant by Lehur et al. [60] are those between the ages of 19 and 84 years with an average of at least two FI episodes a week for 3 weeks, of idiopathic, traumatic, and neuropathic origin, who have previously attempted or were not candidates for conservative therapeutic approaches. Exclusion criteria were the following: history of significant chronic defecatory motility disorder, underlying systemic disease as a source of FI (neurologic disorder, scleroderma, chronic diarrhea, IBD, and irritable bowel syndrome), diabetes requiring oral hypoglycemic agents or insulin, previous

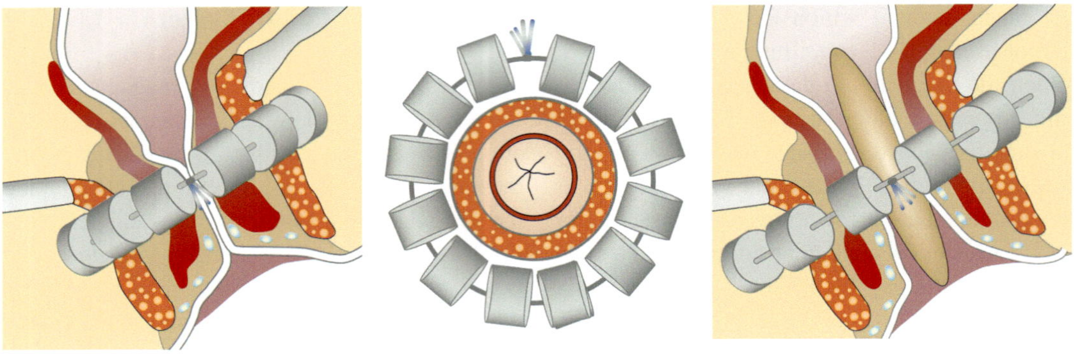

Fig. 7.4 Magnetic anal sphincter augmentation device. Closed (to the left) and open (to the right). (From Thomas and Vaizey [88]. Reprinted with permission)

anorectal posterior compartment surgery and rectal resection, current overt rectal prolapse or vaginal prolapse, complex anal or rectovaginal fistula or active pelvic infection, a history of pelvic radiation or anal, rectal or colon cancer within 2 years, or with an electric or metallic implant within 10 cm of the area of device placement. Excluded also were patients who were pregnant, nursing, or planning to become pregnant and who were unable to comply with the follow-up schedule. At present the indications for MAS installation are less restrictive [64]: at least one fecal leak/week for 3 weeks, a Cleveland Clinic Incontinence Score of at least 10 points, and a FI refractory to dietary advices, biofeedback, perineal re-education, and medication. At the same time, the exclusion criteria are reduced: pregnancy or plan of pregnancy, full-thickness rectal prolapse, IBD, pelvic or perineal infections, previous rectal resection and/or radiation, or colon/rectal/anal cancer within 2 years, whereas every previous surgical treatment of FI is not an exclusion criterion.

The preliminary report of this "magnetic collar" for anal sphincter incontinence [60] showed at 6 months an improvement in only 5 of 14 patients (all females), considering the number of FI episodes /week (from 7.2 to 0.7), the Wexner Continence Score (from 17.2 to 7.8), and the FI Quality of Life Score (FIQoL) in all domains. There were two patients with infections that lead to device removal and creation of a stoma, whereas another one spontaneously passed the device. Other adverse events were perineal pain (2 cases), rectal bleeding (1 case), chronic infection (1 case), and obstructed defecation (2 cases).

In a subsequent study by Barussaud et al. in 2013 [65] on 23 patients (all females) with a median follow-up of 17.6 months (range 6–45), the Cleveland Clinical Florida Incontinence Severity (CCF-IS or CCIS) preoperative score of 15.2 significantly decreased to 6.9 in 19 patients at 6 months, and to 5.3 in only 3 patients at 36 months (Fig. 7.5), whereas the FIQoL median score significantly improved from 1.97 to 3.19 after 6 months in 19 patients, and to 2.93 after 36 months in only 3 patients (Fig. 7.6). There were some *adverse events*. One patient had an intraoperative rectal perforation that prevented the device installation. Two patients had the device removed, one of them for infection, whereas the other passed the device during a straining effort. Seven patients were not satisfied, five for lack of improvement in continence, likely due to a failure in opening up of the device. Two complained of pain at defecation, one with difficulty in evacuation, saying that the device did not open up well on defecation. Three had to take laxatives after the operation for constipation. In these last four cases, it is likely that the "magnetic collar" did not open up regularly.

On the other hand, the experience of Bridoux et al. in 2014 [66] was completely negative, being characterized by several *adverse events*. None of

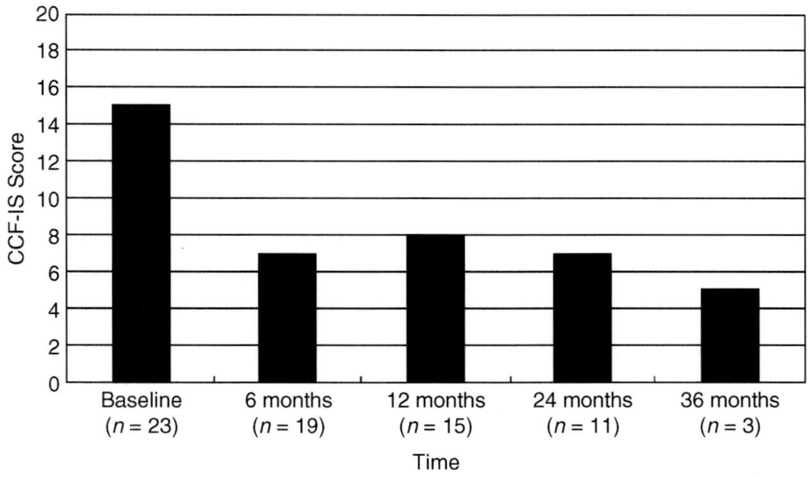

Fig. 7.5 Cleveland Clinic Florida Incontinence Severity (CCF-IS) score before and after magnetic anal sphincter implantation at 6, 12, 24, and 36 months (*n* = number of patients). (From Barussaud et al. [65]. Reprinted with permission from John Wiley and Sons)

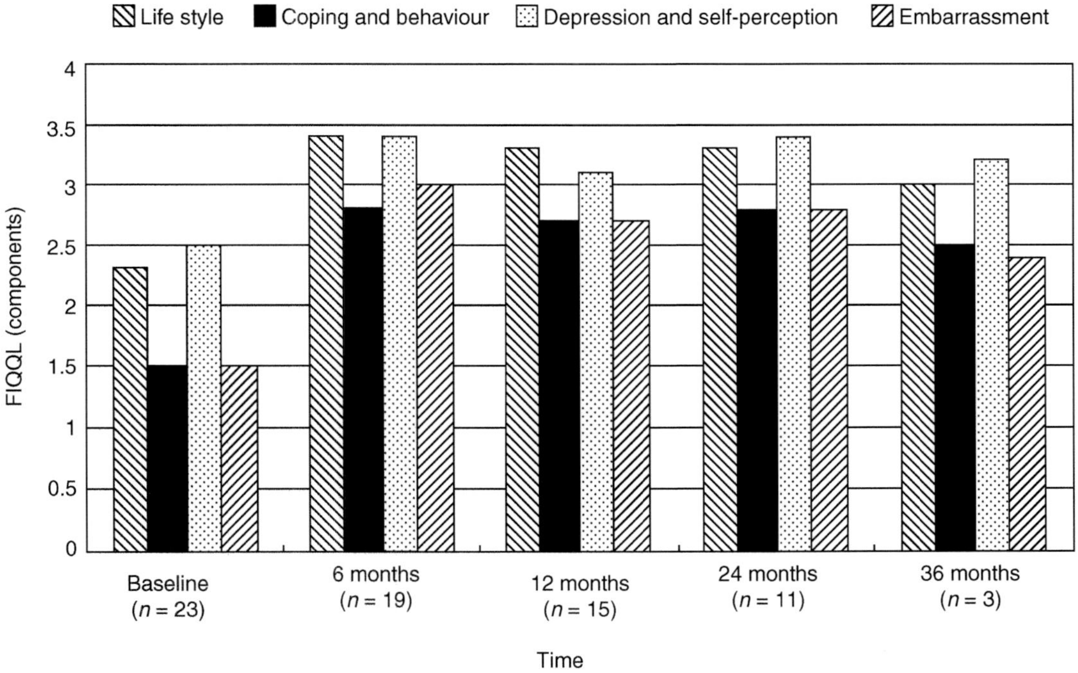

Fig. 7.6 Fecal Incontinence Quality of Life (FIQoL) score (four items) before and after implantation of a magnetic anal sphincter at 6, 12, 24, and 36 months (*n* = number of patients). (From Barussaud et al. [65]. Reprinted with permission from John Wiley and Sons)

the seven patients who underwent implantation of MAS reached a ≥ 50% reduction of CCIS score at 9 months median follow-up, and the FIQoL score did not improve significantly in the four domains at 6 months. In five patients, the device was explanted after some months, in three for severe infections, and in the other two for chronic pain and incontinence.

On the contrary, the study of Pakravan and Helmes in 2015 [67] had a better outcome. The implantation of MAS in 18 patients (15 women), including 7 with previous rectal resection for rectal prolapse, showed a ≥ 50% reduction in the number of FI episodes in 13 patients after a follow-up of 24 months. The CCIS median score significantly decreased from 17.5 (range 14–20) to 7.3 (range 0–12.0), and the FIQoL median score significantly improved in all the domains. In addition, the manometric resting and squeeze mean pressures were increased at 6 months. Regarding *adverse events*, an intraoperative rectal perforation occurred that prevented the implantation of the device, and 29% of patients complained of local pain after operation.

To validate the MAS treatment in comparison to other surgical therapies for FI, Wong et al. performed two small nonrandomized comparative studies of the clinical effects of MAS implantation with the artificial bowel sphincter (ABS) [68] and sacral nerve stimulation (SNS) [69] in patients with severe FI. In the first study, the results of MAS implantation in a group of ten patients were compared with those obtained in another group of ten patients treated with the *artificial bowel sphincter (ABS)* after a mean follow-up of 8 and 22 months, respectively (Table 7.1). Significant improvements of continence and quality of life scores were observed in both groups without significant differences in intergroups, but with better anal pressure scores in patients with ABS. However, both treatments showed various *adverse events*: the MAS device stopped working in one patient and spontaneously extruded in another, whereas ABS failed working in two patients and required an explantation for infection and pain in another two patients, along with four revisions. In addition, two patients with MAS complained, one of fecal impaction and another of constipation, whereas six patients with ABS suffered, two from fecal impaction and four from constipation (Table 7.1). However, it is necessary to consider that the follow-up of patients with ABS was about three times longer than that of patients with MAS.

Table 7.1 Comparison between the clinical outcomes of patients undergoing magnetic anal sphincter and artificial bowel sphincter implantations drawn from the study of Wong et al. 2011 [68] and a comparison between those of magnetic anal sphincter and sacral nerve stimulation from the study of Wong et al. [69]

	Magnetic anal sphincter	Artificial bowel sphincter	Magnetic anal sphincter	Sacral nerve stimulation
Number of patients	10 (10 women)	10 (10 women)	12	16
Mean follow-up (months)	8 (range 6–13)	22.5 (range 6–72)	18 (range 8–30)	22 (range 10–28)
Jorge Waxner Median Score	From 17 to 6[a]	From 16 to 4[a]	From 16.5 to 6[a]	From 15 to 11.5[a]
FIQoL Median Score	From 2.03 to 3.51[a]	From 1.80 to 3.63[a]	Significant improvement in all 4 components	Significant improvement in all 4 components
Resting anal pressure cm H2O (median)	From 35 to 58.5[a]	From 34 to75[a]	From 42.5 to 54[a]	From 34 to 33
Device Explantation Extrusion Nonfunctioning	1 extrusion (spontaneous) 1 nonfunctioning	4 revisions 2 explantations 2 nonfunctioning	1 extrusion (spontaneous)	1 explantation
Fecal impaction or constipation or antidiarrheal	1 impaction 1 constipation	2 impaction 4 constipation	1 impaction 1 constipation 2 antidiarrheal	1 constipation 6 antidiarrheal
Infections		1		1
Bleeding	2		2	
Pain		1		

Note: The scores of incontinence severity and of FIQoL represent the mean values measured before intervention followed by those observed at the end of the study
[a]Statistically significant

The other nonrandomized study [69] compared the clinical outcomes of a group of 12 women with severe FI treated with MAS with those of a group of 16 women with severe FI subjected to *sacral nerve stimulation (SNS)* implantation. Both groups showed, after a mean follow-up of 18 and 22 months, respectively, similar results in improving continence and quality of life (Table 7.1). However, there were some *adverse events*: one device was removed in a patient with SNS for infection, whereas a spontaneous extrusion of the device occurred in a patient with MAS. In addition, four patients with MAS complained: one of fecal impaction, another of constipation, and two of diarrhea, whereas seven patients with SNS suffered: one from constipation and six from diarrhea.

The conclusion of the author in both studies was that MAS in the short term improves fecal continence and quality of life to a similar degree as ABS and SNS. However, SNS device is less invasive and less burdened by complications and explantations than MAS, which in turn is less invasive and with fewer adverse events than ABS. A more complete and extended comparison between the two FI treatments MAS and SNS is the target of two multicenter, prospective, randomized, interventional, controlled trials that are underway: the French MOS STIC [70] and the English SaFaRI [71].

I also wanted to compare the results of a long-term multicenter study on effectiveness and safety of MAS in patients with severe FI [72] with two studies based on *anal canal narrowing techniques*: in one study, the insertion around the anal sphincter of a simple elastic sling made of biocompatible silicone [73], and in the other, the infiltration into the anal sphincter of a bulking agent represented by biocompatible collagen [33] (Table 7.2). I realize that this is a rough comparison, but these three studies did not differ much, considering the number of patients, severity of the FI, and follow-up duration.

The comparison showed that the highest percentage of patients with subjective improvement of symptoms was found in the studies with the insertion of sling and injection of collagen, whereas the incontinence severity median score decreased in an almost similar way in patients who underwent MAS and the others. However, the biggest difference was in the occurrence of *adverse events and complications* that took place early and late after operation. In fact, after *MAS implantation*, 67% of patients experienced 30 adverse events such as defecatory dysfunction (20%), pain at the implant site (14%), erosion due to the device (11%), infection of the implant site (11%), and bleeding (9%). And there was device explantation in seven cases for infection, erosions, or device failure. The defecatory dysfunction (difficult evacuation) was found in seven patients, who were treated with conservative means such as suppositories and enemas, but in one case of obstructed defecation the patient opted for stoma creation without device removal. Conversely, after *sling insertion*, there were 13 adverse events (Table 7.2) which included infections (12%), erosions (6%), and sling rupture (21%), causing sling removal in 13 cases, with reinsertion in 10 cases, and subsequent removal in 3 cases. In patients treated with *injection of collagen*, there were no significant adverse events, but 38% of patients needed another injection after 9–16 months and other 15% required a third injection after 14–20 months. Other studies with slings insertion and bulking agent injections [28, 74–77] had a similar rate of good clinical results and few complications, but prospective, randomized, and comparative studies have not been conducted to date.

Quite recently a single-center study was published by Kim et al. in 2019 [64] collecting 45 patients, with a mean follow-up of 36 months (range 6–84), and with a portion of them previously included in other publications [60, 72] and in the MOS-STIC trial [70]. This paper does not add further significant data regarding CCIS and FIQoL with respect to those in the studies above examined. Both parameters were significantly improved, and 48% of patients declared satisfaction. However, the study was interesting because the authors performed an analysis of the causes of success or failure in patients implanted with MAS and concluded that the origin of FI, previous damage of sphincter, and its manometric values did not influence the outcome, whereas the

Table 7.2 Comparison between the clinical outcomes of patients undergoing magnetic anal sphincter implantation from the study of Sugrue et al. [72], insertion of elastic band perianal sling made of biocompatible silicone from the study of Devesa et al. [73], and collagen intra-anal injection from the study of Maslekar et al. [33]

	Magnetic anal sphincter	Elastic band perianal sling	Collagen intra-anal injection
Number of patients	35 (34 women)	33 (20 women)	100 (70 women)
Mean follow-up (months)	60	65	36
Symptom subjective improvement	53%	97%	68%
Incontinence severity (average scores)	From 15.7 to 7[a] (Cleveland Clinic Incontinence Score)	From 15 to7[a] (Jorge-Wexner Score)	From 14 to 8[a] (Cleveland Clinic Incontinence Score)
FIQoL median index (average of the 4 scales)	From 8.2 to 12.8[a]	From 7.8 to 14.3[a]	Not done
Device explantation or reoperation	7 explantations (infections, erosions, ineffectiveness) 1 creation of stoma for fecal impaction	13 sling removal (sling breakage, infections, erosions), with 10 reinsertions and further removals in 3	38%: second injection 15%: third injection
Adverse events (total)	30	13	None
Difficulty in evacuation	20%	None	None
Pain	14%	None	None
Erosion	11%	6%	None
Infection	11%	12%	None
Bleeding	9%	None	None

[a]statistically significant
Note: The scores of incontinence severity and of FIQoL represent the mean values measured before intervention, followed by those observed at the end of the study

only independent predictive factor for success after MAS implantation was no previous FI surgery.

Comment

The main question is: does the magnetic device to prevent fecal incontinence represent a real progress with respect to other nonmagnetic systems, considering the working mechanism, clinical effectiveness, occurrence of complications, and difficulty in implantation, and last but not least the cost/effectiveness ratio?

The *first attempt* of Willital et al. in 1982 [52] prevented the fecal incontinence by means of an anal plug kept "in situ" with magnets, but, although the authors considered the results in seven patients "satisfactory," it was no longer replicated, probably due to the high risk of local complications and patient intolerance, especially when sitting down.

The only magnetic device on the market today is the "*magnetic collar" system*, that is the *magnetic anal sphincter (MAS)* named FENIX (TORAX Medical, Inc. Share View, Minnesota, USA).

From a *technical point of view*, the conception of the working mechanism of magnets for closing and opening the anal canal denotes a high engineering skill. The device on the bench works perfectly, but once implanted in an organism, things change, because over time the local tissue reaction intervenes, upsetting the plans and putting "the stick in the wheels." In fact, a fibrotic reaction develops around the device, as demonstrated by studies in pigs in which a similar "magnetic collar" implanted around the cardias appeared encapsulated in fibrous tissue at a necropsy carried out after 44 weeks [78]. The fibrosis around the wires and the magnetic beads could likely hamper the detachment and reattachment of the magnetic beads, which must slip along the wires when the "collar" opens and closes [79]. The fibrous encapsulation of the device by a fibrotic reaction was also confirmed in some patients, in whom the esophageal "magnetic collar" was explanted for serious complications [80, 81]. The anal "magnetic collar" follows the same fate of that used for cardias, that is of being encapsulated in fibrous tissue, as observed in a series of canine studies made for establishing its safety [60]. The fibrous tissue become increasingly hard and rigid over time, and it is reasonable to suppose that it could interfere with the movements of the magnetic beads of the device in an open or closed position, leading to incontinence or defecation difficulty. This could explain the poor results of MAS described in some patients in regard to the incontinence and dysfunctions of evacuation.

However, when this fibrotic encapsulation takes place around the "magnetic collar" at the lower esophageal sphincter level, it could be possible that the device continues to exert its antireflux activity through a mechanism similar to that of the notorious Angelkich prosthesis [82]. In fact, the latter one dangling on the cardias may control reflux, not only by preventing unfolding of the lower esophageal sphincter, when challenged by an increase of intragastric pressure [83], but also padding with its weight against the esophago-gastric junction with a protrusion into the lumen like a bar that creates an obstacle to reflux [84]. This phenomenon could take place also with the "magnetic collar" positioned around the anal sphincter. The string of magnetic beads of MAS could pad the wall of the anal canal mimicking the effect of a sling or a bulking agent, favoring fecal continence, even in the unlucky eventuality that it does not work.

Another problem is represented by the difficulty in the choice of the device length, because, if the "collar" is too large, minor and liquid leakage and flatus are not prevented, and if too tight, an obstruction or a difficult defecation may take place. To overcome this problem, a series of three sizing tools have been subsequently designed mimicking the magnetic device, the last of which seeming the most proper [63]. In any case, the measure of the circumference of the annular tunnel around the anal canal requests various measurements, and the measure obtained sometimes is not as precise as the surgeon wants, resulting a little too large or too tight, leading to small liquid leakage or to some difficulty in evacuation, respectively, as sometimes described in abovementioned studies. In the first eventuality, the best results will be obtained for patients with solid stool incontinence [60], and in second one, it is necessary to maintain stool softness to avoid the difficult defecation [65].

As regards the *clinical effectiveness* of MAS, there are studies with very good results [67] and others very negative [66]. But, in general the rate of good results is similar to those of other techniques, such as SNS [68] and ABS [69]. All these systems, however, may not block entirely minor and liquid leakage, as well as flatus [64, 67]. It is interesting to observe that some results of anal slings [73] and bulking infiltrations [33], especially those delivered under ultrasonic guidance [85], are at the level of those of MAS (Table 7.2), although limited in working duration. However, most of these studies show follow-ups shorter than those of MAS, and, therefore, request other more validated studies to be considered as an alternative. The analysis of the *causes* of success or failure in patients implanted with MAS demonstrated that neither the cause of FI, previous damage of the sphincter, or its manometric values influenced the outcome, but only prior surgery, such as SNS, ABS, and injection of bulking agents, may predict a dismal result [64, 67]. Pakravan and Helmes [67] drew attention to the fact that the worst results with MAS, like those of Bridoux et al. [66], were obtained in patients 12 years younger and physically more active than those in his own series, concluding that the MAS implantation does better in older and more sedentary patients.

Considering *adverse events*, in all studies with MAS, there is a more or less high rate of major complications leading to explantations, extrusions of the device, and stoma creations [60, 63–69, 72], which may reach a mean value of 18.3%. This percentage is higher than that of patients treated with SNS (5%) [40], but less than those with ABS (24%) [44]. The operation for MAS implantation is already in itself very complex and at risk of complications, not only during the device implantation, such as rectal perforation that occurred in two patients [65, 67], but also when the device was explanted. In patients explanted and not reimplanted, the defecatory function is compromised and sometimes a stoma creation was necessary [60, 72]. In one patient subjected to stoma, the useless device was left "in situ" to avoid further complications [72]. In addition, in patients implanted with MAS, there are many other complications such as erosions, infections, bleedings, local pain, defecatory dysfunctions, and fecal obstruction, which represent a considerable discomfort for the patient. The incidence of adverse events is higher in patients with previous anorectal surgery, and this is a reason for the suggestion that these patients should be excluded from the MAS implantation by protocol [64]. This fact, together with the worse results in young patients, could represent a non-negligible limitation when choosing MAS in the surgical management of FI. On the other hand, it could be unadvisable to install SNS after MAS explantation if the anal sphincter is too damaged by surgery. After MAS explantation, a stoma may be created [60] even if it could be possible to implant an ABS in some cases. Conversely, after failure of SNS and ABS, MAS implantation may be performed in some patients.

The MAS treatment has been approved by the US FDA as a Humanitarian Device Exemption for use in patients with FI who do not respond to SNS. Consequently, the insertion of MAS should not precede that of SNS. MAS has been proposed as a surgical treatment in selected patients with end-stage FI [60, 65, 67], but uncertainty remains when dealing with patients with idiopathic moderate-severe FI, as can be inferred from the CCIS and Jorge Wexner scores of some patients treated with MAS in previously cited studies and considering that the indications for MAS implantation based on FI severity now are less restrictive [64]. In this type of patient, other fairly effective surgical managements with low or null risk of serious complications could be considered, such as the insertion of silastic slings [73] or the local infiltration of bulking agents [33] (Table 7.2). One can ask if these systems with apparently similar good results, although less efficient in the long term, but easily repeatable and with a good safety level, are preferable to others more complicated and fraught with undesirable consequences (a success expectation not much higher than 50% and burdened by a high cost), which may render the ratio cost/effectiveness unfavorable. Bulking agent injections or perianal elastic slings could compete with MAS in the treatment of borderline severe FI, not so much for effectiveness, but for scarceness of adverse events, simplicity, ease of repeatability, and, last but not least, low cost. MAS is considered a choice in patients with severe incontinence refractory to other major surgical treatments [64]. It is generally accepted that a definite solution to the problem of fecal incontinence has still to be found [86], and I add: "and perhaps for the problem of gastro-esophageal reflux too" [79].

This opinion raises a crucial question. Considering that the success of the devices available today is obtained in a percentage not much higher than 50% of patients, one can ask: Is the magnetic solution for FI the wrong idea or an inadequate realization [87]? I do not believe that it is a wrong idea, but I am convinced that another type of magnetic device more efficient and with at less risks of complications may be realized in the future.

The "Possible" Future

The aforementioned original idea of a *pair of magnetic plaques*, although tested only in animals, but with good results in augmenting the pressure of the anal sphincter, could be taken into consideration for future development. This magnetic system previously described presents some advantages with respect to the MAS system.

- It has a simpler operational activity because it does not have mechanical joints or sliding parts that could be blocked by fibrin deposition, hampering the movements of the magnets. In fact, in the pair of magnetic plaques, the attraction force manifests itself through the lumen of the anal canal, so that the magnets can freely move one versus the other and easily return to the resting position. The fibrin encapsulation of the magnets, instead of impeding their operative activity, may contribute to firmly affix them in the bulk of the gut wall.
- The plaques could be made with different types of magnets with various attraction forces, modeled in various shapes that better fit to their anatomical position and covered with a soft biomaterial on the face toward the anal lumen, to avoid ischemia and erosions of the compressed tissues.
- Because the distance between the two plaques "in situ" may vary from one patient to another, the pressure of closure too may vary and consequently, also the force of attraction necessary to adequately close the lumen. The force of closure could be chosen accurately by testing the effect of plaques of various attraction force on the anal lumen pressure, measuring it by means of manometry or other systems during surgery. We must remember that the force of closure must be sufficient to prevent leakage, especially of liquid feces, but not too strong, to avoid mucosal lesions.
- The surgical procedure for implanting the plaques is easier and less risky than that for MAS, which requires the laborious creation of a tunnel around the anal canal, a procedure that may expose to rectal perforation [67], and a measure of its circumference with a sizing tool [63].
- The plaques may also be easily disinfected and sterilized, thus making the appearance of local infections more difficult, a not uncommon problem during this kind of operations for FI.
- Finally, this system may be less expensive regarding both the magnetic device and the surgical procedure.

Unfortunately, this kind of magnetic device is not yet available, and before considering it as a simple and effective solution for fecal incontinence, it is still necessary to perform further experiments in animals and clinical trials in selected patients. This new road appears long and arduous, but I think it is worth the undertaking.

Acknowledgment The author thanks Romano Bragaglia MD for assistance with translation.

References

1. Nazarko L. Faecal incontinence: investigation, treatment and management. Br J Community Nurs. 2018;23:582–8.
2. Nelson RL. Epidemiology of fecal incontinence. Gastroenterology. 2004;126(1 Suppl 1):S3–7.
3. Macmillan AK, Merrie AE, Marshall RJ, Parry BR. The prevalence of fecal incontinence in community-dwelling adults: a systematic review of the literature. Dis Colon Rectum. 2004;47:1341–9.
4. Talley NJ, O'Keefe EA, Zinsmeister R, Melton LJ 3rd. Prevalence of gastrointestinal symptoms in the elderly. A population-based study. Gastroenterology. 1992;102:895–901.
5. Thekkinkattil DK, Dunham RJ, O'Herlihy S, Finan PJ, Sagar PM, Burke DA. Measurement of anal cushions in idiopathic faecal incontinence. Br J Surg. 2009;96:680–4.
6. Henry MM. Pathogenesis and management of fecal incontinence in the adult. Gastroenterol Clin N Am. 1987;16(1):35–45.
7. Engel AF, Kamm MA, Talbot IC. Progressive systemic sclerosis of the internal anal sphincter leading to passive faecal incontinence. Gut. 1994;35(6):857–9.
8. Swash M. The neurogenic hypothesis of stress incontinence. Ciba Found Symp. 1990;151:156–70; discussion 170-5.
9. Mularczyk A, Basilisco G. Fecal incontinence induced by spontaneous internal anal sphincter relaxation: report of a case. Dis Colon Rectum. 2002;45:973–6.
10. Kusunoki M, Shoji Y, Ikeuchi H, Yamagata K, Yamamura T, Utsunomiya J. Usefulness of valproate sodium for treatment of incontinence after ileoanal anastomosis. Surgery. 1990;107:311.
11. Parès D, Martinez-Vilalta M, Ortiz H, Soriano-Mas C, Maestre-Gonzalez Y, Pujol J, Grande L. Assessment of brain activity during voluntary anal sphincter contraction: comparative study in women with and with-

out fecal incontinence. Neurogastroenterol Motil. 2018;30(9):e13347.
12. Norton C, Chelvanayagam S, Wilson-Barnett J, Redfern S, Kamm MA. Randomized controlled trial of biofeedback for fecal incontinence. Gastroenterology. 2003;125(5):1320–9.
13. Heymen S, Jones KR, Ringel Y, Scarlett Y, Whitehead WE. Biofeedback treatment of fecal incontinence: a critical review. Dis Colon Rectum. 2001;44(5):728–36.
14. Norton C, Cody JD, Hosker G. Biofeedback and/or sphincter exercises for the treatment of faecal incontinence in adults. Cochrane Database Syst Rev. 2006;3:CD002111.
15. Norton C, Gibbs A, Kamm MA. Randomized, controlled trial of anal electrical stimulation for fecal incontinence. Dis Colon Rectum. 2006;49(2):190–6.
16. Scheuer M, Kuijpers HC, Bleijenberg G. Effect of electrostimulation on sphincter function in neurogenic fecal continence. Dis Colon Rectum. 1994;37:590.
17. Arroyo Fernández R, Avendaño Coy J, Ando Lafuente S, Martín Correa MT, Ferri Morales A. Posterior tibial nerve stimulation in the treatment of fecal incontinence: a systematic review. Rev Esp Enferm Dig. 2018;110:577–88.
18. Thin NN, Horrocks EJ, Hotouras A, Palit S, Thaha MA, Chan CL, Matzel KE, Knowles CH. Systematic review of the clinical effectiveness of neuromodulation in the treatment of faecal incontinence. Br J Surg. 2013;100:1430–47.
19. Parisien CJ, Corman ML. The Secca procedure for the treatment of fecal incontinence: definitive therapy or short-term solution. Clin Colon Rectal Surg. 2005;18(1):42–5.
20. Ruiz D, Pinto RA, Hull TL, Efron JE, Wexner SD. Does the radiofrequency procedure for fecal incontinence improve quality of life and incontinence at 1-year follow-up? Dis Colon Rectum. 2010;53:1041–6.
21. Herman RM, Berho M, Murawski M, Nowakowski M, et al. Defining the histopathological changes induced by nonablative radiofrequency treatment of faecal incontinence--a blinded assessment in an animal model. Color Dis. 2015;17:433–40.
22. Kim DW, Yoon HM, Park JS, Kim YH, Kang SB. Radiofrequency energy delivery to the anal canal: is it a promising new approach to the treatment of fecal incontinence? Am J Surg. 2009;197:14–8.
23. Wexner SD, Marchetti F, Jagelman DG. The role of sphincteroplasty for fecal incontinence reevaluated. A prospective physiologic and functional review. Dis Colon Rectum. 1991;34:22.
24. Engel AF, Kamm MA, Sultan AH, Bartram CI, Nicholls RJ. Anterior anal sphincter repair in patients with obstetric trauma. Br J Surg. 1994;81:1231.
25. Zutshi M, Tracey TH, Bast J, Halverson A, Na J. Ten-year outcome after anal sphincter repair for fecal incontinence. Dis Colon Rectum. 2009;52:1089–94.
26. Pinho M, Ortiz J, Oya M, Panagamuwa B, Asperer J, Keighley MR. Total pelvic floor repair for the treatment of neuropathic fecal incontinence. Am J Surg. 1992;163:340–3.
27. Deen KI, Oya M, Ortiz J, Keighley MR. Randomized trial comparing three forms of pelvic floor repair for neuropathic faecal incontinence. Br J Surg. 1993;80:794–8.
28. Larach SW, Vazquez B. Modified Thiersch procedure with silastic mesh implant: a simple solution for fecal incontinence and severe prolapse. South Med J. 1986;79:307–9.
29. Sainio AP, Halme IE, Husa AJ. Anal encirclement with polypropylene mesh for rectal prolapse and incontinence. Dis Colon Rectum. 1991;34:905.
30. Devesa M, Hervas PL, Vicente R, Rey A, Die J, Moreno I, Teruel D. Anal encirclement with a simple prosthetic sling for faecal incontinence. Tech Coloproctol. 2011;15:17–22.
31. Van Koughnett JA, Wexner SD. Current management of fecal incontinence: choosing amongst treatment options to optimize outcomes. World J Gastroenterol. 2013;19:9216–30.
32. Stojkovic SG, Lim M, Burke D, Finan PJ, Sagar PM. Intra-anal collagen injection for the treatment of faecal incontinence. Br J Surg. 2006;93:1514–8.
33. Maslekar S, Smith K, Harji D, Griffiths B, Sagar PM. Injectable collagen for the treatment of fecal incontinence: long-term results. Dis Colon Rectum. 2013;56:354–9.
34. Watson NF, Koshy A, Sagar PM. Anal bulking agents for faecal incontinence. Color Dis. 2012;14(Suppl 3):29–33.
35. Hong KD, Kim JS, Ji WB, Um JW. Midterm outcomes of injectable bulking agents for fecal incontinence: a systematic review and meta-analysis. Tech Coloproctol. 2017;21:203–10.
36. Hussain ZI, Lim M, Stojkovic SG. Systematic review of perianal implants in the treatment of faecal incontinence. Br J Surg. 2011;98(11):1526–36.
37. Yoshioka K, Keighley MR. Clinical and manometric assessment of gracilis muscle transplant for fecal incontinence. Dis Colon Rectum. 1988;31:767–9.
38. Mander BJ, Wexner SD, Williams NS, Bartolo DC, et al. Preliminary results of a multicentre trial of the electrically stimulated gracilis neoanal sphincter. Br J Surg. 1999;86:1543–8.
39. Hull T, Giese C, Wexner SD, Mellgren A, Devroede G, Madoff RD, Stromberg K, Coller JA, SNS Study Group. Long-term durability of sacral nerve stimulation therapy for chronic fecal incontinence. Dis Colon Rectum. 2013;56:234–45.
40. Mellgren AI, Wexner SD, Coller JA, Devroede G, Lerew DR, Madoff RD, Hull T, SNS Study Group. Long-term efficacy and safety of sacral nerve stimulation for fecal incontinence. Dis Colon Rectum. 2011;54:1065–75.
41. Matzel KE. Sacral nerve stimulation for faecal incontinence: its role in the treatment algorithm. Color Dis. 2011;13(Suppl 2):10–4.
42. Indinnimeo M, Ratto C, Moschella CM, Fiore A, Brosa M. Giardina. Sacral neuromodulation for the

treatment of fecal incontinence: analysis of cost-effectiveness. Dis Colon Rectum. 2010;53:1661–9.
43. Devesa JM, Rey A, Hervas PL, Halawa KS, et al. Artificial anal sphincter: complications and functional results of a large personal series. Dis Colon Rectum. 2002;45:1154–63.
44. Hong KD, Dasilva G, Kalaskar SN, Chong Y, Wexner SD. Long-term outcomes of artificial bowel sphincter for fecal incontinence: a systematic review and meta-analysis. J Am Coll Surg. 2013;217:718–25.
45. Wexner SD, Jin HY, Weiss EG, Nogueras JJ, Li VK. Factors associated with failure of the artificial bowel sphincter: a study of over 50 cases from Cleveland Clinic Florida. Dis Colon Rectum. 2009;52:1550–7.
46. Wong WD, Congliosi SM, Spencer MP, Corman ML, et al. The safety and efficacy of the artificial bowel sphincter for fecal incontinence: results from a multicenter cohort study. Dis Colon Rectum. 2002;45:1139–53.
47. Kiely EM, Ade-Ajayi N, Wheeler RA. Caecal flap conduit for antegrate continence enemas. Br J Surg. 1994;81:215.
48. Griffiths DM, Malone PS. The Malone antegrade continence enema. J Pediatr Surg. 1995;30:68.
49. Patton V, Lubowski DZ. Clinical outcome and efficacy of anterograde colonic enemas administered via an indwelling cecostomy catheter in adults with defecatory disorders. Dis Colon Rectum. 2015;58:457–62.
50. Chatoor DR, Taylor SJ, Cohen CR, Emmanuel AV. Faecal incontinence. Br J Surg. 2007;94:134–44.
51. Willital GH, Meier H, Krebs C, Groitl H. Surgical technic to alleviate anal incontinence using a magnetic anal closure. Chir Forum Exp Klin Forsch. 1979:157–9.
52. Willital GH, Meier H. Der kunstliche enddarmverschlub ein neues konzept in der behandlung der analen incontinenz. Med Welt. 1982;33:43/1226–50/1230.
53. Bortolotti M. A novel antireflux device based on magnets. J Biomech. 2006;39:564–7.
54. Cope C. Evaluation of compression cholecystogastric and cholecystojejunal anastomoses in swine after peroral and surgical introduction of magnets. J Vasc Interv Radiol. 1995;6:546–52.
55. Cope C, Clark TW, Ginsberg G, Habecker P. Stent placement of gastroenteric anastomoses formed by magnetic compression. J Vasc Interv Radiol. 1999;10:1379–86.
56. Bortolotti M, Ugolini G, Grandis A, Montroni I, Mazzero G. A novel magnetic device to prevent fecal incontinence (preliminary study). Int J Color Dis. 2008;23:499–501.
57. Hill J, Corson RJ, Brandon H, Redford J, Faragher EB, Kiff ES. History and examination in the assessment of patients with idiopathic fecal incontinence. Dis Colon Rectum. 1994;37:473–8.
58. Bharucha AE. Anorectal testing is useful in rectal incontinence. Am J Gastroenterol. 2006;101:2679–81.
59. Bortolotti M, Grandis A. Mazzero. A novel endoesophageal magnetic device to prevent gastroesophageal reflux. Surg Endosc. 2009;23:885–9.
60. Lehur PA, McNevin S, Buntzen S, Mellgren AF, Laurberg S, Madoff RD. Magnetic anal sphincter augmentation for the treatment of fecal incontinence: a preliminary report from feasibility study. Dis Colon Rectum. 2010;53:1604–10.
61. Bonavina L, DeMeester T, Fockens P, Dunn D, et al. Laparoscopic sphincter augmentation device eliminates reflux symptoms and normalizes esophageal acid exposure: one- and 2-year results of a feasibility trial. Ann Surg. 2010;252:857–62.
62. Mantoo S, Meurette G, Podevin J, Lehur PA. The magnetic anal sphincter: a new device in the management of severe fecal incontinence. Expert Rev Med Devices. 2012;9:483–90.
63. Kim M, Lehur PA. How to size the anal canal circumference when implanting a magnetic anal sphincter for fecal incontinence. Evolution and update of a new surgical technique. Dis Colon Rectum. 2016;59:901–3.
64. Kim M, Meurette G, Ragu R, Wyart V, Lehur PA. Functional results and quality of life following magnetic anal sphincter augmentation in severely incontinent patients. Ann Surg. 2019;269:310–4.
65. Barussaud ML, Mantoo S, Wyart V, Meurette G, Lehur PA. The magnetic anal sphincter in faecal incontinence: is initial success sustained over time? Color Dis. 2013;15(12):1499–503.
66. Bridoux V, Gourcerol G, Leroi AM, Ducrotte P, Michot F, Tuech JJ. Response to Barussaud et al.: the magnetic anal sphincter in faecal incontinence, is initial success sustained over time? Color Dis. 2014;16:145–6.
67. Pakravan F, Helmes C. Magnetic anal sphincter augmentation in patients with severe fecal incontinence. Dis Colon Rectum. 2015;58:109–14.
68. Wong MT, Meurette G, Stangherlin P, Lehur PA. The magnetic anal sphincter versus the artificial bowel sphincter: a comparison of 2 treatments for fecal incontinence. Dis Colon Rectum. 2011;54(7):773–9.
69. Wong MT, Meurette G, Wyart V, Lehur PA. Does the magnetic anal sphincter device compare favourably with sacral nerve stimulation in the management of faecal incontinence? Color Dis. 2012;14:323–9.
70. Lehur PA, Wyart V, Riche VP. SaFaRI: sacral nerve stimulation versus the Fenix® magnetic sphincter augmentation for adult faecal incontinence: a randomised investigation. Int J Color Dis. 2016;31:1505.
71. Williams AE, Croft J, Napp V, Corrigan N, et al. SaFaRI: sacral nerve stimulation versus the FENIX magnetic sphincter augmentation for adult faecal incontinence: a randomised investigation. Int J Color Dis. 2016;31:465–72.
72. Sugrue J, Lehur PA, Madoff RD, McNevin S, et al. Long-term experience of magnetic anal sphincter augmentation in patients with fecal incontinence. Dis Colon Rectum. 2017;60:87–95.

73. Devesa JM, Vicente R. The use of a simple anal sling in the management of anal incontinence. Gastroenterol Rep (Oxf). 2014;2:136–9.
74. Horn HR, Schoetz DJ Jr, Coller JA, Veidenheimer MC. Sphincter repair with a Silastic sling for anal incontinence and rectal procidentia. Dis Colon Rectum. 1985;28:868–72.
75. Tjandra JJ, Tan J, Lim F, Murray-Green C. Long-term results of injectable silicone biomaterial for passive fecal incontinence – a randomized trial. Dis Colon Rectum. 2006;49:730–1.
76. Bartlett L, Ho YH. PTQ anal implants for the treatment of faecal incontinence. Br J Surg. 2009;96:1468–75.
77. Soerensen MM, Lundby L, Buntzen S, Laurberg S. Intersphincteric injected silicon biomaterial implants: a treatment for faecal incontinence. Color Dis. 2009;1:73–6.
78. Ganz RA, Gostout CJ, Grudem J, Swanson W, Berg T, DeMeester TR. Use of a magnetic sphincter for the treatment of GERD: a feasibility study. Gastrointest Endosc. 2008;67:287–94.
79. Bortolotti M. The "magnetic collar": the ultimate solution for gastroesophageal reflux? Scand J Gastroenterol. 2014;49:511–2.
80. Asti E, Siboni S, Lazzari V, Bonitta G, Sironi A, Bonavina L. Removal of the magnetic sphincter augmentation device. Surgical technique and results of a single-center Cohort study. Ann Surg. 2017;265:941–5.
81. Harnsberger C, Broderick RC, Fuchs H, Berducci M, et al. Magnetic lower esophageal sphincter augmentation device removal. Surg Endosc. 2015;29:984–6.
82. Varshney S, Kelly JJ, Branagan G, Somers SS, Kelly JM. Angelchik prosthesis revisited. World J Surg. 2002;26:129–33.
83. Bonavina L, DeMeester T, Mason R, Stein HJ, Feussner H, Evander A. Mechanical effect of the Angelchik prosthesis on the competency of the gastric cardia: pathophysiologic implications and surgical perspectives. Dis Esophagus. 1997;10:115–8.
84. Benjamin SB, Knuff TK, Fink M, Woods E, Castell DO. The Angelchik antireflux prosthesis. Effects on the lower esophageal sphincter of primates. Ann Surg. 1983;197:63–7.
85. Maeda Y, Laurberg S, Norton C. Perianal injectable bulking agents as treatment for fecal incontinence in adults. Cochrane Database Syst Rev. 2010;12(5):CDOO7959.
86. Lehur PA, Barussaud ML. The magnetic anal sphincter: a seductive promise still not kept. Color Dis. 2015;17:452.
87. Bortolotti M. The disappointing performance of the new "Magnetic Sphincters": a wrong idea or a wrong realization? J Gastrointestin Liver Dis. 2015;24:149–50.
88. Thomas G, Vaizey C. Surgery. In: Collins B, Bradshaw E, editors. Bowel dysfunction. Cham: Springer; 2016. p. 225–39.

Magnets for Urinary Incontinence

8

Michel Gagner

Introduction

This chapter is about a sphincter that can prevent the incontinence of urine in patients and is totally different from the recent studies on magnetic stimulation. Indeed, a randomized controlled study evaluated responses to pulsed magnetic stimulation administered twice weekly for 16 weeks, with an option to continue treatment regardless of treatment allocation. Researchers found that women randomized to the pulsed arm were more prone to report significant improvements in urinary incontinence [1]. At 2 months, 45 of 60 subjects (75%) in the pulsed arm versus 13 of 60 (22%) in the controls responded ($p < 0.001$). At 14 months, subjects who received 32 sessions of active pulsed magnetic stimulation had the greatest percentage of treatment responders (18 of 24 or 75%), followed by those who received 16 sessions (26 of 36 or 72% and 28 of 41 or 68%) and those who did not receive any active pulsed magnetic stimulation (4 of 19 or 21%) ($p < 0.001$) [1]. Magnets themselves had an initial enthusiasm but have been disappointing lately and the causes are reconsidered in this literature review [2].

M. Gagner (✉)
Hôpital du Sacré-Cœur de Montréal, Montréal, QC, Canada

Chief of Surgery, Westmount Square Surgical Center, Westmount, QC, Canada

Literature Review

Berry produced an acrylic prosthesis around the bulbous urethra in the 1960s but abandoned it due to "dislocation." Subsequently, Kaufman developed a silicone gel, also applied to the bulbous urethra. Rosen described an inflatable one with a fluid reservoir pump in the scrotum for men. In 1973, Scott invented the AS721 hydraulic silicone artificial sphincter. Most of the subsequent development has been a variant of these, but now applied to the bladder neck [3].

Hajivassiliou et al. have the recent historical development of these devices designed to achieve urinary continence [4]. These devices, "Foley clamp," Kaufman prosthesis, Giori, Summers and Rosen sphincters, Gruneberger and Cleveland Clinic magnetic designs, Craggs sphincter, and the AMS family of sphincters (AMS 721, AMS 761, AMS 742 (A, B, C), AMS 792, AMS 800) were analyzed and discussed. The design of active hydraulic devices was discussed in intricate details in this paper. This review analyzed the problems relating to the application of pressure and the presence of foreign material around the urethra. "Volume set" devices are universally unsuccessful and detrimental for urethral integrity as opposed to "pressure set" hydraulic sphincters (e.g., AMS 800). The implications for the design of artificial implants were discoursed [4].

In 1975, Kwart et al., in Scott's team as mentioned above, introduced a new bladder pump

M. Gagner (ed.), *Magnetic Surgery*, https://doi.org/10.1007/978-3-030-73947-8_8

prosthesis, designed and evaluated in the normal dog bladder. This encompasses a magnetic pump located subcutaneously with internal silicone catheters from bladder to the urethra. The pump is powered from a handheld activator, which is magnetically coupled externally across the skin. This pump was assessed in 12 dogs for an average of 65 days and delivered adequate emptying of the bladder without alteration of the normal urinary tract or pump malfunction [5].

The new magnetic urethral closure system consists of a retropubically implanted magnet and another removable intravaginal magnet, thus gently closing the urethra. The devices from Grüneberger and his team from the University of Ulm revealed its proper utility in 12 sheep during a period of observation of up to 33 weeks, without technical failings. The pressure on the tissue can be regulated by the size and strength of the removable magnet, and the pressure action time can straightforwardly be restrained to the tangible needs of the patient. Necrosis of the vagina wall and urethra have not been witnessed, using smooth-edged magnets [6, 7].

The Ulm magnetic/urethral-closure system comprises of a retropubically implanted magnet, secure to the inner part of the pubic symphysis, and an intravaginal magnet, which, by their reciprocal attraction, close the urethra. Magnetic force/distance features of rare earth/cobalt magnets employed for this function have been probed with distances comparable to those to be expected with the system in situ. Experiments on excised sheep urethra and bladder have revealed correct function of the closure system up to a urethral pressure of more than 120 cm H2O. The system has also been verified in vivo in 16 Merino sheep [8].

As stated earlier, the pioneer Grüneberger and his team from the University of Ulm, Germany, have been in the forefront of this magnetic urinary device, which involves a retropubically implanted magnet (Fig. 8.1). The other removable magnet is positioned in the vagina when the patient is physically active and when continence is preferred. The first experiences with a magnetic urethral closure system in female patients with recurrent urinary incontinence, when surgery usually fails (no descent and extremely hypotonic), were promising. Continence was achieved, and the handling was considered easy and could be managed by intelligent and well-motivated patients. The system has been used successfully in seven patients carrying the magnet in the vagina over 8 h daily for up to 3 years [9]. Following this report, an updated paper showed results after the system has been used in 11 patients with up to 5 years follow-up observation [10]. This prior experience has been supported by animal experience in sheep. The magnetic closure device implanted retropubically, and another removable intravaginal magnet permitted a gentle closure of the urethra. The pressure on the tissue can be adjusted by the size and strength of the removable smooth-edged magnets, and no necrosis of the vaginal wall and urethra could be observed in the earlier periods [11].

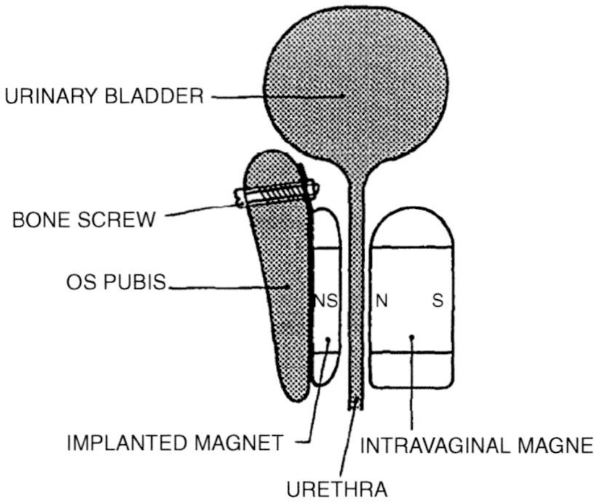

Fig. 8.1 Grüneberger's device. (From Grüneberger et al. [8]. Reprinted with permission from Elsevier)

Fukumura et al. reviewed their experience in 1993 [12]. The artificial urethral sphincter (AUS) had been in clinical use for more than 20 years at that time. A magnetically operated AUS was developed; although the skin between the magnets will be compressed all day long, little information existed on the effects of chronic pressure on the skin structure and blood flow. Two internal magnets and one control metal disk were implanted in five miniature pigs, subcutaneously at three various locations, and external magnets with changing magnetic forces were employed to the skin superimposing the internal magnets for 6 weeks. Contemporaneously, in four pigs, the skin blood flow was gauged by a laser Doppler flow meter applying diverse pressures. Results showed that a prolonged compression of 10 mmHg preserved normal skin morphology in all animals but one, where blood flow had not recovered 2 weeks postoperatively. Dramatic compression of 20 mmHg for 6 weeks, nevertheless, created pressure ulcers in all five cases ($p < 0.05$ vs. 10 mmHg group). The skin blood flow dropped for pressures exceeding 20 mmHg (0 mmHg: 4.3 +/− 1.2, 10 mmHg: 4.3 +/− 3.3, 20 mmHg: 2.6 +/− 2.7 ml/min/100 g). Fukumura concluded that the magnetically managed AUS should use a pressure less than 10 mmHg exerted on the interposed skin [12].

In 2000, Ali-El-Dein et al. invented a new magnetic device for intensifying the urethral resistance to flow in a dog model, to provide a potential mechanical device for the treatment of incontinence in women. In 12 female mongrel dogs, a magnet encased in a silicon layer was positioned on the anterior side of the urethra, 3 cm distal to the bladder neck, and secured with sutures. To increase the urethral resistance, a second magnet was inserted into the vagina and the device triggered. Urethral compression in the middle of the magnets resulted in a twofold amplification of the maximal pressure in the proximal urethra and in a threefold upsurge of the leak-point pressure. After 14 days of incessant compression of the vaginal wall and the urethra between the magnets, there was no measurable tissular damage. Although, the study by Ali-El-Dein confirmed the effect of a magnetic device causing an increase in urethral pressure and that prolonged compression caused no apparent damage to the urethra or vagina in the short term, a longer-term study would be required to comprehend patterns of foreign body migration and erosion [13].

According to Mazzocchi et al., urinary incontinence affects more than 300 million people globally, and they have conceived a magnetically controlled endourethral artificial urinary sphincter, an innovative artificial endourethral urinary sphincter capable to completely restore continence. It can be implanted by a minimally invasive technique in an outpatient fashion, not shifting nearby organs both for women and men. Their described device is fabricated with a unidirectional valve made of polymers with an incorporated magnetically activated system capable of amplifying the opening pressure. Bench tests and ex vivo studies on human cadavers demonstrated that the device is capable to restore continence and possibly allow urination when desired. This proposed new device was promising to restore a normal continence in daily life in patients affected. Human trials and randomized control trials are the necessary next steps nevertheless [14].

Marziale et al. recently reviewed the state of implantation of artificial urinary sphincter (AUS) as the gold standard treatment when conservative and minimally invasive therapies disappoint. In their review, the AUSs (extra-urethral and endo-urethral sphincters) offered globally, both depicted at the research level and filed as patents were examined. The ability of the different solutions to effectively replace the natural sphincter were discussed, and opposed to adverse events, such as tissue atrophy, invasiveness of the implant, and so forth. The future research priorities appear to focus on new materials, compression and closure appliances, implantation methods, with the long-term purpose of developing an successful, reliable, permanent, and minimally invasive AUS, capable of restoring a normal quality of life for incontinent patients [15].

Andig et al. reported a negative outcome case that exemplifies the above apprehensions. The affected urethra constricted over time due to erosion and scarring, and the patient commenced intermittent catheterization, because free micturition was impossible. The magnet was shattered, the bladder neck was eroded, several pieces were found in the bladder, and abundant fragments were scattered throughout the small pelvis. Surgery entailed removing most of the fragments, followed by bladder neck closure and suprapubic diversion. This was a disastrous consequence [16].

Recently, the company Torax Medical, Inc. (based in Minnesota) filed for a patent internationally last October 2019 (PCT/IB2019/059193) by inventors Huster C, Taylor K, Grudem JK, Bullitt BD, and DeMarchi J, for a sphincter augmentation device that looks essentially the same as the LINX device for GERD, except that this one is used to constrict the urethra (Figs. 8.2 and 8.3). The US patent was filed on October 26, 2018, published recently on April 30, 2020, and now available to the general public.

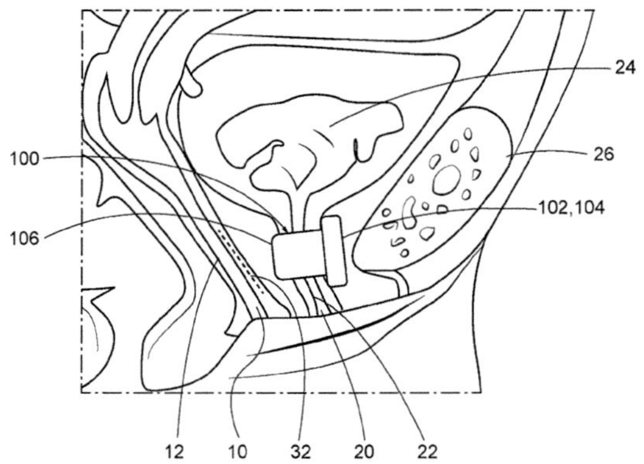

Fig. 8.2 Position in the pelvis. (From WIPO IP Portal – Patent Scope. WO2020084598 – Magnetic Sphincter Augmentation Device for Urinary Incontinence. Available at: https://patentscope.wipo.int/search/en/detail.jsf?docId=WO2020084598)

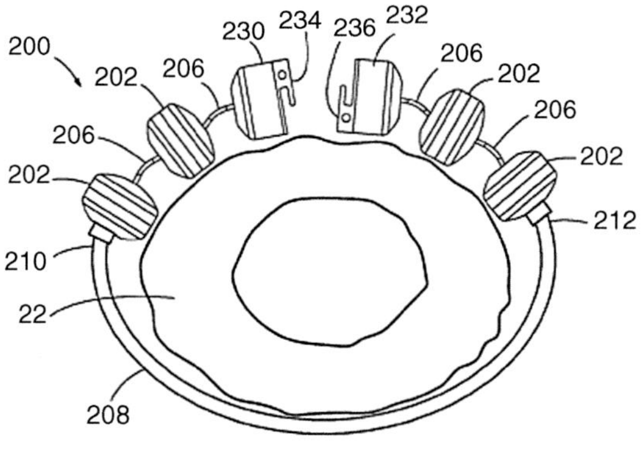

Fig. 8.3 Reproduced from the patent PCT/IB2019/059193, showing a collar of oval magnets around the urethra. Magnets are circumferential on one side only, 180 degrees. From WIPO IP Portal – Patent Scope. WO2020084598 – Magnetic Sphincter Augmentation Device for Urinary Incontinence. (Available at: https://patentscope.wipo.int/search/en/detail.jsf?docId=WO2020084598)

The device is sized to be positioned externally around the urethra, so that the array of small magnets flexing inward toward the urethra lumen. It is not clear to me how you can urinate if the collar is constantly in the closing states. There must be a fine line between the opening pressure and closing one; this is possible I suppose with a catheter (in and out) or by forceful intraabdominal pressure [17]. One is awaiting clinical studies in humans to see if this will pass the test of time, and to see the erosion rates, as the tissue around the urethra is much thinner than what is seen with the esophagogastric junction. The urethra in females is usually only 4 cm long, and MRI studies have measured a 2.5–4 mm muscular component around the urethra. The intraabdominal esophagus thickness is usually 5–6 mm; this may confer a lower rate of erosions to the esophagus [18, 19].

Biardeau et al. from McGill University have proposed a modification of the AMS 800 device, electromagnetically controlled but with a Bluetooth application to remotely control the system, incorporating a lithium battery of 10 months duration [20]. This hydraulic pressure system device will likely continue to be used clinically and will serve as a fierce competitor to renewed surgically implanted magnets around the urethra; clinical results must be seen in the next decade.

References

1. Lim R, Liong ML, Leong WS, Karim Khan NA, Yuen KH. Pulsed magnetic stimulation for stress urinary incontinence: 1-year Followup results. J Urol. 2017 May 01;197(5):1302–8.
2. Bortolotti M. The disappointing performance of the new "Magnetic Sphincters": a wrong idea or a wrong realization? J Gastrointestin Liver Dis. 2015;24(2):149–50.
3. Montague DK. Evolution of implanted devices for urinary incontinence. Cleve Clin Q. 1984;51(2):405–9.
4. Hajivassiliou CA. The development and evolution of artificial urethral sphincters. J Med Eng Technol. 1998;22(4):154–9.
5. Kwart AM, Hughes B, Scott WW. Evaluation of a magnetic bladder pump for neurogenic bladders. Investig Urol. 1975;12(6):442–5.
6. Grüneberger AD, Hennig G, Bollemer F. Das Magnetsystem eines Harnröhrenverschlusses [A

magnet-system for urethral closure]. Biomed Tech (Berl). 1982;27(10):238–42.
7. Grüneberger AD, Hennig GR. A magnetic urethral closure device: preliminary report of an experimental study. J Urol. 1983;130(4):798–801.
8. Grüneberger AD, Hennig GR, Bullemer F. A magnet system for urethral closure in females. J Biomed Eng. 1984;6(2):102–6.
9. Grüneberger AD. Klinische Erfahrungen mit einem magnetischen Harnröhrenverschluss [Clinical experiences with magnetic urethral closure]. Geburtshilfe Frauenheilkd. 1990;50(2):150–4.
10. Grüneberger AD. Entwicklung eines magnetischen Urethralverschlusses und erste klinische Erfahrungen [Development of a magnetic urethral closure and initial clinical experiences]. Urologe A. 1987;26(3):106–11.
11. Grüneberger AD, Hennig GR. Entwicklung eines magnetischen Urethralverschlusses--eine tierexperimentelle Studie [Development of a magnetic urethral closure device--an animal experiment study]. Zentralbl Gynakol. 1993;115(7):328–31.
12. Fukumura F, Harasaki H, Fukamachi K, et al. Development of a magnetically operated artificial urethral sphincter. Chronic effects of compression on the skin structure and blood flow. ASAIO J. 1993;39(3):M283–7.
13. Ali-El-Dein B, El-Demerdash R, Kock NG, Ghoneim MA. A magnetic device for increasing the urethral resistance to flow: an experimental study in female dogs. BJU Int. 2000;85(1):150–4.
14. Mazzocchi T, Ricotti L, Pinzi N, Menciassi A. Magnetically controlled Endourethral artificial urinary sphincter. Ann Biomed Eng. 2017;45(5):1181–93.
15. Marziale L, Lucarini G, Mazzocchi T, et al. Artificial sphincters to manage urinary incontinence: a review. Artif Organs. 2018;42(9):E215–33.
16. Anding R, van Ahlen H, Müller SC, Latz S. Magnetisches Harnröhrenverschlusssystem. Desaströser Verlauf nach Implantation zur Behandlung der weiblichen Belastungsinkontinenz [Magnetic urethral closure device. Negative outcome after implantation for the treatment of female urinary incontinence]. Urologe A. 2015;54(7):1010–3.
17. WIPO IP Portal – Patent Scope. WO2020084598 -- Magnetic sphincter augmentation device for urinary incontinence. Available at: https://patentscope.wipo.int/search/en/detail.jsf?docId=WO2020084598.
18. Macura KJ, Genadry R, Borman TL, Mostwin JL, Lardo AC, Bluemke DA. Evaluation of the female urethra with intraurethral magnetic resonance imaging. J Magn Reson Imaging. 2004;20(1):153–9.
19. Xia F, Mao J, Ding J, Yang H. Observation of normal appearance and wall thickness of esophagus on CT images. Eur J Radiol. 2009;72(3):406–11.
20. Biardeau X, Hached S, Loutochin O, Campeau L, Sawan M, Corcos J. Montreal electronic artificial urinary sphincters: our futuristic alternatives to the AMS800™. Can Urol Assoc J. 2017;11(10):E396–404.

The Use of Magnets in the Treatment of Congenital Disorders

9

Bethany Slater and Russell K. Woo

Introduction

Drs. Hendren and Hale at Boston Children's Hospital first reported the use of electromagnetic bougienage to lengthen the esophageal ends in a patient with esophageal atresia in order to facilitate later repair [1]. Since then pediatric specialist have employed magnets to treat a variety of congenital disorders. The published experience with using magnets to treat congenital disorders falls into two categories: magnets used to facilitate the treatment of atresias of the alimentary tract and magnets used to guide the growth and remodeling of bone for the treatment of musculoskeletal disorders (Table 9.1). In general, the use of magnets to treat congenital disorders has been aimed at the gradual distraction of malformed tissue to achieve a more anatomically and physiologically normal state. In this chapter, we will highlight the various congenital defects for which magnets have been employed and review worldwide published experience with the use of magnets to treat these pediatric conditions.

B. Slater
Department of Pediatric Surgery, University of Chicago Medicine, Chicago, IL, USA

R. K. Woo (✉)
Department of Surgery, Division of Pediatric Surgery, University of Hawaii, John A. Burns School of Medicine, Honolulu, HI, USA
e-mail: russell.woo@kapiolani.org

Table 9.1 Published surgical applications of magnets to treat congenital disorders

Congenital disorder	Use of magnets	Magnetic systems employed
Pectus Excavatum	Gradual distraction of malformed chest wall	3MP device: Magnimplant and Magnatract (Hayes Manufacturing, Sunnyvale, CA and Hantel Technologies, Hayward, CA)
Congenital scoliosis	Spinal distraction with magnetically controlled growing rods	MAGEC® System (NuVasive, San Diego, CA)
Esophageal atresia	Esophageal lengthening, compression anastomosis, and stricturoplasty	Flourish™ (Cook Medical, Bloomington, IN) Commercially available magnets
Anal atresia	Rectal lengthening and compression anoplasty	Commercially available magnets

The Use of Magnets for the Treatment of Pectus Excavatum

Pectus excavatum is a congenital, anterior chest wall deformity that results in a posterior depression of the sternum (Fig. 9.1). It accounts for 90% of all anterior chest wall disorders, affecting 1 in every 300–400 live births [2, 3]. The concave

M. Gagner (ed.), *Magnetic Surgery*, https://doi.org/10.1007/978-3-030-73947-8_9

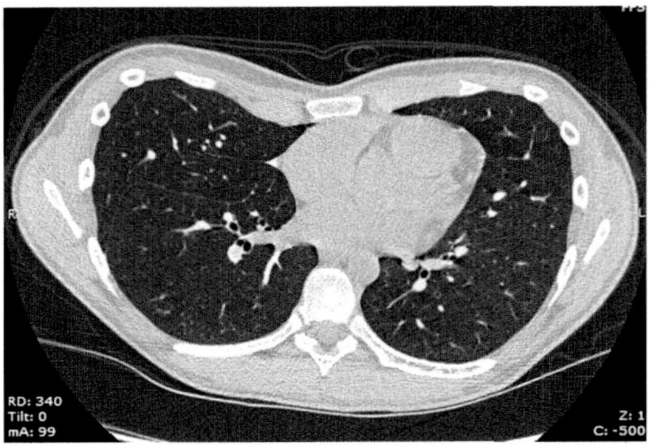

Fig. 9.1 Pectus excavatum or "funnel chest"

appearance is noticeable at birth and worsens during rapid bone growth experienced during adolescence. Many cases result in psychological distress, with some reports of cardiopulmonary limitation.

The standard surgical treatments for pectus excavatum involve major surgical reconstruction of the anterior chest. The modified Ravitch procedure involves exposure of the sternum and cartilage junctions via a large midline or transverse incision. The abnormal cartilaginous segments connecting the ribs to the sternum are then resected, and the sternum may be remodeled by wedge osteotomy and then fixed to a more normal position with an underlying metal bar which remains in the patient for at least a year. More recently, the thoracoscopic-assisted Nuss procedure has become the most widely used surgical approach to treat pectus excavatum. This requires the placement of one or more custom-shaped metal bars across the retrosternal position of the defect under thoracoscopic guidance. The bars serve to push the sternal defect outward and are generally left in place for 2 or more years before removal.

While both the Ravitch and Nuss procedures are effective with multiple studies demonstrating favorable outcomes, they involve a significant surgical event with the purpose of completely correcting the chest wall deformity at one time. This necessarily requires general anesthesia and is associated with a potentially significant postoperative recovery period and possible complications. With this in mind, Dr. Harrison and colleagues from the University of California San Francisco have reported the development and evaluation of a magnetic system designed to treat pectus excavatum deformities in a more gradual manner using minimal force applied over a longer period of time. Their method, called the Magnetic Mini-Mover Procedure or 3MP, is designed to achieve reformulation of the malformed pectus excavatum chest wall cartilage gradually, without hospitalization or major surgery.

In their first report, published in 2007, they detailed the development and design of the magnetic system. The system utilizes an implantable device (Magnimplant, Hayes Manufacturing, Sunnyvale, CA and Hantel Technologies, Hayward, CA) that is inserted and fixed to the sternum through a small incision at the sternal xiphoid junction. This is then coupled with an external magnet attached to a custom-designed and fitted externally worn brace (Magnatract, Hayes Manufacturing, Sunnyvale, CA and Hantel Technologies, Hayward, CA) to generate a sustained outward force sufficient to gradually remodel the pectus excavatum deformity (Fig. 9.2). They also reported the results of the testing simulations that they performed to assess the feasibility and safety of the devices [4].

In a follow-up publication in 2010, the group reported the interim findings of a Food and Drug Administration-sponsored clinical trial evaluating the 3MP procedure. In this report, the group detailed the initial procedures and testing for 10 otherwise healthy patients with moderate to severe pectus excavatum deformities who underwent initiation of the 3MP procedure. The patients ranged from 8 to 14 years of age and all had a Haller index of greater than 3.5. They did not detect any significant effects of the persistent magnetic field on wound healing or cardiopulmonary function and found no detectable complications associated with wearing the external brace. Most of the patients underwent insertion of the magnetic implant as an outpatient procedure requiring approximately 30 minutes of operating time. They attempted to measure changes in pectus severity with treatment using serial imaging but found that this was difficult

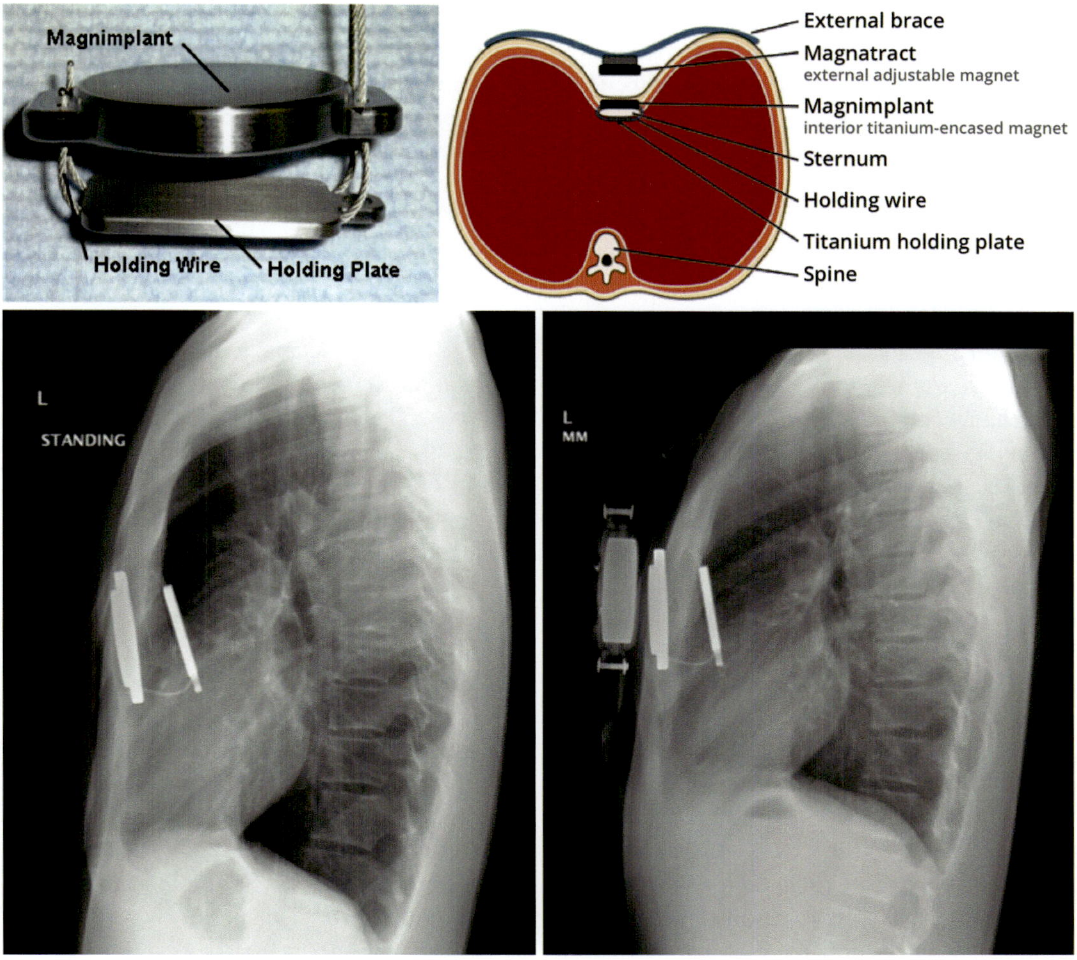

Fig. 9.2 3MP device: A titanium-enclosed magnet is implanted onto the anterior sternum. Externally, patients wear a custom-fitted brace designed to correct the deformity using magnetic force. On lateral CXR, the implant alone is shown on the left; on the right, the implant is coupled with the external brace. (From Graves et al. [7]. Reprinted with permission from Elsevier)

due to variability in patient positioning and respiratory cycle during serial images as well as from interference due to the implant itself. They also reported modifications to the device that were identified and connected during the course of this initial trial period [5].

In 2012, the group published a follow-up report of the FDA-sponsored clinical trial. This was designed to report the safety and efficacy of the 3MP procedure and devices. They monitored safety by post implant and post explant electrocardiograms and monthly chest x-rays performed while the patients were being treated. They found no detectable ill effect from the devices and 18 months treatment duration. Device failure or improper positioning/migration required revision in 5 of the 10 patients. They found that pectus severity as measured by the pectus index improved in the younger patients who are undergoing early or mid-puberty. However, older patients with less compliant chests did not see improvement. They also evaluated the cost-effectiveness of the 3MP procedure. They found an average cost of $46,859 for the 3MP procedure compared to $81,206 for the Nuss procedure and $81,022 for the Ravitch procedure. They concluded that the 3MP procedure was a safe and cost-effective outpatient treatment option for patients in the stages of early to mid-puberty to treat pectus excavatum [6].

Most recently Dr. Harrison and collaborators from other institutions reported the results of an FDA-sponsored multicenter trial designed to supplement the safety and efficacy data from the earlier pilot trial. Fifteen patients underwent the 3MP procedures and treatment with an average age of 12 years and treatment duration of 25 months. For this trial, the authors lengthened the treatment period to 2 years, after which point the implants were removed. They also utilized an improved magnetic implant which was simpler to place and less prone to breakage. They measured efficacy by Haller index determined by post-operative imaging in 13 patients and found a decrease or improvement in the Haller index in 5 patients, an unchanged Haller index in 2 patients, and an increased or worsened Haller index in 6 patients. Patient satisfaction surveys were also administered and demonstrated that 8 of 13 patients were satisfied with the results of the treatment. Of note, 7 out of 15 of the study patients experienced device failure from breakage of the implant's titanium cables due to fatigue fracture. The authors felt that this likely affected the efficacy of the treatment in these patients. Overall the authors highlighted the lessons learned from the design, development and testing of this technology and procedure and concluded that the 3MP was a safe outpatient procedure capable of treating prepubertal patients with pectus excavatum [7].

The Use of Magnets for the Treatment of Congenital Scoliosis

Congenital scoliosis refers to a spectrum of anomalies of the spine resulting from abnormal vertebral development during the fourth to sixth weeks of gestation and has an overall incidence of 1 in every 1000 live births [8]. Congenital scoliosis is classically divided into failures of vertebral segmentation, failures of vertebral formation, and mixed forms. While congenital scoliosis can occur in isolation, it can also be associated with other congenital anomalies. Specifically, anomalies of the genitourinary, musculoskeletal, and cardiovascular systems have been reported as these systems undergo significant development in utero at the same time as the spine [9]. Congenital scoliosis results in asymmetric growth of the spine that causes an abnormal curvature at an early age [10].

In general, the treatment for congenital scoliosis requires surgery. As opposed to idiopathic scoliosis and older children, the spinal curvatures are usually inflexible and are therefore unresponsive to bracing therapy. Surgical treatments for congenital scoliosis are aimed at stopping the progression of the deformity while optimizing the potential for the ongoing growth of the child. Surgery is indicated in children who have defects that are predicted to be at high risk for progression and defects that are increasing in severity. Treatment options include in situ fusion and hemiepiphysiodesis, hemivertebra resection, and growth-friendly surgery. Growth-friendly surgery options include the implantation of Vertical Expandable Prosthetic Titanium Rib (VEPTR) devices and possible expansion thoracoplasty as well as growing rods [9].

Growing rods are generally used to treat early onset scoliosis and had been reported as a safe and effective treatment in this population. As opposed to spinal fusion, growing rods treatments do not inhibit the further growth of the spine or thoracic cavity. Conventional growing rods systems are made up of telescopically distractible rods anchored to the spine by proximal and distal pedicle screws or hooks. These rods are serially lengthened at 6-month intervals with a minor surgical procedure. These serial distraction procedures are typically outpatient surgeries involving a small incision over the rod connectors [11]. More normal spinal alignment is achieved through constant and regularly adjusted spinal distraction that corresponds with the growth of the child.

Recently, magnetically controlled growing rods have been employed to provide growing rod therapy in children with early onset scoliosis without the need for multiple invasive adjustment procedures. First reported in 2012 by Cheung and colleagues [12], magnetically controlled growing rod systems consist of specialized nonreusable titanium spinal distractible rods. These rods feature an enlarged midportion containing a magnetically drivable lengthening mechanism that allows for remote noninvasive distraction (Fig. 9.3). Since this initial report, multiple authors have reported the results with the use of single or dual system magnetically controlled growing rods in children with early onset scoliosis [13, 14]. In addition, authors have reported relative safety with respect to the use of magnetic resonance imaging in patients with magnetically controlled growing rods in place [15].

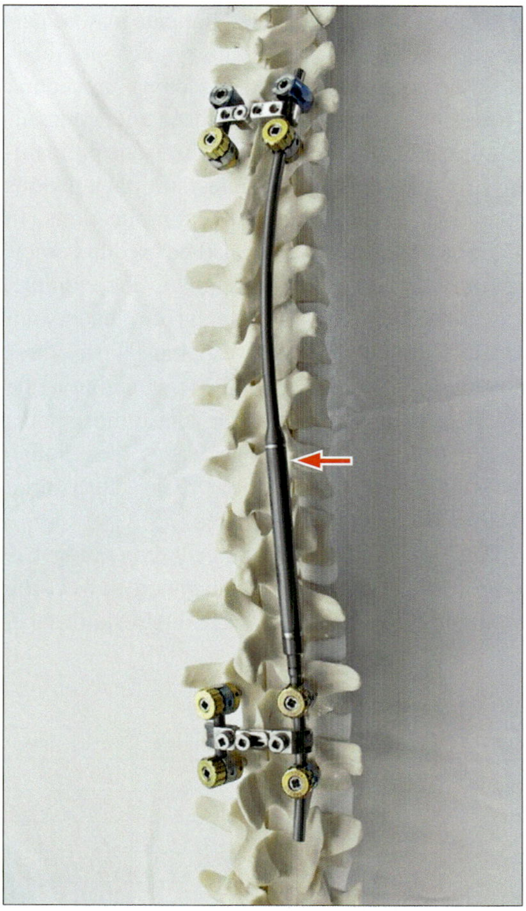

Fig. 9.3 A single magnetically controlled growing rod fixed to a spine model. (From Cheung et al. [41]. Reprinted with permission from Elsevier)

The published experience with magnetically controlled growing rods is predominantly of children with early onset scoliosis. A few of the published studies include patients with congenital scoliosis. Specifically, Akbarnia and colleagues published a series of 14 patients treated with magnetically controlled growing rods in patients with congenital scoliosis. This series demonstrated comparable results to conventional growing rods with a significant reduction and return trips to the operating room [12]. Currently the MAGEC® System (NuVasive, Sand Diego, CA) is commercially available in the United States. While the published experience with magnetically controlled growing rods in patients with congenital scoliosis is very limited, future reports and application are anticipated.

The Use of Magnets for the Treatment of Esophageal Atresia

Esophageal atresia (EA), with and without tracheoesophageal fistula (TEF), is the most common congenital anomaly of the esophagus with an incidence of 1:3500 live born infants [16]. Other congenital anomalies are often associated with EA, with cardiac defects being the most frequent, and affect the survival and treatment of these patients. EA is often classified according to the Gross classification by anatomic patterns with type C, proximal atresia with distal TEF, as the most common. Type A is a pure esophageal atresia without fistula and has the greatest likelihood of being associated with a long gap. Patients with EA typically present with excessive salivation, difficulty feeding, and may have respiratory distress. The diagnosis is confirmed with a chest radiograph demonstrating a feeding tube coiled in the upper esophageal pouch [17].

Most patients with EA undergo surgical repair with esophageal anastomosis and ligation of the tracheoesophageal fistula if present soon after birth. However, factors due to the patient's characteristics, such as congenital anomalies or prematurity, surgical issues, or anatomic concerns, can restrict the ability to obtain esophageal continuity. Patients with long gap EA, in which a primary repair is unable to be achieved without significant tension, comprise a group of technically challenging patients in which no consensus for management has been reached. Most pediatric surgeons proceed with operative gastrostomy tube placement and a period of observation to allow for spontaneous growth of the esophageal ends. Long gap EA is commonly based on a gap assessment during fluoroscopy after gastrostomy creation, and there is no standard accepted distance defining it [18]. Multiple operative strategies have been described for these patients including delayed primary anastomosis [19, 20], extensive mobilization, circular myotomies [21], esophageal flaps, and internal or external traction of the segments [22, 23]. More recently, thoracoscopic approaches have been employed to improve visualization, obtain significant mobilization, and for elongation and internal traction procedures [20, 24, 25]. Although gastric transposition and colonic interposition are also options if esophageal replacement is required, it is optimal to preserve the native esophagus if possible [26].

The use of magnets is a nonsurgical alternative for esophageal anastomosis in selected patients [27]. Magnets have been described in the literature for various types of anastomoses since the 1970s [1, 28, 29]. As described in our introduction, Hendren and Hale first reported the use of electromagnetic bougienage to lengthen the esophageal ends in a patient with EA, facilitating later surgical repair [1]. Catheter-based magnetic anastomosis was initially described in five infants with EA in Argentina [30]. Anastomosis was achieved in all the patients in an average of 4.8 days. A later series was published describing achievement of primary esophageal anastomosis in an additional four patients with EA using catheter based bullet-shaped magnet pairs [31]. A recent study described a two-stage approach whereby young infants had an initial esophageal approximation without luminal continuity followed by magnamosis (Table 9.2) [32].

The magnets situated in the proximal and distal esophageal pouches have opposite polarity and thus once aligned attract one another leading to lengthening of the ends. Once the magnets connect or couple, the central, intervening tissue becomes ischemic and sloughs off while the outer rim heals establishing the anastomosis. The length of the gap must be within the magnetic field achievable by the two magnets to attain attraction and connection.

The use of magnets in EA patients may be particularly beneficial for patients who cannot tolerate thoracotomy or a thoracoscopic procedure. These patients might include those with congenital anomalies, respiratory issues from prematurity, or who have undergone multiple previous operations or have had prior complications. In addition, the magnets may also be used in combination with surgery as an adjunct. For example, they may be used in patients that underwent repair with postoperative esophageal strictures not amenable to dilation [33, 34]. In addition, the magnets can be utilized for anastomosis in a staged fashion for esophageal gaps longer than the strength of the magnetic field after initial operative stretching procedures [35].

The US Food and Drug Administration has approved a catheter-based magnetic device, the Flourish™ Pediatric Esophageal Atresia Device,

Table 9.2 Summary of studies using magnets for patients with esophageal atresia

Study	No. of EA pts	Use of magnet	Average no. of days to anastomosis	% stricture
Takamizawa 2007 [34]	1	Stricture	34	100
Zaritzky 2009 [30]	5	Anastomosis	4.8	80
Zaritzky 2014 [31]	9	Anastomosis	4.2	89
Lovvorn 2014 [32]	2	Staged anastomosis	7.5	100
Dorman 2016 [35]	1	Staged anastomosis	13	100
Woo 2017 [33]	2	Stricture	8.5	100
Greenstein 2018 [27]	1	Anastomosis	10	100
Slater 2019	13	Anastomosis	6.3	100

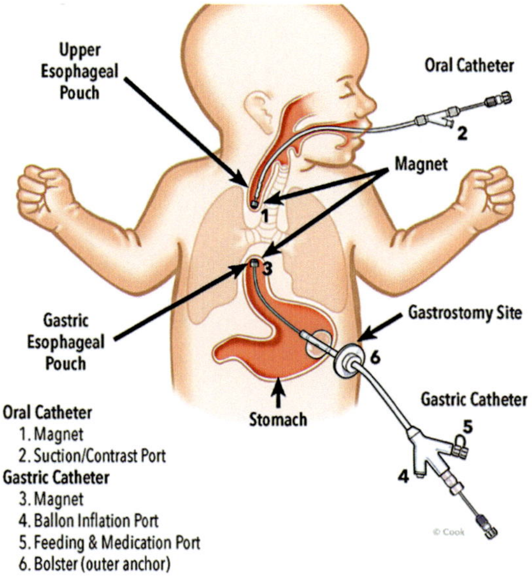

Fig. 9.4 Flourish™ device with proximal suction port and distal port for feeds. (Permission for use granted by Cook Medical, Bloomington, IN)

for use in lengthening atretic esophageal ends and creating an anastomosis in patients up to 1 year of age (Cook Medical, Bloomington, IN). It has been federally authorized as a humanitarian use device. The device consists of an esophageal and gastric catheter each containing an inner catheter fitted with a bullet-shaped neodymium iron boron magnet (Fig. 9.4). The proximal portion has a central hole for insertion of a guide wire and a suction port for removal of saliva and for injection of contrast to confirm anastomosis. The distal catheter has a channel for enteral feeds and a 5 ml balloon. The distance between the upper and lower pouches must be less than 4 cm in length to use the flourish device.

The magnetic anastomosis procedure may be performed under anesthesia or sedation and is done under fluoroscopic guidance. After completion, daily chest radiographs are done to verify proper alignment of the magnets. Successful anastomosis is confirmed by esophagram, saliva in the gastrostomy catheter, or feeds in the esophageal catheter. After a day, the magnets may be removed and replaced with an oro- or nasogastric tube over a wire (Fig. 9.5). A prospective, single-arm, observational study is currently enrolling patients to evaluate the safety and benefit of the Flourish Device.

Areas for research to improve the results of magnamosis for EA include modifying the shape and strength of the magnets to minimize postprocedure stenosis and potentially facilitate esophageal growth more accurately. Creating a mechanism to decrease the magnetic strength as the pouches approach one another might allow greater control and flexibility of the lengthening portion. This may also decrease the risk of tearing from too much force as the esophageal ends get closer. Finally, early stent placement after the magnamosis might be another way to minimize stricture formation.

The Use of Magnets for the Treatment of Anal Atresia

Anorectal malformation (ARM) has an average worldwide incidence of 1 in 5000 live births [36]. The classification system uses anatomic descriptions and is an important factor in the therapeutic and prognostic implications for infants with ARMs. Other congenital anomalies are also common in these patients. Rectal atresia is a rare congenital malformation, comprising approximately 1% of all anorectal malformations [37]. Unlike other anorectal malformations, patients with rectal atresia usually have a short stenosis or fibrous band in the distal rectum, an anal opening within the normal sphincter complex, and no fistulous connection to the urinary system. This defect may be associated with a presacral mass. As such, a full evaluation with imaging must be performed to assure that a mass is not missed preoperatively. Similar to long gap esophageal atresia, there are multiple reported treatment strategies with no clear consensus on operative approach. These repair techniques have consisted of circumferential rectoanal anastomosis, pull-through of proximal rectum, or posterior sagittal approaches [37–39]. Some of the methods attempt to retain part of the anorectum to minimize distortion of the sphincter complex and sensation within it. The published literature reports satisfactory outcomes for these patients [37–39].

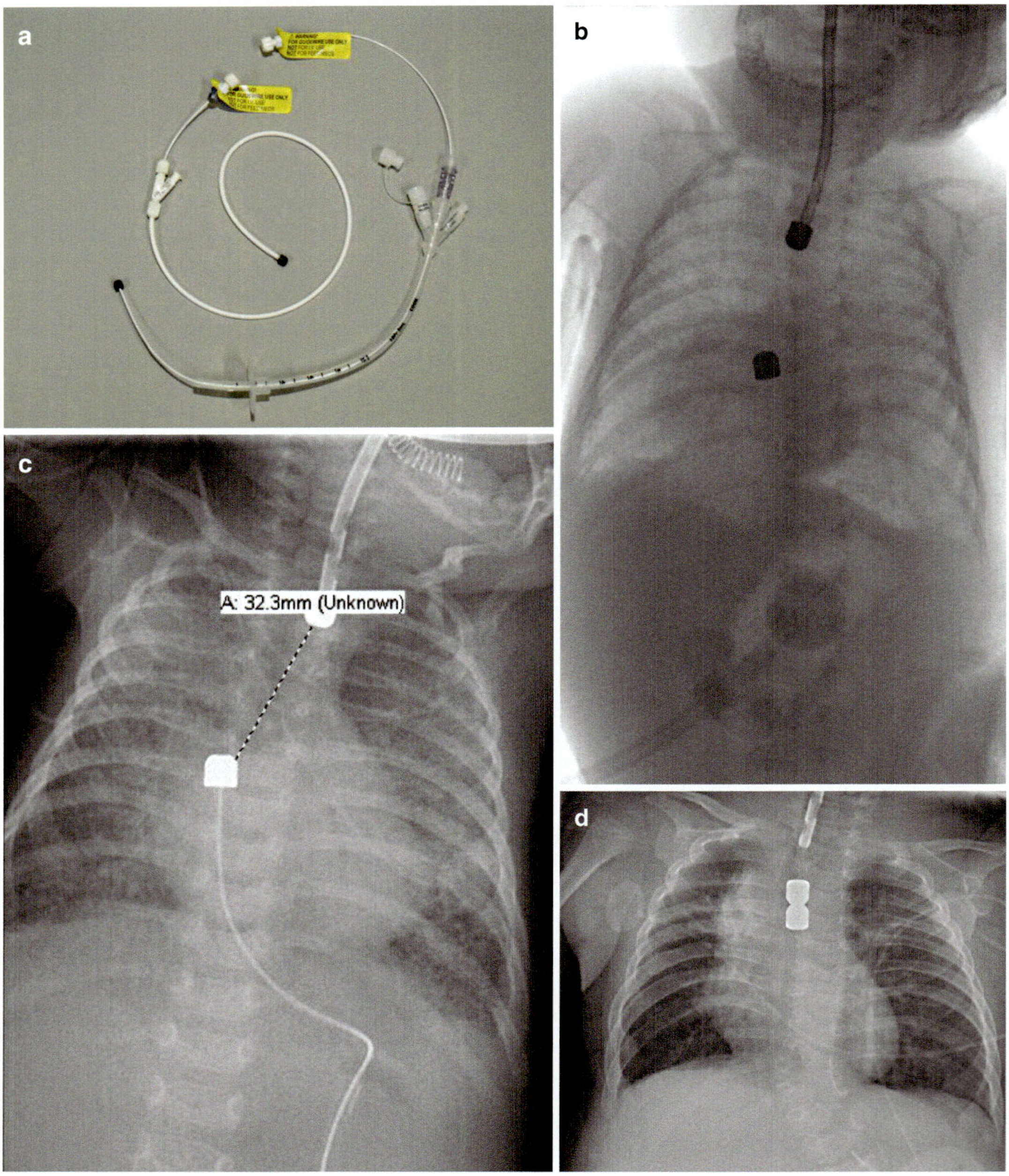

Fig. 9.5 (**a**) Flourish™ device used for esophageal atresia. (**b**) Fluoroscopic image of device after insertion. (**c**) CXR after insertion of catheter-based magnets. (**d**) CXR with magnets coupled together

However, most include small series or case reports, and many do not have long-term results.

The anatomy of rectal atresia or stenosis allows for magnamosis to be performed. A case report has described the use of magnets to successfully achieve anastomosis of the proximal and distal pouches in a patient with rectal atresia that had undergone creation of an end colostomy and mucous fistula [40]. The magnets were introduced through the mucous fistula under fluoroscopic guidance and through the anus. After 4 days, the two magnets with a disc of tissue between them were passed per rectum. This minimally invasive approach allows for avoidance of disruption of the sphincter mechanism and associated nerves. Given that patients with rectal atresia or stenosis have an excellent prognosis in regards to bowel control, this is particularly important. In addition, the lack of dissection prevents inadvertent injury to the rectal wall, vagina, or urethra.

References

1. Hendren WH, Hale JR. Electromagnetic bougienage to lengthen esophageal segments in congenital esophageal atresia. N Engl J Med. 1975;293(9):428–32.
2. Fokin AA, Steuerwald NM, Ahrens WA, Allen KE. Anatomical, histologic, and genetic characteristics of congenital chest wall deformities. Semin Thorac Cardiovasc Surg. 2009;21(1):44–57.
3. Morikawa N, Laferriere N, Koo S, Johnson S, Woo R, Puapong D. Cryoanalgesia in patients undergoing nuss repair of pectus excavatum: technique modification and early results. J Laparoendosc Adv Surg Tech A. 2018;28(9):1148–51.
4. Harrison MR, Estefan-Ventura D, Fechter R, Moran AM Jr, Christensen D. Magnetic mini-mover procedure for pectus excavatum: I. development, design, and simulations for feasibility and safety. J Pediatr Surg. 2007;42(1):81–5; discussion 5-6.
5. Harrison MR, Curran PF, Jamshidi R, Christensen D, Bratton BJ, Fechter R, et al. Magnetic mini-mover procedure for pectus excavatum II: initial findings of a food and drug administration-sponsored trial. J Pediatr Surg. 2010;45(1):185–91; discussion 91-2.
6. Harrison MR, Gonzales KD, Bratton BJ, Christensen D, Curran PF, Fechter R, et al. Magnetic mini-mover procedure for pectus excavatum III: safety and efficacy in a food and drug administration-sponsored clinical trial. J Pediatr Surg. 2012;47(1):154–9.
7. Graves CE, Hirose S, Raff GW, Iqbal CW, Imamura-Ching J, Christensen D, et al. Magnetic mini-mover procedure for pectus excavatum IV: FDA sponsored multicenter trial. J Pediatr Surg. 2017;52(6):913–9.
8. Giampietro PF, Blank RD, Raggio CL, Merchant S, Jacobsen FS, Faciszewski T, et al. Congenital and idiopathic scoliosis: clinical and genetic aspects. Clin Med Res. 2003;1(2):125–36.
9. Pahys JM, Guille JT. What's new in congenital scoliosis? J Pediatr Orthop. 2018;38(3):e172–e9.
10. Hedequist D, Emans J. Congenital scoliosis: a review and update. J Pediatr Orthop. 2007;27(1):106–16.
11. Bekmez S, Dede O, Yazici M. Advances in growing rods treatment for early onset scoliosis. Curr Opin Pediatr. 2017;29(1):87–93.
12. Akbarnia BA, Cheung K, Noordeen H, Elsebaie H, Yazici M, Dannawi Z, et al. Next generation of growth-sparing techniques: preliminary clinical results of a magnetically controlled growing rod in 14 patients with early-onset scoliosis. Spine (Phila Pa 1976). 2013;38(8):665–70.
13. Tang N, Zhao H, Shen JX, Zhang JG, Li SG. Magnetically controlled growing rod for early-onset scoliosis: systematic review and meta-analysis. World Neurosurg. 2019.
14. Figueiredo N, Kananeh SF, Siqueira HH, Figueiredo RC, Al Sebai MW. The use of magnetically controlled growing rod device for pediatric scoliosis. Neurosciences (Riyadh). 2016;21(1):17–25.
15. Woon RP, Andras LM, Noordeen H, Morris S, Hutchinson J, Shah SA, et al. Surgeon survey shows no adverse events with MRI in patients with magnetically controlled growing rods (MCGRs). Spine Deform. 2018;6(3):299–302.
16. Harmon CM, Coran AG. Congenital anomalies of the esophagus. In: Coran AG, editor. Pediatric surgery. 7th ed. Philadelphia: Elsevier; 2012.
17. Lee S. Basic knowledge of tracheoesophageal fistula and esophageal atresia. Adv Neonatal Care. 2018;18(1):14–21.
18. Baird R, Lal DR, Ricca RL, Diefenbach KA, Downard CD, Shelton J, et al. Management of long gap esophageal atresia: a systematic review and evidence-based guidelines from the APSA outcomes and evidence based practice committee. J Pediatr Surg. 2019;54(4):675–87.
19. Friedmacher F, Puri P. Delayed primary anastomosis for management of long-gap esophageal atresia: a meta-analysis of complications and long-term outcome. Pediatr Surg Int. 2012;28(9):899–906.
20. Rothenberg SS, Flake AW. Experience with thoracoscopic repair of long gap esophageal atresia in neonates. J Laparoendosc Adv Surg Tech A. 2015;25(11):932–5.
21. Lai JY, Sheu JC, Chang PY, Yeh ML, Chang CY, Chen CC. Experience with distal circular myotomy for long-gap esophageal atresia. J Pediatr Surg. 1996;31(11):1503–8.
22. Kimura K, Soper RT. Multistaged extrathoracic esophageal elongation for long gap esophageal atresia. J Pediatr Surg. 1994;29(4):566–8.
23. Nasr A, Langer JC. Mechanical traction techniques for long-gap esophageal atresia: a critical appraisal. Eur J Pediatr Surg. 2013;23(3):191–7.
24. van der Zee DC, Gallo G, Tytgat SH. Thoracoscopic traction technique in long gap esophageal atresia: entering a new era. Surg Endosc. 2015;29(11):3324–30.
25. Bogusz B, Patkowski D, Gerus S, Rasiewicz M, Gorecki W. Staged thoracoscopic repair of long-gap esophageal atresia without temporary gastrostomy. J Laparoendosc Adv Surg Tech A. 2018.
26. Zani A, Cobellis G, Wolinska J, Chiu PP, Pierro A. Preservation of native esophagus in infants with pure esophageal atresia has good long-term outcomes despite significant postoperative morbidity. Pediatr Surg Int. 2016;32(2):113–7.
27. Greenstein J, Elios M, Tiernan K, Hageman JR, Zaritzky M. Magnetic anastomosis as a minimally

invasive treatment for esophageal atresia. NeoReviews. 2018;19(9):533–8.
28. Cope C, Ginsberg GG. Long-term patency of experimental magnetic compression gastroenteric anastomoses achieved with covered stents. Gastrointest Endosc. 2001;53(7):780–4.
29. Takao S, Matsuo Y, Shinchi H, Nakajima S, Aikou T, Iseji T, et al. Magnetic compression anastomosis for benign obstruction of the common bile duct. Endoscopy. 2001;33(11):988–90.
30. Zaritzky M, Ben R, Zylberg GI, Yampolsky B. Magnetic compression anastomosis as a nonsurgical treatment for esophageal atresia. Pediatr Radiol. 2009;39(9):945–9.
31. Zaritzky M, Ben R, Johnston K. Magnetic gastrointestinal anastomosis in pediatric patients. J Pediatr Surg. 2014;49(7):1131–7.
32. Lovvorn HN, Baron CM, Danko ME, Novotny NM, Bucher BT, Johnston KK, Aritzky MF. Staged Repair of Esophageal Atresia: Pouch Approximation and Catheter-based Magnetic Anastomosis. Journal of Pediatric Surgery Case Reports. 2014;2:170–5.
33. Woo R, Wong CM, Trimble Z, Puapong D, Koehler S, Miller S, et al. Magnetic compression stricturoplasty for treatment of refractory esophageal strictures in children: technique and lessons learned. Surg Innov. 2017;24(5):432–9.
34. Takamizawa S, Yamanouchi E, Muraji T, Nishijima E, Satoh S, Tsugawa J. MCRA of an anastomotic stenosis after esophagoesophagostomy for long gap esophageal atresia: a case report. J Pediatr Surg. 2007;42(5):769–72.
35. Dorman RM, Vali K, Harmon CM, Zaritzky M, Bass KD. Repair of esophageal atresia with proximal fistula using endoscopic magnetic compression anastomosis (magnamosis) after staged lengthening. Pediatr Surg Int. 2016;32(5):525–8.
36. Levitt M, Pena A. Anorectal malformations. In: Coran AG, editor. Pediatric surgery. 7th ed. Philadelphia, PA: Elsevier; 2012.
37. Hamrick M, Eradi B, Bischoff A, Louden E, Pena A, Levitt M. Rectal atresia and stenosis: unique anorectal malformations. J Pediatr Surg. 2012;47(6):1280–4.
38. Luo CC, Ming YC, Chu SM, Chao HC. Individualized management of upper rectal atresia. J Pediatr Surg. 2009;44(12):2406–9.
39. Upadhyaya P. Rectal atresia: transanal, end-to-end, rectorectal anastomosis: a simplified, rational approach to management. J Pediatr Surg. 1990;25(5):535–7.
40. Russell KW, Rollins MD, Feola GP, Scaife ER. Magnamosis: a novel technique for the management of rectal atresia. BMJ Case Rep 2014;2014.
41. Cheung KM, Cheung JP, Samartzis D, Mak KC, Wong YW, Cheung WY, et al. Magnetically controlled growing rods for severe spinal curvature in young children: a prospective case series. Lancet. 2012;379(9830):1967–74.

Use of Magnets in Flexible Endoscopy

10

C. Roberto Simons-Linares and John J. Vargo

Abbreviations

3D	three dimensional
AUC	area under the curve
BBS	benign biliary strictures
CE	capsule endoscopy
C-ESD	conventional ESD
Ct	contractions
EGD	esophagogastroduodenoscopy
EGJ	esophagogastric junction
EMR	endoscopic mucosal resection
ERCP	endoscopic retrograde cholangiopancreatography
ESD	endoscopic mucosal dissection
EUS	endoscopic ultrasound
FB	foreign body
FCSEMS	fully covered self-expandable metal stent
FNA	fine-needle aspiration
GERD	gastroesophageal reflux disease
GES	gastric emptying study
GI	gastrointestinal
GOO	gastric outlet obstruction
IAS	incisionless anastomosis system
IR	interventional radiology
LAMS	lumen-apposing metal stent
MACE	magnetically assisted capsule endoscopy
MACL	magnetically aided colonoscopic localization system
MAD	magnet-assisted diverticuloplasty
MAFBORE	magnetic-aided foreign body removal
MAG	magnetic compression anastomosis
MAGBIS	magnets for gastrointestinal and biliary strictures
MAG-ESD	magnetic-assisted endoscopic submucosal dissection
MAGLES	magnetic augmentation of the lower esophageal sphincter
MAG-MEUS	magnetic-aid microendoscopic ultrasound
MATCAP	magnetically assisted therapeutic capsule
MCA	magnetic compression anastomosis
MEI	magnetic endoscope imaging
MGEC	magnets for gastroenterostomy creation
MI	motility index
NPO	nil per os
PSC	primary sclerosing cholangitis
PTHC	percutaneous transhepatic cholangiogram
RCT	randomized clinical trials

C. R. Simons-Linares
Gastroenterology, Hepatology and Nutrition Department, Cleveland Clinic, Cleveland, OH, USA

J. J. Vargo (✉)
Enterprise Endoscopy Operations, Endoscopic Research and Innovation, Section of Therapeutic, Gastroenterology, Hepatology and Nutrition, Cleveland Clinic, Cleveland, OH, USA
e-mail: vargoj@ccf.org

M. Gagner (ed.), *Magnetic Surgery*, https://doi.org/10.1007/978-3-030-73947-8_10

SAMSEM	smart self-assembling magnet for endoscopy
SCs	standard colonoscopies
SEMS	self-expandable metal stent
W-ESD	waterjet-assisted ESD

Introduction

The use of magnets in endoscopy is of great interest, as they allow the endoscopist to remotely control endoscopic tools or devices by exerting magnetic force over the distance. Importantly, there are multiple gastrointestinal tract lesions that are challenging to reach endoscopically, and magnets could overcome this issue. Magnets can improve the care of multiple diseases that involve endoscopic procedures, giving an amazing opportunity for research, patient care improvement, and to advance the field of endoscopy. In recent years, there have been multiple emerging applications for magnets in gastrointestinal endoscopy and although, in most cases, randomized clinical trials (RCT) are lacking; the current evidence come from multiple prospective observational studies that have demonstrated the safety and efficacy of endoscopic magnetic devices. In this chapter, we review the evidence-based use of magnets in flexible endoscopy of the gastrointestinal (GI) tract.

Magnetic-Aided Foreign Body Removal (MAFBORE)

MAFBORE is probably the most pioneering implementation of magnets in endoscopy that started in the 1990s. In 1997, Seo et al. reported a pediatric series of foreign body (FB) removal (disk batteries and coins) safely with a powerful magnet attached to the tip of the scope [1]. Most recently, Coash et al. reported the endoscopic removal of a long sharp metallic FB by a magnet snare [2]. Multiple case reports and series have reported the use of magnets in forceps, snares, or attached magnets to the tip of the endoscope and have reported to be safe and of great utility to remove the metallic FB [3–7]. They are particularly helpful for the removal of circular flat metallic FBs (coins and round batteries) because circular flat metallic FB is very difficult to grasp, snare, or remove with nonmagnetic endoscopic tools. In conclusion, having magnetized endoscopic tools such as snares and forceps are very useful and should be part of a foreign body removal toolbox.

Table 10.1 MAFBORE remarks

Advantages	Disadvantages
Could reduce endoscopy time and sedation	Additional cost
In some cases, no need for endoscopy and sedation[a]	Cannot be used in patients with cardiac devices
Avoid surgery for challenging circular, metallic, and flat foreign body removal	

For pancreatobiliary stents

Another similar use of magnets is magnetic pancreatobiliary stent removal. This technique is an interesting use of this technology as currently standard removal of pancreatobiliary stents is with esophagogastroduodenoscopy (EGD) that requires sedation and patient's nil per os (NPO) status. Magnetic removal of pancreatobiliary stents without requiring EGD or endoscopy was reported in an animal study of five porcine models [8]. The investigators successfully removed endoscopically placed ferromagnetic biliary stents by using an external powerful magnet. This is an attractive concept and could reduce endoscopy-related risks when removing the stents endoscopically, does not require sedation, and could be cost saving to our health system [9] (Table 10.1).

Magnetically Assisted Capsule Endoscopy (MACE) (Fig. 10.1)

Manipulation of capsule endoscopy (CE) was not possible before the implementation of magnet technology. The possibility of manipulating the CE is a big game changer for its utility as there is extensive evidence that CE works very well for diagnostic purposes, but its main limi-

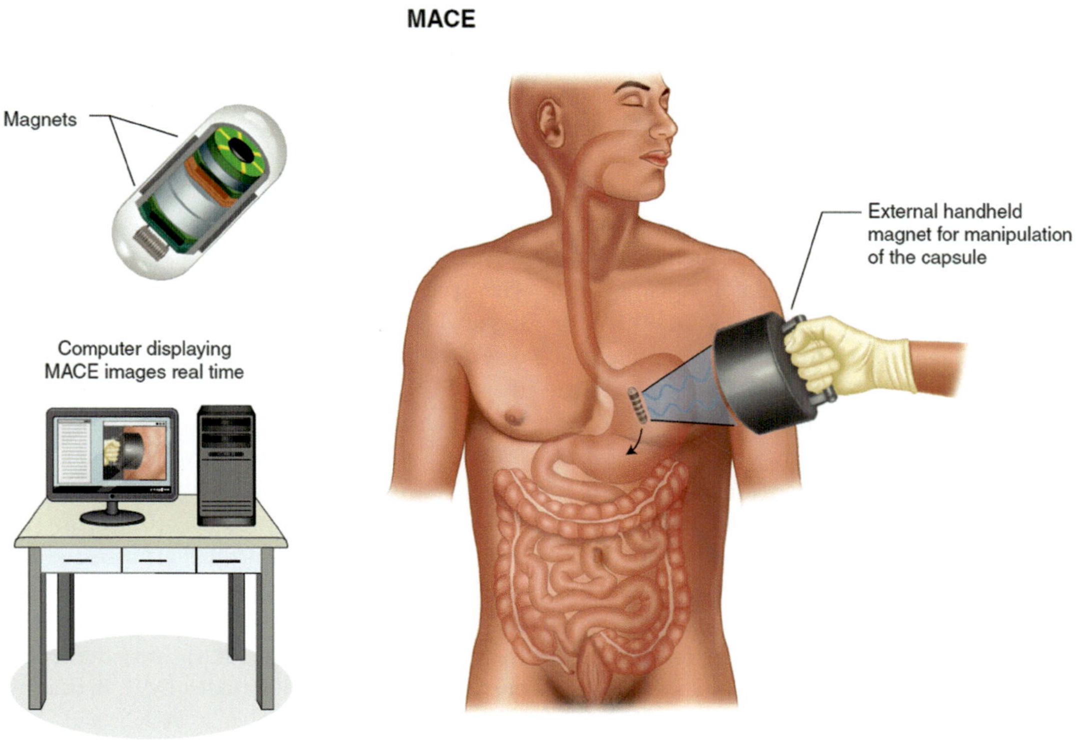

Fig. 10.1 Magnetically assisted capsule endoscopy (MACE). Manipulation of capsule endoscopy (CE) is now possible with capsules that contain magnets and with the help of an external magnetic handle for maneuverability of the internal capsule

tation is that it does offer therapeutic interventions. Since the creation of CE in 1999 by Swain, CE has been increasing in popularity due to its noninvasive approach, tolerability, and great diagnostic yield. In recent years, rare magnet technology has been incorporated to the regular capsule endoscopy and multiple studies have already proven its feasibility and safety of MACE maneuverability [10]. Besides the therapeutic potential with maneuverable MACE, there are other potential benefits such as better exploration of the luminal GI tract areas that are passed too quickly by a standard CE due to the normal GI motility. Moreover, this add-on benefit could potentially allow MACE to become the test of choice for accurate, maneuverable, and less-invasive GI tract exploration in multiple diseases for diagnostic as well as for screening purposes. There are four MACE device systems that have been developed, and some others are currently under development. Importantly, all these devices use similar technology: magnets built-in the capsule endoscope and this is externally controlled by a magnetic field guidance system [11–15]. One of the largest prospective, blinded comparative trials was performed by Denzer et al. The study included 189 individuals comparing MACE versus standard upper endoscopy; the study found 23 major lesions in 21 patients. The MACE accuracy was 90.5% (95%CI, 85.4–94.3%), specificity of 94.1% (95%CI, 89.3–97.1%), and sensitivity of 61.9% (95%CI, 38–82%). Interestingly, the study also showed that MACE is clearly preferred by patients over standard upper endoscopy [16]. A study with 10 healthy volunteers was performed to assess safety and feasibility of MACE. The study concluded that MACE is safe, feasible, and very well tolerated by patients [11]. Interestingly, another study of healthy volunteers showed that the assessment of the esophagus was suboptimal, raising concern that the magnetic force of that device to be weaker and overcome by the potent esophageal motility, hence, leading to the very rapid passage of the capsule through the esophagus and obscuring proper endoscopic assessment [12]. Recent studies have shown that the esophagogastric junction (EGJ) is appropriately visible for assessment in 92% of cases [17–19]. With regard to diagnostic yield, there was an interesting animal study by Hale et al. that showed that MACE was noninferior to upper endoscopy assessment [20]. The study was a randomized trial in porcine models and found that MACE had comparable diagnostic yield of presewn beads in the stomach. Flexible endoscopy identified 90/90 beads (88%) and MACE identified 80/90 (89%). The difference in sensitivities was 1.11 (95%, 0.06–28.26) and the study concluded that MACE was noninferior to standard upper endoscopy. Importantly, no study reported a MACE-related adverse event, although one study reported device malfunctioning and technical failure in one individual.

MACE for GI Motility

Gastroparesis is characterized by delayed gastric emptying without mechanical obstruction and is most common in diabetic patients. Gastric emptying study (GES) with radioactive material has been traditionally used to help diagnose gastroparesis. In the last decade, wireless capsule endoscopy with magnets has been adapted as a noninvasive, nonradioactive test to measure the stomach and GI tract pressure as well as the transit times [21–24]. A study in 2008 by Kuo et al. compared GES with MACE in 87 healthy subjects and 61 gastroparesis patients; the investigators found that the correlation between MACE and GES at 4 hours was 0.74 and at 2 hours was 0.63 [22]. This was the first study that showed MACE correlates with GES and importantly, it discriminates between healthy and gastroparesis subjects. In addition, a recent study was performed to validate the diagnostic and performance capacity of MACE for patients with suspected gastroparesis [25]. Investigators performed a multicenter prospective study of 167 patients with gastroparesis, from which 53 had diabetes and 114 non-daibetic controls. Interestingly, delayed gastric emptying was detected in a higher proportion of subjects by MACE (34.6%) than by GES (24.5%) ($p = 0.009$). The study concluded that MACE provides a higher diagnostic yield than GES and that MACE detects delayed gastric emptying more frequently than GES and identifies extragastric transit abnormalities.

MACE for GI tract motility assessment can also assess other parts of the GI tract, not only the stomach. A study of 188 subject (107 healthy, 23 gastroparesis, and 58 constipation) assessed the small bowel–fed response captured with MACE. The assessment was made by measuring frequency of contractions (Ct), area under the curve (AUC), and motility index (MI). In healthy subjects, all parameters (Ct, AUC, and MI) increased significantly ($p < 0.01$) after a meal ingestion. In subjects with gastroparesis, all motility parameters failed to increase significantly when compared to healthy subjects. Constipated subjects had similar motility (small bowel–fed response) when compared to healthy subjects [26]. Thanks to MACE, scientists are also able to test the small and large bowel motility, which makes MACE a very good initial test of choice. For example, a study found that domperidone prolongs oral to duodenal transit time as demonstrated by MACE. They tested 31 patients who received domperidone and 33 patients who did not. Median oroduodenal transit was 13 and 30 minutes in the untreated and domperidone groups, respectively ($p < 0.001$) [27].

In summary, MACE has great potential for many reasons: There are multiple uses that a maneuverable capsule can be applied to, for example, for substances or compounds transportation (powder, liquid, granules, beads, and fecal transplantation) to target medication delivery, chemotherapy/radiotherapy, and further interventions (Fig. 10.2). In addition, it can improve the visual endoscopic assessment and allow possible therapeutic interventions such as clipping

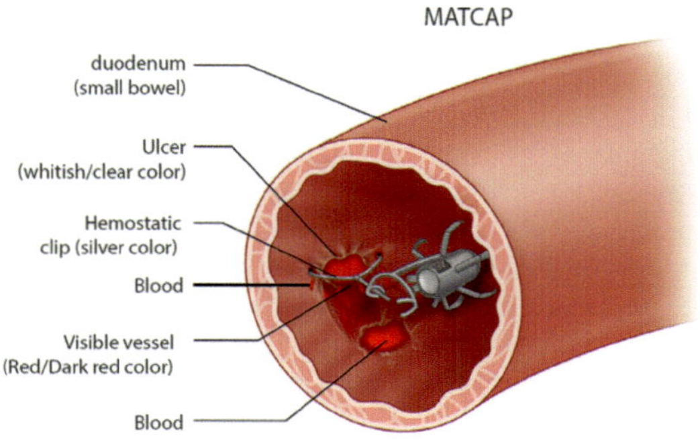

Fig. 10.2 Magnetically assisted therapeutic capsule (MATCAP). In the future, a capsule could be easily maneuverable for targeted delivery of compounds (nanoparticles, drugs/chemotherapy, tools, clips, and hemostatic spray), interventions, and allows fast proper triage and screening of luminal lesions. This robotic capsule could be equipped with medications and tools such as hemostatic clips to treat a gastrointestinal bleed from an ulcer or arteriovenous malformations in the small bowel or anywhere in the luminal gastrointestinal tract

of bleeding lesions or even taking tissue for a biopsy or needle aspiration. Another interesting concept is the delivery of nanotechnology that could enable greater matter/tools manipulation and perhaps to perform diagnostic procedures within the luminal tract such as magnetic-aid microendoscopic ultrasound (MAG-MEUS), biopsies, or aspiration of tissue or other therapeutic procedures in challenging areas of the luminal GI tract, new working space or compartments (subadventitial space), and pancreatobiliary ducts (Table 10.2).

Table 10.2 MACE remarks

Advantages	Disadvantages
Wireless virtual examination with multiple passes	Limited visulaization due to rapid passage in the esophagus
Maneuverable device	Therapeutics still needs to be developed (tissue sampling and accurate clipping)
No sedation	Time consuming/needs learning curve to maneuver
Triage for acute GI bleed	Lack of RCTs
Screening for luminal cancers or precancerous conditions (Barrett's esophagus)	
Potential targeted delivery of compounds	
Noninvasive nonradioactive (compared to gastric emptying study)	
New use for GI motility assessment	
Growing evidence/studies	

Magnetic-Assisted Endoscopic Submucosal Dissection (MAG-ESD) (Fig. 10.3)

MAG-ESD was first described by Kobayashi et al. when the investigators proposed that a magnetic microforceps could potentially generate sufficient traction force of the desired mucosal surface during endoscopic mucosal resection (EMR). For this experimentation, the investigators develop a magnetic anchoring system that

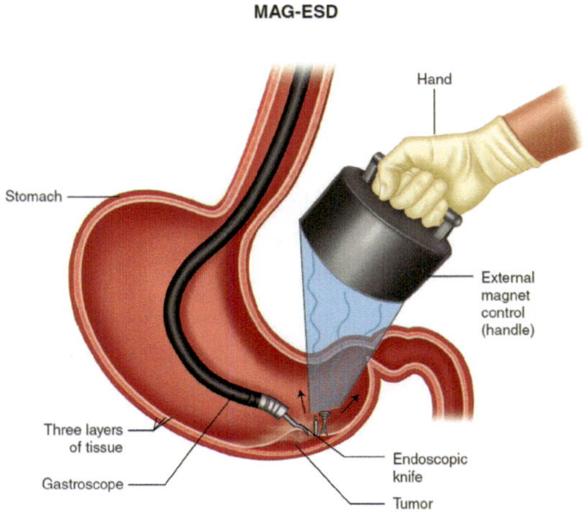

Fig. 10.3 Magnetic-assisted endoscopic submucosal dissection (MAG-ESD). MAG-ESD refers to the technique of endoscopic resection of a lesion (i.e., tumor) in the gastrointestinal tract with the assistance of a magnetic microforceps or anchoring device that generate sufficient traction force of the desired mucosal surface during endoscopic resection/dissection of the tumor. The magnetic anchoring device that is attached to the lesion of interest is manipulated through an external magnetic handle

was composed of three parts: a handmade magnetic weight composed of magnetic stainless steel, a microforceps, and a connecting thread. Subsequently, the investigators demonstrated the successful use of their device in a porcine model [28].

Endoscopic mucosal dissection (ESD) allows en bloc resection and accurate histologic diagnosis. One of its big challenges is that it is time-consuming and lifting devices or tools to facilitate more rapid dissection and resection are lacking. New magnetic devices to facilitate traction during ESD can enhance safety and efficiency of the procedure [29, 30]. Internal and external magnetic traction devices for ESD (MAG-ESD) have been recently developed. Recently, a group of investigators developed an internal magnet traction device for ESD that was tested in a porcine model. The investigators studied the new device versus conventional ESD (C-ESD) and found that MAG-ESD was significantly shorter than C-ESD (median 6.4 minutes vs. 14.4 minutes; $p < 0.05$), and the number of muscularis propria per lesion was significantly lower in the MAG-ESD than C-ESD (median: 0 vs. 1; $p < 0.05$). Investigators concluded that MAG-ESD is effective and safe when compare to conventional techniques [31]. Another animal study in Japan showed the feasibility of combining both external and internal neodymium magnets for anchoring during ESD. The external magnet device was a handheld magnet and it could move or lock by a flexible arm, which is a great advantage because it does not require an extra assistant or person to handle/hold the external magnet. The internal magnetic anchoring system consisted of a magnet that was attached to a hemoclip by using a 3-0 silk. The study found that this magnetic anchoring technique was safe, feasible, and efficient in all 10 resected lesions. Remarkably, the actual preparation and setting up of the magnetic anchoring system have a median time of only 4 minutes (range 2–7 minutes) [32].

A study by Rodriguez-Sanchez et al. compared MAG-ESD to waterjet-assisted ESD (W-ESD) and conventional ESD (C-ESD) in an animal prospective nonrandomized trial. Forty-six ESD procedures were performed (MAG-ESD = 10, W-ESD = 12, and C-ESD = 24) [31]. There was no difference between the three techniques in terms of safety and efficacy of the resection. But the investigators found that MAG-ESD was faster when compared to the other techniques (minutes per cm^2 = 10.85 vs. 7.43 vs. 3.41; $p = 0.001$). They concluded that MAG-ESD is more efficient than the other two alternative techniques [31] (Table 10.3).

Table 10.3 MAG-ESD remarks

Advantages	Disadvantages
Decreases procedure duration[a]	Additional training required
Shorter procedure = shorter anesthesia time	May require additional assistance or training of endoscopy personnel
Expand reachable locations for resection	Device adds extra cost
Optimize performance of endosciopically directed mucosal resection in patients in whom singificant co-morbidities would increas the risk of morbidity via operative route	Magnetic force decay over distance
Theoretically flatten ESD learning curve	

[a]The duration of MAG-ESD decreases not only in experienced endoscopists but also in junior endoscopists

Magnets for Gastroenterostomy Creation (MGEC) (Fig. 10.4)

Yamanouchi et al. developed a magnetic compression anastomosis (MCA) technique by using two magnets as the mean to create a nonsurgical sutureless enteric fistula or anastomosis [33]. Clinical application of this technique could be of great benefit for gastrointestinal obstruction, which can happen anywhere in the GI tract and is common at the pyloric channel and proximal duodenum; most commonly known as gastric outlet obstruction (GOO). The etiology of GOO can be benign or malignant, and the structural impedance can be extrinsic or intrinsic to the GI luminal tract. Depending on the etiology, GOO primary therapy involves endoscopic dilation or

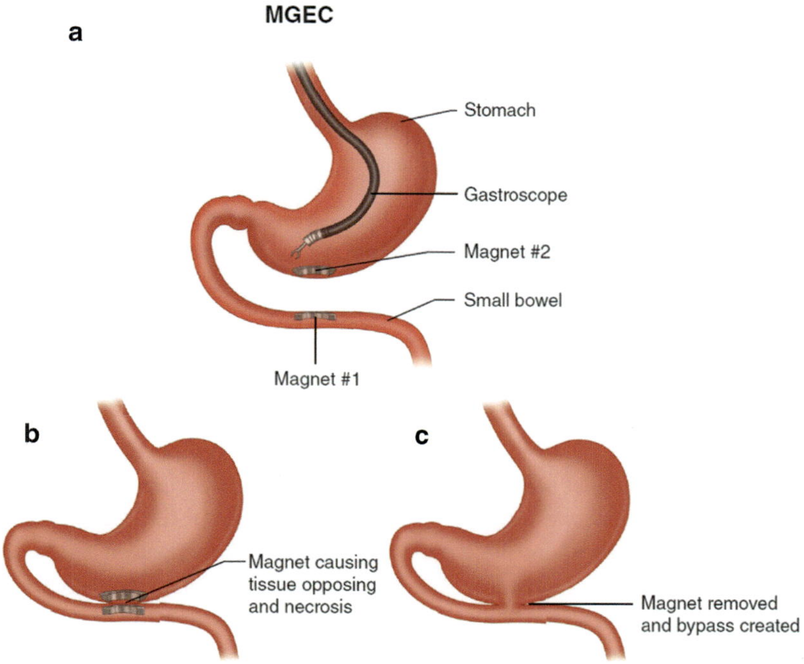

Fig. 10.4 (a–c) Magnets for gastroenterostomy creation (MGEC). MGEC refers to the endoscopic technique that utilizes two potent magnets as the mean to create a nonsurgical sutureless enteric fistula or anastomosis (or new tract between the two luminal surfaces)

endoscopic placement of a self-expandable metal stent (SEMS), or lumen-apposing metal stent (LAMS) [34]. Surgical enteroenteric bypass is an alternative approach but is more invasive and morbid. In recent years, endoscopic ultrasound (EUS)-guided gastroenterostomy creation, commonly from the stomach to the jejunum, has been successfully performed with the use of LAMS placement as a bridge for the bypass and future epithelialization and maturation of the new tract [35, 36].

EUS-guided or surgical gastroenterostomy creation requires anesthesia and is also associated with higher risks and complications for patients with multiple comorbidities who are unfit for these procedures. EUS-guided LAMS placement is less invasive than surgery, but can have complications (LAMS migration, bleeding, and anesthesia intolerance) [35]. In recent years there has been growing literature of a new minimal invasive technique using magnets to create gastroenteric anastomosis or bypass.

Gastroenteric or enteroenteric anastomosis by magnetic compression has been described since early 2000 by Cope et al. An animal study evaluated the efficacy of a prototype for magnetic compression of gastroenteric fistulas [37]. The magnets were introduced perorally with endoscopic and fluoroscopy guidance. The two magnets were approached across the gastric and jejunal walls of five dogs successfully and they had formation of fistula at a mean of 5.5 days (12 mm diameter). The investigators monitored the fistulas at 1 and 2 months endoscopically, and found no morbidity associated with this procedure. Authors concluded that this prototype and technique are safe, efficient, and could be used in the palliation of malignant GOO [37]. In 2011, Thompson et al. described a smart self-assembling magnet for endoscopy (SAMSEM) device for transoral endoscopic creation of gastrojejunostomy in pig models [38]. The technique uses compression anastomosis technology through the delivery of the endoscopic SAMSEM device but requires fluoroscopy aid for the completion of the gastrojejunostomy. In this study, an endoscope was advanced into the peritoneal cavity through the gastrotomy and a segment of small bowel was grasped and put close to the stomach. Then, an enterotomy was created endoscopically and an overtube was advanced into the small bowel where the fist magnet is deployed.

Table 10.4 M-GEC remarks

Advantages	Disadvantages
Once natural fistula is formed, magnets are removed without any need for permanent stent or prosthesis utilization	Learning curve of new technology can be harder to implement (compared to EUS knowledge +30 years)
Potential access of more challenging GI tract (jejunoileal bypass) areas than other approaches	Endoscopic approach not yet tested in humans (only animals)
Could be best to approach mobile organs such as the gallbladder (where LAMS placement can fail)	

Next, a second magnet is deployed into the stomach and finally the two magnets (stomach and jejunum) are mated under fluoroscopy guidance [38–41]. In another study, the same group of investigators has also described the use of this technology and technique for the creation of a jejunoileal bypass and other intestinal bypasses by using an incisionless anastomosis system (IAS) in animal models [42] (Table 10.4).

Magnets for Gastrointestinal and Biliary Strictures (MAGBIS)

Magnetic Compression Anastomosis (MAG) for Benign Biliary Strictures (BBS)

Magnetic compression anastamosis of tight biliary strictures has been used in anastomotic BBS, which is a complication of liver donor transplant. It usually involves placement of two magnets: in one end through endoscopic retrograde cholangiopancreatography (ERCP) and the other end through a percutaneous transhepatic cholangiogram (PTHC), with the goal of achieving approximation of the two stenotic ends in order to allow recanalization of the bile duct [43–46]. A study of 12 patients [44] reported that successful magnet approximation duct to duct was achieved in 10 of 12 patients (90%). The results were excellent, with 10 of the 10 patients (100%) having recanalization of the stricture. The mean time for magnet removal was 74.2 days (range 14–181 days). One of the 10 patients had recurrence of the biliary stricture and one case was complicated with mild cholangitis at 331 days follow-up of the study [44]. The same group of investigators recently reported similar outcomes in another study of 39 patients [47], where MAG was successfully achieved in 35 of 39 patients (90%). Interestingly, the rate of BBS recurrence was lower than conventional methods and this could be likely because MAG allows the creation of a new fistulous tract rather than the dilation of a previously stenotic tract [47].

Another study of seven patients that used MAG for recanalization of BBS showed that recanalization was successful in five of the seven patients. Two patients failed this approach, which was due to very long strictures or stenotic segments which could not be initially approximated [46]. Similar results were obtained in a Turkish study, where 100% of patients (six) achieved recanalization of the BBS [48].

Overall, the outcomes of MAG for BBS are very promising, as recanalization occurs in 100% of patients who had successful magnet biliobiliary approximation (90%). MAG for benign anastomotic biliary strictures is an attractive alternative to surgical intervention and should be at least considered as a backup approach to conventional methods (ERCP and IR intervention). This technique is yet to be tested in primary sclerosing cholangitis (PSC) or malignant biliary stenosis.

Magnetic Enhance Gastrointestinal Luminal Patency

Similar to biliary anastomosis for severe refractory esophageal strictures, magnets have been successfully used. The technique involves the positioning of two magnets endoscopically and with fluoroscopy aid with the goal of approximation of both stenotic ends. This approach has been only used when other standard-of-care

Table 10.5 MAGBIS remarks

Advantages	Disadvantages
Alternative therapy (rescue strategy)	Bidirectional access required (percutaneous/surgical and endoscopic/luminal)
Allows formation of a new fistula or fistulization of tissue, instead of mucosa disruption and scaring (endoscopic dilation)	Lack of RCTs
Magnets can be removed after satisfactory opening of the stricture	Similar outcomes to FCSEMS stents (for biliary strictures)
	Similar outcomes to endoscopic fluoroscopy guidewire technique or EUS-guided FNA (esophageal or luminal anastomotic strictures)

FCSEMS fully covered self-expandable metal stent

interventions (endoscopic dilation and stent placement) have failed. In a case series of two pediatric patients with esophageal atresia where both patients were suffering from refractory recurrent esophageal strictures, the investigators reported successful magnetic compression of the stricture and stricturoplasty. Recanalization was achieved in both cases (100%) and no leaks or early complications were reported. At 31 months of follow-up after magnetic stricturoplasty, both patients had durable esophageal patency without symptoms [49] (Table 10.5).

Magnetically Aided Colonoscopic Localization System (MACL)

This is a revolutionary approach to improve colonoscopy training and performance. Thanks to the magnetic rings in the scope implemented by this technology, it allows real-time three-dimensional (3D) representation of the shape, position, progression, and loop of the endoscope in a bedside monitor (ScopeGuide system, Olympus, Center Valley, PA) [50, 51]. It was originally used as a magnetic probe through the scope, but the newer models have magnetic rings built-in the Olympus scopes. It also offers multiple benefits such as assisting the endoscopist to reduce looping of the scope throughout the colon, it can visually reflect the external pressure application (at the loop site), no doubt this offers a great training advantage for trainees, and is available for pediatric colonoscopies, adult colonoscopies, and push colonoscopies. Unfortunately, the technology is not available for retrograde balloon enteroscopy or balloon colonoscope, which would be of tremendous help to reach deeper distances in the small bowel. There are multiple randomized controlled trials (RCTs) that have evaluated magnetic endoscope imaging (MEI) over standard colonoscopies (SCs) [51–55]. Also, two meta-analyses have been performed in this topic. The first meta-analysis by Chen et al. assessed the theoretical advantages of MEI over SCs and compared their efficacies. Eight RCTs comprising 2967 patients were included. The main outcome was cecal intubation rate and time. The MEI group had almost twice higher change in cecal intubation (OR: 1.92; 95% CI: 1.13–3.27) when compared with SC, but there was no significant difference for cecal intubation time [56]. The second meta-analysis by Mark-Christensen et al. evaluated the performance of MEI in colonoscopy. This study included a total of 13 randomized studies, accounting for 4470 patients. The MEI group was associated with significantly lower risk of failed cecal intubation as reflected by the risk difference 4% (95%CI: 0–7%) as well as lower cecal intubation time with a mean difference of half a minute (0.58 minutes) (95%CI 0.28–0.88) [57].

In summary, MACL is a better alternative to its counterpart, colonoscopy simulator station. MACL offers a unique advantage of improving patient care in real time while performing the colonoscopy and has been well studied by multiple RCTs and two meta-analyses. It is associated with higher chances for cecal intubation which is

Table 10.6 MACL remarks

Advantages	Disadvantages
Higher rates of cecal intubation[a]	Not available for balloon enteroscopy
Shorter time to reach cecum[a]	No retrofit
Multiple RCTs and two meta-analysis	Extra investment/cost to acquire equipment
Potential to improve procedure-related patient comfort	Studies did not show benefit for experienced endoscopist.
Noninvasive and no radiation or fluoroscopy	

[a]The rates of cecal intubation improve among inexperienced endoscopists or trainees

a quality marker for colonoscopy as well as shorter time to cecal intubation during elective colonoscopy. Finally, MACL is of great benefit for training and educating future or early career endoscopists (Table 10.6).

Other Recent Utilizations of Magnets in Endoscopy

Magnet-Assisted Diverticuloplasty (MAD) for the Closure of a Zenker's Diverticulum

A 48-year-old man with a progressive, worsening dysphagia from a large Zenker's diverticulum underwent endoscopic diverticulotomy, but after 5 months the diverticulum had not disappeared. The authors performed a magnet-assisted diverticuloplasty (MAD), which involves the placement of a first ring-shaped magnet in the esophagus, 2 cm proximally from the base of the diverticulum using a clip. The second magnet was placed at the base of the diverticulum to allow the diverticulum wall and esophageal wall to approach each other and complete compression of the septum. At 1-month follow-up, significant improvement of the diverticulum was confirmed by upper endoscopy and barium swallow [58]. MAD is a new and alternative approach if other endoscopic techniques are not successfully treating a Zenker's diverticulum or when surgical intervention is not desired by the patient.

Magnetic Augmentation of the Lower Esophageal Sphincter (MAGLES)

A recent animal study was performed to assess this innovative concept for gastroesophageal reflux disease (GERD) [59]. In this approach, a long submucosal tunnel is made in the mid-to-lower esophagus and the muscularis propria is incised within the submucosal tunnel. A subadventitial tunnel is made by biliary balloon catheter blunt dissection and a magnet is deployed in the subadventitial space. The second magnet is placed within the opposing esophageal wall. The investigators found that submucosal tunnels were successfully formed without perforation in all cases (100%) and subadventitial tunnels in 9 of 10 cases (90%). The study concluded that subadventitial tunnels are feasible endoscopically and represent a new working space for endoscopic therapy. Magnetic lower esophageal sphincter augmentation is an interesting concept to treat GERD and, importantly, it could be performed endoscopically through endoscopic placement of magnets within the subadventitial space. However, the effectiveness of this new endoscopic intervention for GERD is still to be compared to other surgical approaches [60–62].

Conclusions and Take-Home Points

- The application of magnets in endoscopy is in its infancy and has a bright future.
- There are many applications for magnets in the GI tract and most have already demonstrated safety and efficacy.
- Development of MACE, where the capsule could be easily maneuverable for targeted delivery of compounds (nanoparticles, drugs/chemotherapy, tools, clips, and hemostatic spray) and allow fast proper triage and screening, would be of excellent use.
- MGEC that allows compression anastomosis or nonsurgical bypass creation has great potential benefit that needs to be explored in humans.
- Other magnetically controlled endoscopic tools such as traction devices for ESD, or large

Table 10.7 Magnets in endoscopy remarks

Advantages	Disadvantages
Less likely to migrate compared to other devices/tools/stents (theoretically)	Magnetic force decay over distance
Potential use without narcotics or anesthesia	Depends on patient's abdominal wall thickness (fat pad)
Facilitates access to challenging GI tract areas (small bowel)	Interaction between magnets and other metal instruments
Maneuverable for targeted delivery of compounds	Interaction between magnets and patient's ferromagnetic foreign bodies (pacemakers and orthopedic prosthesis)
No radiation or fluoroscopy involved	Larger and more powerful magnets are costly

resections, need to be improved (efficacy, safety, and cost) to be widely implemented.

- Magnets in endoscopy is an exciting field with promising preliminary evidence and it offers large opportunities for device development and research (Table 10.7).

References

1. Seo JK. Therapeutic endoscopy: removal of gastrointestinal foreign bodies in children. Zhonghua Min Guo Xiao Er Ke Yi Xue Hui Za Zhi. 1997;38(3):183–6.
2. Coash M, Wu GY. Endoscopic removal of a long sharp metallic foreign body by a snared magnet: an attractive solution. J Dig Dis. 2012;13(4):239–41.
3. Aslinia FM, Flasar MH. Endoscopic ferromagnetic object retrieval by use of a simple magnet (with video). Gastrointest Endosc. 2012;76(3):667–8.
4. Laff HI. Use of the alnico magnet in bronchoscopy and esophagoscopy. Laryngoscope. 1949;59(2):186–93.
5. Latraverse V. Use of an endoscopic electromagnet for the extraction of foreign bodies from the stomach. Union Med Can. 1951;80(3):377–9.
6. Ofosu A, Ramai D, Reddy M. Overtube-assisted foreign body removal: a review of endoscopic management and case illustration. Cureus. 2017;9(9):e1730.
7. Seo TJ, et al. Endoscopic removal of impacted magnetic foreign bodies in the gastroesophageal junction. Surg Laparosc Endosc Percutan Tech. 2011;21(6):e313–5.
8. Ryou M, et al. Magnetic pancreaticobiliary stents and retrieval system: obviating the need for repeat endoscopy (with video). Gastrointest Endosc. 2012;75(4):888–892.e1.
9. Cantillon-Murphy P, et al. A magnetic retrieval system for stents in the pancreaticobiliary tree. IEEE Trans Biomed Eng. 2010;57(8):2018–25.
10. Swain CP, Gong F., Mills TN. Wireless transmission of a colour television moving image from the stomach using a miniature CCD camera, light source and microwave transmitter. Gut 1997;45:AB40.
11. Keller J, et al. Inspection of the human stomach using remote-controlled capsule endoscopy: a feasibility study in healthy volunteers (with videos). Gastrointest Endosc. 2011;73(1):22–8.
12. Keller J, et al. Remote magnetic control of a wireless capsule endoscope in the esophagus is safe and feasible: results of a randomized, clinical trial in healthy volunteers. Gastrointest Endosc. 2010;72(5):941–6.
13. Keller JFC, Volke F, et al. Remote magnetic control of a wireless capsule endoscope in the esophagus is safe and feasible: results of a randomized, clinical trial in healthy volunteers. Gastrointest Endosc. 2010;72:941–6.
14. Shamsudhin N, et al. Magnetically guided capsule endoscopy. Med Phys. 2017;44(8):e91–e111.
15. Liao Z, Duan XD, Xin L, et al. Feasibility and safety of magnetic-controlled capsule endoscopy system in examination of human stomach: a pilot study in healthy volunteers. J Interv Gastroenterol. 2012;2(4):155–60.
16. Denzer UW, et al. Magnetically guided capsule versus conventional gastroscopy for upper abdominal complaints: a prospective blinded study. J Clin Gastroenterol. 2015;49(2):101–7.
17. Kim HM, Choi JS, Cho JH. A pilot trial of ambulatory monitoring of gastric motility using a modified magnetic capsule endoscope. J Neurogastroenterol Motil. 2014;20(2):261–4.
18. Liao Z, et al. Accuracy of magnetically controlled capsule endoscopy, compared with conventional gastroscopy, in detection of gastric diseases. Clin Gastroenterol Hepatol. 2016;14(9):1266–1273.e1.
19. Ohta H, Katsuki S. Subject-friendly entire gastrointestinal screening with a single capsule endoscope by magnetic navigation and the internet. Conf Proc IEEE Eng Med Biol Soc. 2014;2014:6997–7000.
20. Hale MF, et al. Magnetically steerable gastric capsule endoscopy is equivalent to flexible endoscopy in the detection of markers in an excised porcine stomach model: results of a randomized trial. Endoscopy. 2015;47(7):650–3.
21. Diaz Tartera HO, et al. Validation of SmartPill((R)) wireless motility capsule for gastrointestinal transit time: intra-subject variability, software accuracy and comparison with video capsule endoscopy. Neurogastroenterol Motil. 2017;29(10):1–9.
22. Kuo B, et al. Comparison of gastric emptying of a nondigestible capsule to a radio-labelled meal in healthy

and gastroparetic subjects. Aliment Pharmacol Ther. 2008;27(2):186–96.
23. Rauch S, et al. Gastric pH and motility in a porcine model of acute lung injury using a wireless motility capsule. Med Sci Monit. 2011;17(7):Br161–4.
24. Rouphael C, et al. Role of wireless motility capsule in the assessment and management of gastrointestinal dysmotility in patients with diabetes mellitus. Neurogastroenterol Motil. 2017;29(9):e13087.
25. Lee AA, et al. Validation of diagnostic and performance characteristics of the wireless motility capsule in patients with suspected gastroparesis. Clin Gastroenterol Hepatol 2019;17:1770–9.
26. Surjanhata B, et al. Small bowel fed response as measured by wireless motility capsule: comparative analysis in healthy, gastroparetic, and constipated subjects. Neurogastroenterol Motil. 2018;30(5):e13268.
27. McFarlane M, Liu B, Nwokolo C. Domperidone prolongs oral to duodenal transit time in video capsule endoscopy. Eur J Clin Pharmacol. 2018;74(4):521–4.
28. Kobayashi T, et al. Magnetic anchor for more effective endoscopic mucosal resection. Jpn J Clin Oncol. 2004;34(3):118–23.
29. Matsuzaki I, et al. Simplified magnetic anchor-guided endoscopic submucosal dissection in dogs (with videos). Gastrointest Endosc. 2014;80(4):712–6.
30. Mortagy M, et al. Magnetic anchor guidance for endoscopic submucosal dissection and other endoscopic procedures. World J Gastroenterol. 2017;23(16):2883–90.
31. Rodriguez Sanchez J, et al. Electromagnetic assisted endoscopic submucosal dissection is more efficient than water-jet assisted and conventional ESD in experimental model. Endosc Int Open. 2018;6(4):E498–e504.
32. Dobashi A, et al. Efficacy and safety of an internal magnet traction device for endoscopic submucosal dissection: ex vivo study in a porcine model (with video). Surg Endosc. 2019;33(2):663–8.
33. Muraoka N, et al. Yamanouchi magnetic compression anastomosis for bilioenteric anastomotic stricture after living-donor liver transplantation. J Vasc Interv Radiol. 2005;16(9):1263–7.
34. Hamada T, et al. Covered versus uncovered metal stents for malignant gastric outlet obstruction: systematic review and meta-analysis. Dig Endosc. 2017;29(3):259–71.
35. Irani S, et al. Endoscopic gastroenterostomy: techniques and review. Curr Opin Gastroenterol. 2017;33(5):320–9.
36. Kato H, Tsutsumi K, Okada H. Recent advancements in stent therapy in patients with malignant gastroduodenal outlet obstruction. Ann Transl Med. 2017;5(8):186.
37. Cope C, Ginsberg GG. Long-term patency of experimental magnetic compression gastroenteric anastomoses achieved with covered stents. Gastrointest Endosc. 2001;53(7):780–4.
38. Ryou M, et al. Smart Self-Assembling MagnetS for ENdoscopy (SAMSEN) for transoral endoscopic creation of immediate gastrojejunostomy (with video). Gastrointest Endosc. 2011;73(2):353–9.
39. Fong DG, et al. Transcolonic ventral wall hernia mesh fixation in a porcine model. Endoscopy. 2007;39(10):865–9.
40. Ryou M, Agoston AT, Thompson CC. Endoscopic intestinal bypass creation by using self-assembling magnets in a porcine model. Gastrointest Endosc. 2016;83(4):821–5.
41. Ryou M, Aihara H, Thompson CC. Minimally invasive entero-enteral dual-path bypass using self-assembling magnets. Surg Endosc. 2016;30(10):4533–8.
42. Machytka E, et al. Partial jejunal diversion using an incisionless magnetic anastomosis system: 1-year interim results in patients with obesity and diabetes. Gastrointest Endosc. 2017;86(5):904–12.
43. Du X, et al. Application value of magnetic compression anastomosis in digestive tract reconstruction. Zhonghua Wei Chang Wai Ke Za Zhi. 2014;17(5):512–5.
44. Jang SI, et al. Magnetic compression anastomosis is useful in biliary anastomotic strictures after living donor liver transplantation. Gastrointest Endosc. 2011;74(5):1040–8.
45. Okajima H, et al. Magnet compression anastomosis for bile duct stenosis after duct-to-duct biliary reconstruction in living donor liver transplantation. Liver Transpl. 2005;11(4):473–5.
46. Jang SI, et al. Recanalization of refractory benign biliary stricture using magnetic compression anastomosis. Endoscopy. 2014;46(1):70–4.
47. Jang SI, et al. Treatment of completely obstructed benign biliary strictures with magnetic compression anastomosis: follow-up results after recanalization. Gastrointest Endosc. 2017;85(5):1057–66.
48. Ersoz G, et al. Magnetic compression anastomosis for patients with a disconnected bile duct after living-donor related liver transplantation: a pilot study. Endoscopy. 2016;48(7):652–6.
49. Woo R, et al. Magnetic compression stricturoplasty for treatment of refractory esophageal strictures in children: technique and lessons learned. Surg Innov. 2017;24(5):432–9.
50. Leung JW, et al. Magnetic endoscope imaging (ScopeGuide) elucidates the mechanism of action of the pain-alleviating impact of water exchange colonoscopy – attenuation of loop formation. J Interv Gastroenterol. 2012;2(3):142–6.
51. Shah SG, et al. Effect of magnetic endoscope imaging on patient tolerance and sedation requirements during colonoscopy: a randomized controlled trial. Gastrointest Endosc. 2002;55(7):832–7.
52. Corbett GD, et al. Safety of the colonoscope magnetic imaging device (ScopeGuide) in patients with implantable cardiac devices. Endoscopy. 2014;46(2):135–8.
53. Ellul P, et al. Colonic tumour localization using an endoscope positioning device. Eur J Gastroenterol Hepatol. 2011;23(6):488–91.

54. Kaltenbach T, et al. Use of the colonoscope training model with the colonoscope 3D imaging probe improved trainee colonoscopy performance: a pilot study. Dig Dis Sci. 2011;56(5):1496–502.
55. Teshima CW, et al. Magnetic imaging-assisted colonoscopy vs conventional colonoscopy: a randomized controlled trial. World J Gastroenterol. 2014;20(36):13178–84.
56. Chen Y, et al. Magnetic endoscopic imaging vs standard colonoscopy: meta-analysis of randomized controlled trials. World J Gastroenterol. 2013;19(41):7197–204.
57. Mark-Christensen A, Brandsborg S, Iversen LH. Magnetic endoscopic imaging as an adjuvant to elective colonoscopy: a systematic review and meta-analysis of randomized controlled trials. Endoscopy. 2015;47(3):251–61.
58. Ye L, et al. Magnet-assisted diverticuloplasty for treatment of Zenker's diverticulum. Endoscopy. 2018;50(7):E170–e171.
59. Dobashi A, et al. Endoscopic magnet placement into subadventitial tunnels for augmenting the lower esophageal sphincter using submucosal endoscopy: ex vivo and in vivo study in a porcine model (with video). Gastrointest Endosc. 2019;89(2):422–8.
60. Bell R, et al. Laparoscopic magnetic sphincter augmentation versus double-dose proton pump inhibitors for management of moderate-to-severe regurgitation in GERD: a randomized controlled trial. Gastrointest Endosc. 2019;89(1):14–22.e1.
61. Asti E, et al. Magnetic sphincter augmentation for gastroesophageal reflux disease: review of clinical studies. Updat Surg. 2018;70(3):323–30.
62. DeVault KR. Refractory regurgitation responds to magnetic sphincter augmentation but not to increased proton pump inhibitor dose. Gastrointest Endosc. 2019;89(1):23–4.

Magnetic Retraction for Laparoscopic Cholecystectomy and Other General Surgical Interventions

11

Homero Rivas

Background

During the last three to four decades, minimal access surgery has greatly changed the way we perform surgery and also how patients perceive disease and have expectations toward their surgical management. Not only has laparoscopic surgery come a long way but also other innovative techniques and technologies, including advanced energy platforms, robotic surgery, endoluminal surgery, and endovascular surgery among other nonsurgical innovative therapies involving genomics, precision medicine, etc. Magnetic surgery is yet another promising technology that may reduce the incidence of surgically related trauma by using coupling forces across body tissues (abdominal wall, thoracic wall, etc.), without an incision or trauma, in order to move or activate surgical instruments.

Throughout this book, we can see the implementation of magnets in many different surgical specialties. In the same way that many innovations in minimal access surgery have been initially implemented in basic gynecological and general surgical procedures, magnetic surgical techniques have also been initially implemented in those general specialties. Only until after such initial evaluations prove new technologies to be safe and feasible, then they would be implemented in more complex surgical procedures of different subspecialties.

Beginnings

As early as the beginning of last decade, surgeons around the world were implementing magnets in laparoscopic surgery. Perhaps the first surgeon to propose this concept in laparoscopy and to extensively research it was Dr. Jeff Cadeddu and his group from UT Southwestern in Dallas, Texas [1–3]. He proposed the use of a magnetic anchoring system in laparoscopic surgery. This platform comprised a number of different instruments, including a video camera, endoscopic lighting system, laparoscopic retractor, graspers, and even a robotic endoscopic cautery device, which can be manipulated using external magnets across the abdominal wall. Some of these magnets would also rely on fine-needle transabdominal anchoring in order to provide increased stability at a given point across the abdominal wall. This initial platform had some limitations, especially the tethering of electrically active instrumentation (i.e., cautery, camera, lighting, etc.). This system, however, gave very promising hope of magnetic laparoscopic surgery as it proved efficient, mainly for trocar-less grasping tissue retraction across the abdominal wall (i.e., gallbladder). A substantial part of this work took

H. Rivas (✉)
Department of Surgery, Innovation and the Future, Mohammed Bin Rashid University of Medicine and Healthcare Sciences, Dubai, United Arab Emirates
e-mail: homero.rivas@mbru.ac.ae

M. Gagner (ed.), *Magnetic Surgery*, https://doi.org/10.1007/978-3-030-73947-8_11

place in the animal lab, where several different instrumentations were designed following this concept of transabdominal magnetic retraction. Its main value proposition included attaining a much more extensive surgical field and access, with minimized trauma during laparoscopic surgery (reduced portsurgery). Dr. Cadeddu's proposal translated first from a successful animal lab experience into a limited number of patients who underwent laparoscopic surgery safely, facilitated by magnetic anchoring instrumentation. This limited clinical experience included mainly cholecystectomies, where a retracting grasper was being replaced by magnetic anchoring instrumentation. Furthermore, this team evaluated the use of a tethered magnetic, anchored endoscopic camera. At that time, the more complex nature of this later instrumentation made its implementation and use much more cumbersome, and, until now, it has been mainly left aside.

Almost parallel to Dr. Cadeddu's efforts are those of other scholars like Dr. Guillermo Dominguez from Argentina who, through similarly self-designed and produced instrumentation, utilized neodymium magnets to implement laparoscopic graspers and retractors in several basic and advanced general surgical procedures, including cholecystectomy, appendectomy, gastroesophageal fundoplication, and hysterectomy, among others. His main breakthrough was the clinical implementation on actual patients at a larger scale with very promising results [4]. Certainly, during the last decade, other groups around the world have implemented highly customized devices and utilized them in both the animal and clinical settings for many different applications, yet with only local or regional implementation and exposure at best.

Only a few years ago, the US Food and Drug Administration (FDA) approved the first magnetic surgical system (Levita Magnetics Corp., San Mateo, CA, USA) for clinical use, with an initial single indication for laparoscopic cholecystectomies. This was a result of extensive animal evaluation and a large prospective, multicenter, single-arm, open-label study that was conducted to assess the safety and feasibility of this magnetic surgical system. No device-related serious adverse events were reported, and the use of this magnetic retraction provided, in a majority of cases, excellent surgical exposure of the triangle of Calot, which is a crucial requirement for any safe cholecystectomy [5, 6]. Upon FDA approval, limited commercial dissemination of this technology resulted in the implementation of this magnetic platform in local clinical trials across selected academic centers throughout the USA and around the world. The dissemination of this magnetic platform served as a steppingstone for some of those centers around the world to explore on their own, alternative clinical indications using the same magnetic platform on an off-label basis. Presently, there are two different clinical applications approved by the FDA: laparoscopic cholecystectomies and laparoscopic bariatric surgical procedures [5–7].

Lastly, several other scholars have designed and implemented homemade magnetic surgical devices in animal and clinical conditions in different centers around the world. Throughout this chapter, we will review different clinical applications for magnets in laparoscopic surgery [8–11].

Cholecystectomy

Much as with laparoscopic surgery, the implementation of magnetic surgery was first used in basic surgical procedures such as a cholecystectomy. This is a very common operation, with a large market and where animal models, either live pigs or blocks of bovine tissue, are easily available and at relatively low cost. Additionally, there are many surgeons well experienced in this procedure and with a mindset rather suitable to implement subtle changes in technique that in theory would provide as good exposure, with less invasion, less wound-related challenges (i.e., pain, scar, bleeding, hernia, etc.), and, in an ideal world, with very low additional cost.

From a technical point of view, magnetically anchored instruments are mainly suited to reproduce static retraction, without requiring much dynamic manipulation. This is quite important as magnetic forces are still, at best, a bit unpredictable and rely mainly on the size of an external magnet, the size of the grasping surfaces, and the distance of magnets' coupling. With forces not being easy to control or adjust, the tissue being retracted is usually the tissue to be discarded as part of the surgical specimen. This removes some potential concerns, such as the lack of finesse, which may not be relevant when retracting the fundus of the gallbladder. On the contrary, the same could not be said when manipulating magnetically a dissecting instrument, where precision and control are essential.

Among the paucity of clinical papers published in magnetic surgery, the great majority of them involve laparoscopic cholecystectomy. For the purpose of FDA approval for the Levita Mag platform perhaps, a landmark paper supporting laparoscopic magnetic surgery came from the author of this chapter and his collaborating group in Chile [5]. A prospective clinical trial enrolled a randomly selected sample of 50 patients in order to compare the use of conventional laparoscopic cholecystectomy and the use of a magnetic laparoscopic technique in reducing the number of trocars. This positive study not only proved the technique's feasibility and provided excellent surgical exposure but also boasted the absence of device-related serious adverse events, thus supporting the safety of this magnetic platform.

Foregut Surgery

As mentioned earlier, once feasibility and safety of magnetic instrumentation was attained in general basic surgical procedures, many scholars began to implement the procedure in foregut and bariatric surgery. In the case of foregut surgery, due to the unpredictable force that magnetic instrumentation can provide, magnetic instruments have been mainly utilized for purposes of liver retraction either by mimicking laparoscopic fan retraction (Caddedu), grasping the diaphragmatic crura (Dominguez), or by grasping the edge of the liver (Levita Mag). Additionally, magnetic instruments have been utilized for gastric retraction because the stomach can withstand more pressure and retraction, especially in the case of sleeve gastrectomies, when the grasped and retracted area is part of the specimen being resected. Lastly, as an important technical point, the upper abdominal wall usually has a lower thickness than in the lower abdomen and pelvis. This allows for more coupling capacity, which as we will discuss later may be an important limitation in some individuals (i.e., morbidly obese) or given anatomical areas (lower abdomen, pelvis, etc.) where there is an increased thickness of the abdominal wall.

Colorectal Surgery

During most colorectal surgeries, there will be a specimen to be removed. Again, for such retracted anatomical areas, likely to be part of the surgical specimen, magnetic retraction seems ideal. Additionally, most colon surgery would require multiquadrant abdominal exposure. Laparoscopic trocars have a fixed location and are not versatile when access to other areas of the abdomen is needed, resulting in a need for the placement of further ports for instrument utilization and, therefore, further surgical trauma. In laparoscopic colorectal surgery, magnetic instrumentation, especially for retraction or exposure, offers unique advantages when compared with conventional laparoscopic instrumentation. Additionally, some groups have advocated and reported the use of endoscopic localization of colonic lesions with magnetic coupling clips that can assist intraoperatively with the identification of colonic lesions either by the use of external magnets through the abdominal wall or by laparoscopic instruments with magnetic tips capable enough to create magnetic coupling through colonic tissue. Once the specimen is removed, the endoscopically placed magnetic reference is removed as well. While this technique has been reported by a few groups, it still has not gained wide acceptance, likely due to limited access to such specialized endoscopic and laparoscopic instrumentation.

Gynecological Surgery

Gynecologists have always been pioneers and innovators in laparoscopic surgery. From the common implementation of diagnostic laparoscopy to leading the way in therapeutic laparoscopy with appendectomy by Dr. Semm, and so on, gynecologists have historically embraced innovation [12]. In this case, and when feasible, much like in other types of abdominal surgery, magnetic coupling instrumentation can also be utilized during laparoscopic surgery to facilitate retraction and exposure. One must take into consideration that when finesse is required, such as when handling fallopian tubes or ovaries, magnetic retraction may not be a good option. On the other hand, when tissue is being excised, some liberties may be safely taken when using such magnetic forces. By now, hysterectomy techniques, adnexal removal, polypectomy, and other procedures have safely implemented the use of magnetic instrumentation.

Urological Surgery

While being a surgical subspecialty and mainly due to the pioneering work of urologist Dr. Cadeddu, some initial work on magnetic surgery has been done in urology. From the basic surgical proposal in laparoscopy to the design and implementation of diverse magnetic surgical devices, these were implemented in urological surgical procedures in animal and human settings. Once again, perhaps the best applications include organ or tissue retraction in reduced port laparoscopic procedures in urology.

Robotic Surgery

Robotic surgery has been a magnificent innovation in the world of surgery. Much of it, however, has been limited to surgical subspecialties like urology, gynecology, or reconstructive and complex surgical procedures. Important technological advances during the last 20 years have somewhat reduced the large physical footprint of most robotic platforms. Here, the real state space is rather important and having a fourth or fifth working arm is ideal, yet often not feasible. Magnetic platforms could potentially ameliorate this problem, as a simple external magnet could obviate the need for an additional arm, especially when this would be utilized for retraction purposes only. Limited clinical experience has been already presented and published by a paucity of scholars with promising results. Furthermore, novel robotic platforms are being developed with one or more robotic arms with magnetic capabilities.

General Benefits of Magnetic Instrumentation

Perhaps the most relevant benefit of magnetic instrumentation is the expansion of surgical access to more difficult areas of the abdomen during laparoscopic surgery.

Benefits of magnetic surgical instrumentation

- Improved surgical access to most different parts of the abdomen
- Less abdominal wall trauma related to instrumentation
- Less trocar-related complications (i.e., bleeding, infection, hernia, scars, pain, etc.)
- Versatility of instrument location
- Improved ergonomics
- Less reliance on additional surgical assistance
- Relatively low learning curve
- Improved cosmesis

During conventional laparoscopic or even robotic surgery, fixed and restricted surgical fields are the result of the stationary points where the surgical ports are initially placed. Moreover, once placed, if they are not conducive to optimal ergonomics, then their ill position would likely affect the flow of the surgical procedure. Magnets, on the other hand, allow dramatic expansion of those surgical fields, as external magnets can travel great distances along the abdominal wall regardless where they were introduced into the abdomen. Their versatility of being able to travel with instruments in multiple different quadrants across the abdomen is unique to magnetic surgery, even when compared with robotic surgery. Their biggest limitation with regard to access of location within the abdomen is their need to stay close to the abdominal wall in order to maintain active coupling with an external magnet. Additionally, as magnetic instruments do not require a constantly devoted trocar for their use once they are inserted into the abdomen, active coupling across the abdominal wall results in levitation of instruments with minimal contact and pressure to the abdominal wall, thus reducing the associated surgical trauma to very little if any. All potential benefits of reduced port laparoscopic surgery are experienced as well when using magnetic retraction [13–16]. Other potential benefits, yet not well studied, include being able to perform surgery with minimal assistance from a second or third surgeon, and a relatively low learning curve.

Persistent Challenges of Magnetic Instrumentation

Most of the previously described benefits come with a cost, which could be technical as well as economic.

Challenges of magnetic surgical instrumentation

- Unpredictability of magnetic forces
- Unintentional internal and external coupling potentially resulting in accidental injuries
- Poor coupling directly related to thicker abdominal walls (i.e., obesity)
- Unintentional decoupling resulting in instrument loss
- Additional economic cost
- Heat production from electromagnets (not clinically used)

One of the most relevant and persistent challenges that we have when using magnetic instrumentation is the unpredictability of their forces. Magnets cannot be easily controlled other than by gradually separating or bringing them closer to the abdominal wall and, therefore, to the internal magnetic counterparts. Some devices, like the ones proposed by Dr. Dominguez, have ways to adjust this distance with minimal effort, yet magnetic forces remain unpredictable. Only electromagnets can be switched on and off; however, they generate significant heat that presents a hazard and prohibits their use in the operating theater. External magnets cause attraction not only to internal magnetized surfaces from endoscopic magnetic retractors but also to many metal surfaces normally located in most operating theaters. This remains a big challenge that demands great awareness of the surgical team of all these potential magnetically attractive surfaces, as unintended coupling can result in accidents and/or injuries to anyone inside the operating theater, including the patient, but quite especially to those handling the external magnet. Isolation cases used to transport the magnet have decreased this potential risk as do external retractors (i.e., Murdoch retractor, Iron Intern, etc.). Even then, the handling of magnets requires special attention and knowledge of potential unintended coupling. Other challenges include unintentional internal coupling to magnetized devices such as other laparoscopic graspers or retractors. When using more than one magnet, internal coupling can be a challenge as sometimes in may be quite difficult to separate them, or they could also cause internal injury when random tissue becomes entrapped in between the two coupled magnets. Once again, unpredictable forces can cause sudden transabdominal coupling, causing tissue injury that can result in hematomas, etc. when the external magnet is too strong and/or too close in relation to the thickness of the abdominal wall. Coupling, in general, is more optimal in areas with a thin abdominal wall, such as the upper abdomen, and quite challenging when the wall is thick (i.e., obese patients, lower abdomen, etc.). Moreover, unintentional decoupling may result in internal loss of small instrumentation, which in obese abdomens may prove to be quite difficult to find even with the aid of more powerful magnets. This challenge, and the one with unintentional internal coupling, could be ameliorated by use of primitive tactics like using tethering sutures attached to internal magnetic instrumentation. Lastly, for any surgical equipment innovation there is an inherent additional economic cost that is especially notable during the early stages of its implementation. This can represent frustrating challenges commonly encountered by surgeons such as stringent criteria from value analysis committees, reluctance of reimbursement by insurance companies, and others.

Future Directions

As readers will discover throughout this book, magnetic instrumentation in laparoscopic and endoscopic surgery has many promising applications from simple surgical retraction to endoscopic magnetic compression anastomosis, use in complex robotic surgery, and many others. The use of sophisticated neural network algorithms may someday help predict and manage magnetic forces when used in surgery. As this instrumentation crosses the chasm of innovation, it will likely be implemented in many different types of surgery, simple and complex. Once economies of scale and scope are attained, the cost and pricing structures would be more conducive to universal adoption.

Conclusions

Magnets have been extensively used in numerous different industries for many years. While in medicine there are a number of applications that utilize magnets, in surgery, only a few have leveraged the use of magnets as an essential part of their mechanism of action. In general, magnetic instrumentation can provide great benefits in laparoscopic surgery across different specialties including general, gynecological, gastrointestinal, and colorectal surgery, among others. This also applies to robotic surgery and endoscopic procedures. Currently, magnetic instrumentation has been safely implemented in basic and complex surgical procedures and has produced notable benefits such as improved access to surgical fields, less trocar-related complications, improved versatility of trocar placement, improved ergonomics, and more optimal cosmesis, among others. Existing technological limitations include unpredictable magnetic force effects between internal or external objects and unintended coupling or decoupling, leading to accidental trauma. Other inherent challenges, and typical of most innovations, include additional economic costs and reimbursement challenges among several others. In general, there are many promising future applications on the horizon for the use of magnets in surgery.

References

1. Park S, Bergs RA, Eberhart R, et al. Trocar-less instrumentation for laparoscopy: magnetic positioning of intra-abdominal camera and retractor. Ann Surg. 2007;245:379–84.
2. Cadeddu J, Fernandez R, Desai M, et al. Novel magnetically guided intraabdominal camera to facilitate laparoendoscopic single-site surgery: initial human experience. Surg Endosc. 2009;23:1894–9.
3. Morgan M, Olweny EO, Cadeddu JA. LESS and NOTES instrumentation: future. Curr Opin Urol. 2014;24:58–65.
4. Dominguez G, Durand L, De Rosa J, et al. Retraction and triangulation with neodymium magnetic forceps for single-port laparoscopic cholecystectomy. Surg Endosc. 2009;23:1660–6.
5. Rivas H, Robles I, Riquelme F, Vivanco M, Jiménez J, Marinkovic B, Uribe M. Magnetic surgery: results from first prospective clinical trial in 50 patients. Ann Surg. 2018;267(1):88–93.
6. Haskins IN, Strong AT, Allemang MT, et al. Magnetic surgery: first U.S. experience with a novel device. Surg Endosc. 2018;32(2):895–9.
7. Davis M, Davalos G, Ortega C, Chen S, Schimpke S, Jain-Spangler K, Yoo J, Seymour K, Sudan R, Portenier D, Guerron AD. Magnetic liver retraction: an incision-less approach for less invasive bariatric surgery. Obes Surg. 2019;29(3):1068–73.
8. Guerron A, Ortega C, Park C, et al. Magnetic robot-assisted single-incision cholecystectomy. CRSLS. 2018;00073:e2017.
9. Uematsu D, Akiyama G, Magishi A, et al. Single-access laparoscopic left and right hemicolectomy

combined with extracorporeal magnetic retraction. Dis Colon Rectum. 2010;53(6):944–8.
10. Davalos G, Lan BY, Diaz R, Welsh LK, Roldan E, Portenier D, Guerron AD. Single-center experience with magnetic retraction in colorectal surgery. Obes Surg. 2019;29(3):1068–73.
11. Brancadoro M, Tognarelli S, Ciuti G, Menciassi A. A novel magnetic-driven tissue retraction device for minimally invasive surgery. Minim Invasive Ther Allied Technol. 2017;26(1):7–14.
12. Semm K. Die endoskopische appendektomie. Gynakol Prax. 1983;7:131–40.
13. Fuller J, Ashar BS, Carey-Corrado J. Trocar-associated injuries and fatalities: an analysis of 1399 reports to the FDA. J Minim Invasive Gynecol. 2005;12:302–7.
14. Lurje G, Raptis DA, Steinemann DC, et al. Cosmesis and body image in patients undergoing single-port versus conventional laparoscopic cholecystectomy: a multicenter double-blinded randomized controlled trial (SPOCCtrial). Ann Surg. 2015;262:728–35.
15. Brown BC, McKenna SP, Siddhi K, et al. The hidden cost of skin scars: quality of life after skin scarring. J Plast Reconstr Aesthet Surg. 2008;61:1049–58.
16. Golkar FC, Ross SB, Sperry S, et al. Patients' perceptions of laparoendoscopic single-site surgery: the cosmetic effect. Am J Surg. 2012;204:751–61.

12 Magnetic Retraction for Laparoscopic Sleeve Gastrectomy and Other Bariatric Procedures

Marcos Berry, Lionel Urrutia, Rodrigo Lynch, and Juan Pablo Barros

- Laparoscopic sleeve gastrectomy is currently the most common procedure performed worldwide, equivalent to 60% of bariatric procedures, followed by laparoscopic gastric bypass [1].
- In minimally invasive surgery, the magnetic retraction system decreases the number of trocars and facilitates triangulation-enabling reduced port techniques [2].

Obesity is considered a chronic multifactorial disease and is an important risk factor for the development of other diseases responsible for high morbidity and mortality in adulthood [3]. During the last 35 years, principles of minimally invasive surgery have radically changed the way of performing most abdominal operations like cholecystectomy, gastric bypass, and colon resection. Although laparoscopic techniques have not significantly changed in the last 10 years, several advances have been made in visualization devices and instrumentation. Thanks to minimization of surgical trauma, it offers the benefits of less postoperative pain, early ambulation, and shorter hospital stay, as well as better cosmetic results [4].

Recently, there has been a lot of interest in the surgical community to reduce the invasiveness of laparoscopic surgery. To achieve this goal, surgeons are either decreasing the number of trocars placed through the abdominal wall or eliminating them completely [5]. Minimizing the invasiveness of surgery has created its own challenges. Widely used current technology still requires the placement of multiple ports through the abdominal wall and these ports often must be spaced in such a way as to accommodate the reduced working space of laparoscopy.

Surgeons have had to use multiple port sites to perform their operations, and each of these transabdominal punctures is associated with morbidity and risks such as hernias, bleeding, damage to internal organs, as well as more scars and, thus, decreased cosmesis. These side effects have inspired surgeons to work on developing even less invasive techniques through reduction in the number of transabdominal ports needed to two, one, or even none. Reducing the number of transabdominal incisions to one site, called laparoendoscopic single-site surgery (LESS), often involves the use of multiple separate ports through the same incision, or increasingly, the use of one of the several industry-created multiport systems that are currently available in the marketplace [6].

M. Berry (✉)
Bariatric Surgery, Department of Surgery, Clinica Las Condes, Santiago, Chile

L. Urrutia
Department of Surgery, Clinica Las Condes, Santiago, Chile

R. Lynch
Surgery Department, Hospital San Jose de Melipilla, Santiago, Chile

J. P. Barros
Department of Surgery, Hospital Regional de Copiapó, Copiapó, Atacama, Chile

M. Gagner (ed.), *Magnetic Surgery*, https://doi.org/10.1007/978-3-030-73947-8_12

Advanced laparoscopic surgery, especially in bariatric patients, requires great skill on the part of the surgeon due to the size of the organs and intraabdominal structures, as well as the large amount of body fat that often prevents the correct visualization of the surgical field. Usually, an assistant is required to facilitate retraction. Acquiring an adequate field of view must be balanced against the risk of inflicting injury and undermining the benefits of laparoscopy [7]. Today there are many devices and instruments that help improve the results, both technical and aesthetic. In bariatric surgery, the retraction of the liver is essential to ensure adequate visualization of the surgical field. Many instruments are currently used for this purpose, but in general they require the constant use of a port or an additional incision (Fig. 12.1).

Magnetic technology provides a novel solution by allowing the retraction of the liver, stomach, and omentum during bariatric procedures without requiring a port or an additional incision [2]. The aim of this technology is to mitigate the limitations of conventional laparoscopic instruments. The ability to reach any place inside the abdominal cavity without extra trocar placement and with a larger range of movement during surgery is an excellent solution for reduced or single-port techniques.

The exposure of the surgical field is an integral part of all surgeries. The need for a good exposure is more accentuated in minimally invasive surgery, where the objective of limiting invasiveness may affect the ability of the surgeon to ensure adequate exposure in the surgical field. Throughout the evolution of minimally invasive surgery, many different techniques have been employed to achieve adequate exposure, while remaining within the limits of being less invasive [8].

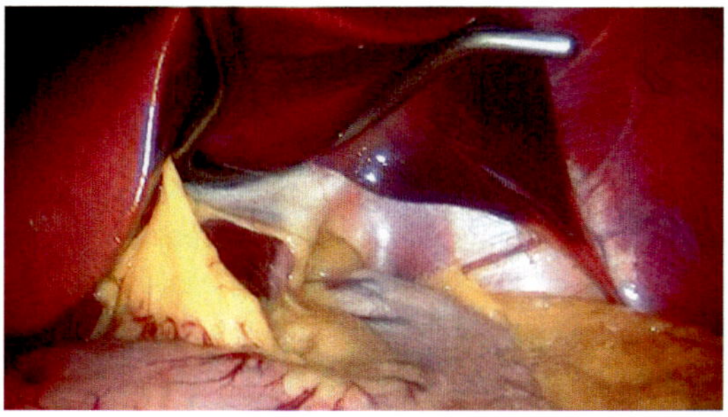

Fig. 12.1 Liver retraction using the Nathanson retractor

In bariatric surgery, the visualization of the stomach and the gastroesophageal junction is essential to adequately evaluate the anatomy. This requires retraction of the left liver, which often covers most of the stomach and esophageal hiatus. Over the years, many commercial products have been developed to achieve this retraction. To achieve this goal there are several ways to do it. Years ago there were methods such as suturing the liver to the abdominal wall, aspirating the left hepatic lobe, or using the nondominant hand to elevate the liver. All these techniques improve the visualization, but all require an exclusive port, the hand of the assistant surgeon, or generate trauma in the liver. Innovation in creating new ways to achieve the goal of having a perfect method of elevating the liver has led to the use of magnets for direct retraction of the liver without using a port.

The magnetic surgical system (Levita Magnetics, San Mateo, CA, USA) (Fig. 12.2) is the first magnetic retractor that received marketing authorization from the FDA. Recently, this device was successfully used during laparoscopic cholecystectomies in the USA and in combination with single-incision platforms assisted by robot [9]. Since this retractor does not require a port, or the hand of the assistant surgeon, it is less invasive during the surgical procedure. In addition, it is minimally traumatic to the liver and provides good exposure of the proximal stomach and gastroesophageal junction.

This magnetic surgical system is an innovative technological platform that utilizes a magnetic retractor designed to grasp and retract tissue and organs. It is composed of a grasper device with a

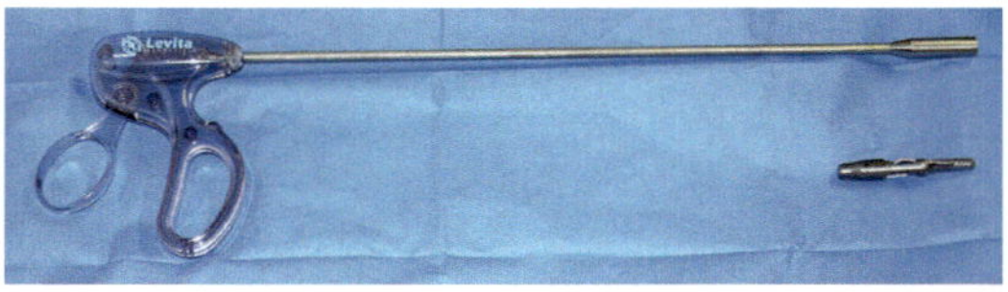

Fig. 12.2 Levita Magnetics™, San Mateo, CA, USA

detachable tip and an external magnet. The grasper is designed similar in shape and function to a regular laparoscopic grasper, with a delivery/retrieval shaft that allows the application of a detachable tip to tissues and organs. It can be used with 10 mm or larger trocars. The detachable tip in the distal part of the grasper is deployed by squeezing the grasper ring once it is positioned on the tissue that must be retracted. After release in the abdominal cavity, the retraction angles and motion are free and can be repositioned as many times and ways as needed. The external magnet is positioned externally on the abdominal wall to magnetically attract the detachable grasper tip. It can be repositioned with a standard rail-mounted arm across the abdominal wall to reach the desired retraction and position.

Our surgical team considers the magnetic retraction a viable option for advanced laparoscopic surgery in the obese population since it allows operating on this type of patient while maintaining the normal flow of the procedure. It is significantly better for patients from an aesthetic point of view, as well as reducing postoperative pain and the risk of infection of the surgical site by avoiding an epigastric incision.

The cosmetic benefit of having one less incision may seem insignificant and is often neglected and underestimated, but it is an important aspect from the patient's perspective (Fig. 12.3). Fewer incisions decrease the risk of infections at the surgical site, one of the main causes of morbidity and financial burden. While the actual reduction in risk of a minor incision has not been fully evaluated, the benefits for patient comfort, less pain, and faster recovery are aligned with the established principles of enhanced recovery after minimally invasive surgery.

Magnetic Retraction for Laparoscopic Sleeve Gastrectomy (LSG)

Laparoscopic sleeve gastrectomy is currently the most common procedure performed in the USA, followed by gastric bypass (RYGB) [10–18]. Sleeve gastrectomy is a restrictive type procedure, resulting in a narrow and tubular stomach.

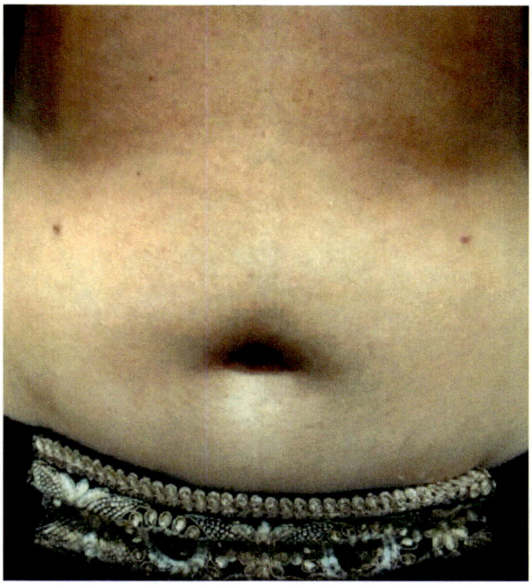

Fig. 12.3 Cosmetic benefit

The concept is simple but some steps of the procedure, if performed incorrectly, can lead to serious complications [11].

In the traditional technique, five ports are placed in the middle and upper part of the abdomen. If exposure is difficult due to a large amount of perigastric fat or a large liver, a sixth port can be placed in the upper left quadrant for the assistant surgeon [12].

Reduced Port Technique Using Magnetic-Assisted Surgery

By modifying the above technique for a less invasive procedure, our team has developed the following surgical steps. First, the patient is placed in French position. The first surgeon is located between the patient's legs. The total number of trocars are three: a first 15 mm umbilical, a second 5 mm at the level of the right midaxillary line, and a third 5 mm in the midline of the left clavicle. We use a 30°/5 mm scope.

This technology with assisted magnetic surgery met the Chilean National Health Institute requirements for its use and commercialization in Chile. It underwent a previous clinical trial in Chile [13]. Feasibility of the procedure was evaluated by intraoperative time, procedure achievement with a reduced port technique, and by ability to adequately mobilize organs without needing an extra trocar insertion.

In our private health center, Clínica Las Condes in Santiago, Chile, our surgical team selected 23 patients who had laparoscopic sleeve gastrectomy indication; 16 women and 7 men, ages ranging between 17 and 62, with an average age of 36 years. The BMI range was between 30 and 38.3 with a median of 33.4 kg/m^2. All of them had signed a written consent form before the surgery. All of them had comorbidities such as insulin resistance, dyslipidemia, arterial hypertension, hypothyroidism, polyarthralgia, nonalcoholic fatty liver disease, or obstructive sleep apnea.

The mean operative time was 1.42 hours. All operations were fully performed by a reduced port technique. There were no complications or side effects related to the device during surgery. None of them had any postoperative complications related to the magnetic system. One of them had abdominal wall bleeding in the right flank trocar wound that was resolved with a skin stitch [13].

We recommend placing the arm of the magnet once the surgical field has been prepared and covering the arm with a sterile plastic drape. Once this is done, it is necessary to adjust the arm joints to the comfort of the surgeon. Thanks to the use of the magnetic surgical system, we reduced from 5 to 3 trocars (reduced port technique) (Fig. 12.4).

The magnetic retraction system consists of an internal metal grasper with a detachable tip that is coupled with an external magnet controller. The external magnet is placed using a specialized articulated arm mounted on the bar of the surgical bed. Due to its size it can be easily maneuvered through the abdominal wall externally. The clamp that will attract the external magnet is introduced through the existing port of 15 mm and is attached to the middle part of the free edge of the left lobe of the liver, in the omentum, or in the stomach, depending on the surgical procedure. The external magnet is then placed on the abdominal wall and attached to the clamp, and the magnetic attraction allows external manipulation of the clamp. Once the procedure is completed, the external magnet is decoupled, and the tip of the clamp is removed from the abdominal cavity using the introducer instrument.

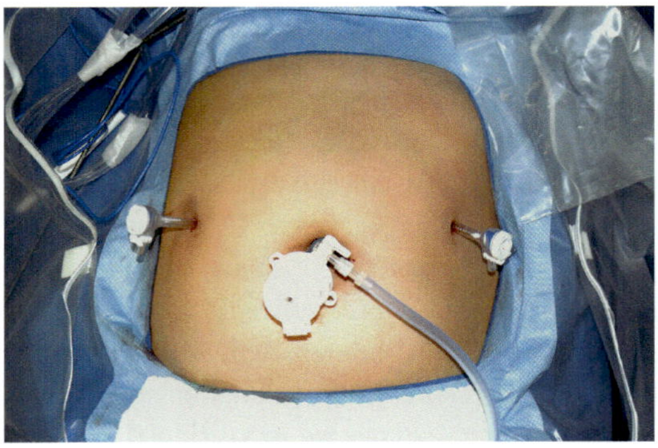

Fig. 12.4 Reduced port technique

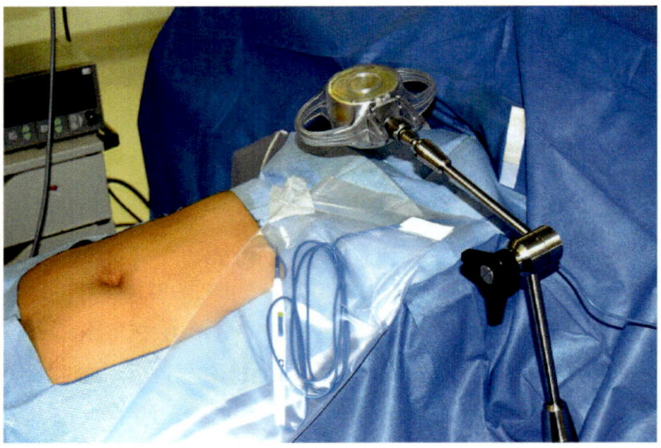

Fig. 12.5 Magnet located on the left side of the patient (standard bedrail-mounted arm)

The external magnet is positioned using a standard bedrail-mounted arm facilitating the support of the magnetic clamp in the liver, stomach, or omentum, according to the comfort of the surgeon (Fig. 12.5). Care should be taken when preparing the surgical field as to not place the magnet near metallic instruments that could be attracted.

In some patients showing cholelithiasis in their preoperative study, we begin the surgery with the laparoscopic magnetic-assisted cholecystectomy (Fig. 12.6). The magnetic clamp pulls the vesicular fundus and facilitates the dissection of the Calot's triangle. At the end of cholecystectomy, the LSG continues.

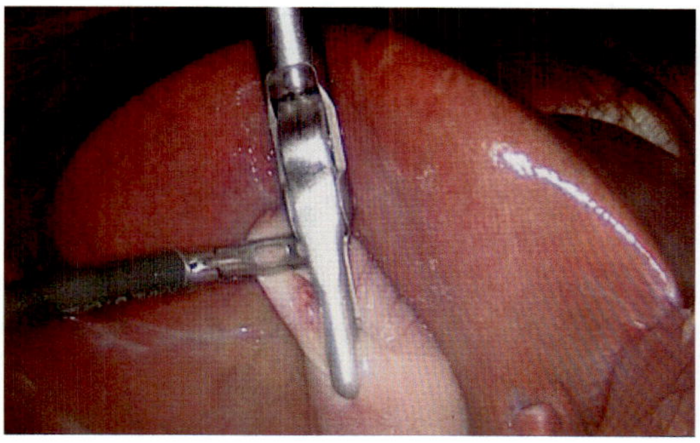

Fig. 12.6 The magnetic clamp pulls up gallbladder fundus

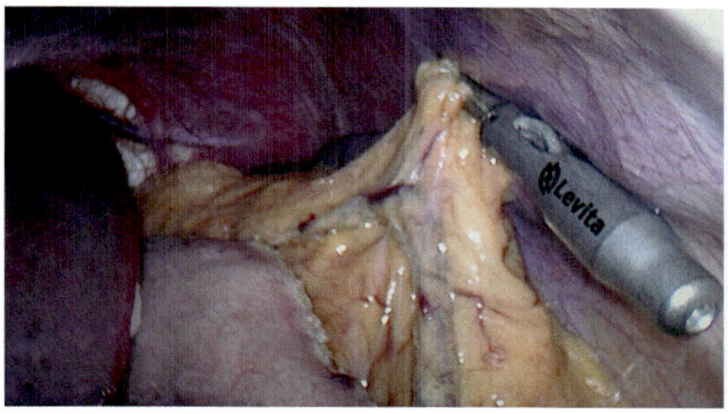

Fig. 12.7 The magnetic grasper pulling the omentum

The next step is to identify the gastroepiploic vessels and begin to release the stomach from the omentum. To achieve this, the magnetic clamp grabs the omentum and pulls it laterally (Fig. 12.7).

The traction can be lateral or superolateral according to the comfort of the surgeon. Once the vessels are identified, the dissecting instrument is inserted (we use ultrasonic dissector). The magnetic clamp should move more superolateral to produce the necessary traction, and with the left hand the surgeon takes the stomach and pulls it to facilitate exposure. In this stage of the surgery, the function of the magnetic clamp is to grasp the omentum to facilitate the dissection of the greater curvature of the stomach (Fig. 12.8).

The goal at this stage is to maintain a smooth and effective dissection until the left crus of the diaphragm and the short vessels are identified. If the left lobe of the liver prevents the visualization of these structures, the magnetic clamp must

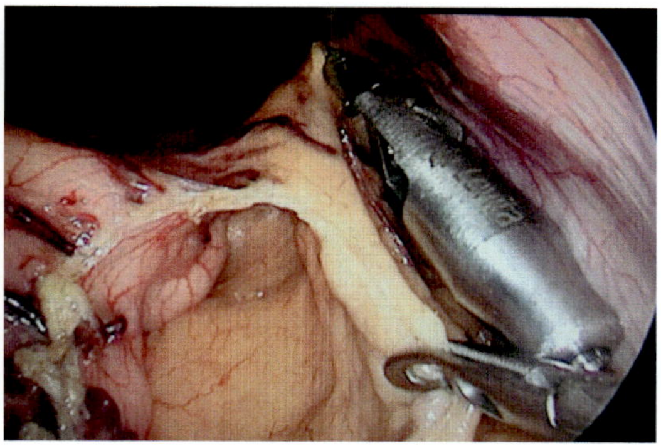

Fig. 12.8 The magnetic grasper tractioning the omentum

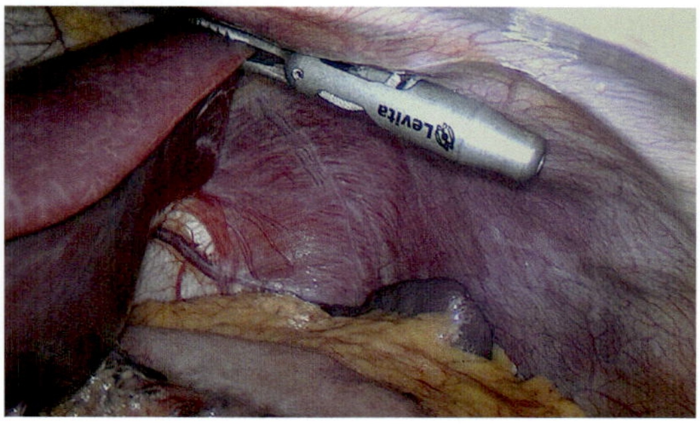

Fig. 12.9 The magnetic grasper lifts the left lobe of the liver

hold and lift the edge of the liver (Fig. 12.9). It is important that the magnetic grasp must be complete to avoid any injury and lift the liver as much as possible. Once the proximal dissection has been completed, it is continued distally to the pylorus, maintaining the surgical steps. When the stomach is completely separated from the omentum, the next step is the stapling and cutting of the stomach to complete the vertical sleeve gastrectomy (Figs. 12.10 and 12.11).

To make the visualization easier and dissection of the vertical sleeve, the magnetic clamp holds the edge of the stomach sequentially from distal to proximal. This position prevents the stomach from bending back, facilitating the first stapling at 4–5 cm from the pylorus. The flexible external arm coupled with the magnet facilitates and helps to perform a straight and symmetrical stapling line.

The visualization of the esophageal hiatus is of particular interest especially for cases of

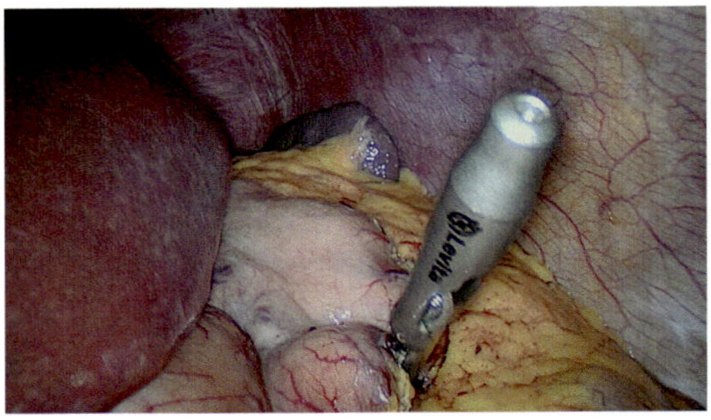

Fig. 12.10 The magnetic grasper grabs the stomach

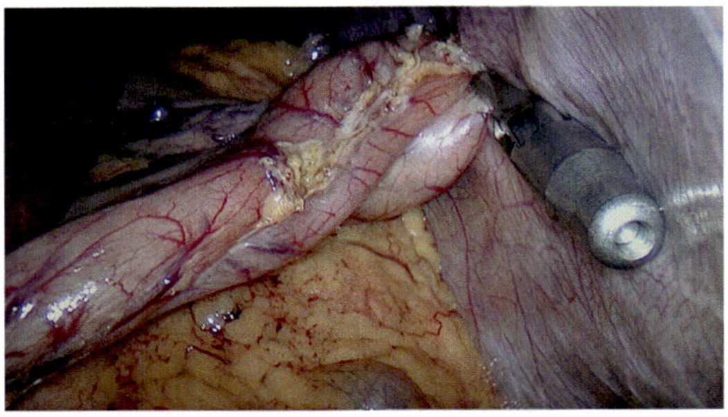

Fig. 12.11 The magnetic grasper grabs the greater curvature of the stomach

sleeve gastrectomy. In our own experience, the device provides an adequate visualization of the structures required in most of our procedures. Large, floppy livers can be more challenging, as they tend to lean in the upper-posterior aspect and cover the hiatus.

Roux-en-Y Gastric Bypass with Magnetic Retraction

The RYGB is a mixed surgery that combines a restrictive procedure with a malabsorptive one [14]. Like the sleeve gastrectomy, it is very important to visualize the esophageal hiatus and the angle of His. To obtain a clear visual, the left lobe of the liver should be lifted up, which in most cases covers the gastroesophageal junction. For this purpose, we use the magnetic clamp that holds the edge of the liver and, thus, a complete visualization of the structures is achieved.

The first step is the creation of the gastric pouch. In this case, the magnetic clamp can be used by lifting the liver or by pulling the stomach to the left of the patient for the safe passage of the stapler. The next step is to vertically divide the omentum in two in order to ascend a jejunal loop through this canal to perform the gastrojejunal anastomosis. In this surgical step, the magnetic clamp assists by pulling the omentum to the left of the patient while the surgeon pulls to the right, generating the necessary traction for the optimal use of dissection and hemostasis instruments. Once the jejunal loop is pulled up, the gastrojejunal anastomosis is performed.

Other Applications of Magnetic Device for Bariatric Surgery

There are a few other reports that describe the use of magnetic retraction for other bariatric procedures such as:

- Adjustable gastric band removal
- Duodenal switch
- Gastrojejunostomy revision
- Sleeve gastrectomy conversion to RYGB

Use of the Magnetic Surgical System

Minimally invasive surgery requires a set of advanced skills as well as innovative devices to achieve excellent results. In bariatric patients, this is even more important since the size, weight, and shape of the intraabdominal organs add an additional degree of difficulty. Given that obese patients are at greater risk of postoperative complications, bariatric surgeons are constantly working to improve their ability to manage these patients through less traumatic approaches.

For our team, constant innovation in surgical instrumentation is welcome, to allow us to perform surgical procedures safely and in the most efficient way. Our goal is to enable patients to recover faster and better, especially in bariatric surgery.

The magnetic surgical system decreases the number of trocars and, most importantly, facilitates the ability to triangulate in laparoscopy. The lack of triangulation leads to inadequate visualization or exposure and poor organ mobilization, which may increase the risk of iatrogenic injury, makes the procedure more difficult, and prolongs surgical time.

This magnetic device system compensates for all these problems, especially in bariatric surgery, in which large intraabdominal organs plus abundant abdominal fat tend to make the tissue management more difficult. On the other hand, the magnetic clamp not only facilitates the traction of the liver but also reduces the use of trocars and the placement of the liver retractor, which often leaves patients with epigastric abdominal pain.

The set-up of the external magnet takes usually less than 2 minutes. The external magnet is reusable and is covered by a sterile bag throughout the procedure, which eliminates the need for sterilization after each surgery. The magnetic clamp is made of metal, similar to any other laparoscopic instrument, and is not reusable.

Discussion

An ideal method of retraction should have certain characteristics to achieve the main objectives of minimally invasive surgery. First, it must be easy to use. Second, it must be able to be in one place but also be able to move. And third, it should not require the use of the hands of the surgeon or assistant. The external magnet used by our surgical team achieves all these objectives.

This chapter shows an innovative solution to the challenges encountered in bariatric surgery through the use of devices that are coupled and mobilized by external magnetic fields through the abdominal wall.

Magnetic-assisted retraction is a novel approach that allows a safe, reproducible, and noninvasive technique for intraabdominal mobilization without restrictions and without ports. We successfully use the device to obtain an optimal retraction of the liver during laparoscopic bariatric procedures as it improves surgical exposure and decreases the number of incisions, in addition to using it to pull other structures such as omentum, stomach, and gallbladder (Fig. 12.12).

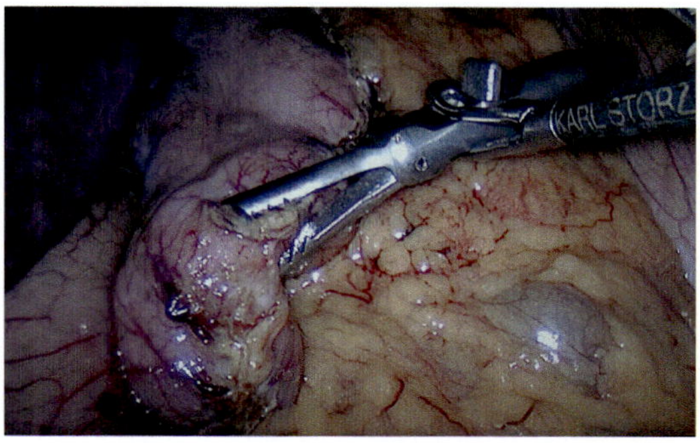

Fig. 12.12 The magnetic surgical system

In general, this type of technology could offer great advantages, including the restoration of triangulation, the improved mobilization of tissues and organs, and a decreased need for trocars due to the nature of the magnetic coupling through the abdominal wall. While performing a conventional laparoscopy with a small number of trocars would face significant limitations, the use of magnetically coupled instrumentation can overcome these challenges with elegance [15–17].

Use of these tools can improve the ergonomics of laparoscopic surgery, allowing positioning of intraabdominal instruments that do not require a separate transabdominal trocar. Further developments of this technology have occurred in multiple surgical fields, broadening their utility, and improving the instrumentation.

This novel technology allows a great exposure in laparoscopic surgery and it can be applied with a short learning curve. It is an excellent tool to facilitate and enable reduced port technique and can also be used in single-port technique.

We believe that magnetic surgery is a significant contribution to MIS and bariatric surgery because it facilitates the exposure of intraabdominal structures by effectively separating the liver in addition to pulling other organs (such as the stomach and omentum), which are mobilized from the outside of the abdominal cavity with less trauma and without the need for extra ports [16].

Conclusion

The use of magnetic retraction in bariatric surgery contributes effectively to achieve the necessary traction of intraabdominal structures for the correct dissection of tissues. It also achieves the retraction of the liver without the need of a port, which allows performing bariatric procedures through minimally invasive surgery, decreasing the possibility of hernias, improving cosmetics, and achieving faster and enhanced recovery of patients into daily life [18].

Magnetic surgery is an innovative tool that enables the development and evolution of laparoscopic surgery while maintaining high standards and has proven to be successful in bariatric surgery.

References

1. Jimenez A, Ibarzabal A, Mize V, Pane A, Andreu A, Molero J, De Hollanda A, Flores L, Ortega E, Lacy A, Vidal J. Ten-year outcomes after Roux-en-Y gastric bypass and sleeve gastrectomy: an observational nonrandomized cohort study. Surg Obes Relat Dis. 2019;15(3):382–8.
2. Davis M, Davalos G, Ortega C, et al. Magnetic liver retraction: an incision-less approach for less invasive bariatric surgery. Obes Surg. 2019;29(3):1068–73.
3. WHO. Obesity: preventing and managing the global epidemic. Report of a WHO consultation. Technical report series 894. Geneva: WHO; 2000.
4. Di Lorenzo N, Canci L, Simi M, Arcudi C, Tognoni V, Gaspari AL, Valdastri P. A magnetic levitation robotic camera for minimally invasive surgery: useful for NOTES? Surg Endosc. 2017;31(6):2529–33.
5. Raman JD, Scott DJ, Cadeddu JA. Role of magnetic anchors during laparoendoscopic single site surgery and NOTES. J Endourol. 2009;23(5):781–6.
6. Best SL, Cadeddu JA. Use of magnetic anchoring and guidance systems to facilitate single trocar laparoscopy. Curr Urol Rep. 2010;11(1):29–32.
7. Vargas-Palacios A, Hulme C, Veale T, Downey CL. Systematic review of retraction devices for laparoscopic surgery. Surg Innov. 2016;23(1):90–101.
8. Rahman R, Azagury DE. Novel technologies and techniques in bariatric surgery. Minerva Chir. 2017;72(2):125–39.
9. Rivas H, Robles I, Riquelme F, et al. Magnetic surgery: results from first prospective clinical trial in 50 patients. Ann Surg. 2018;267(1):88–93.
10. Esquivel CM, Garcia M, Armando L, Ortiz G, Lascano FM, Foscarini JM. Laparoscopic sleeve gastrectomy resolves NAFLD: another formal indication for bariatric surgery? Obes Surg. 2018;28(12):4022–33.
11. Benaiges D, Más-Lorenzo A, Goday A, et al. Laparoscopic sleeve gastrectomy: more than a restrictive bariatric surgery procedure? World J Gastroenterol. 2015;21(41):11804–14.
12. Morales-Conde S, Dominguez G, Gomez JC, et al. Magnetic-assisted single-port sleeve gastrectomy. Surg Innov. 2013;20(4):NP9–NP11.
13. Berry M, Urrutia L, Jose DM. Magnetic grasper technology for laparoscopic gastric sleeve surgery. Oral presentation. SAGES; 2016.
14. Kothari SN, Borgert AJ, Kallies KJ, Baker MT, Grover BT. Long-term (>10-year) outcomes after laparoscopic Roux-en-Y gastric bypass. Surg Obes Relat Dis. 2017;13(6):972–8.
15. Haskins IN, Strong AT, Allemang MT, Bencsath KP, Rodriguez JH, Kroh MD. Magnetic surgery: first U.S. experience with a novel device. Surg Endosc. 2018;32(2):895–9.
16. Diaz R, Davalos G, Welsh LK, Portenier D, Guerron AD. Use of magnets in gastrointestinal surgery. Surg Endosc. 2019;33(6):1721–30.
17. Dominguez G, Durand L, De Rosa J, Danguise E, Arozamena C, Ferraina PA. Retraction and triangulation with neodymium magnetic forceps for single-port laparoscopic cholecystectomy. Surg Endosc. 2009;23(7):1660–6.
18. Małczak P, Pisarska M, Piotr M, Wysocki M, Budzyński A, Pędziwiatr M. Enhanced recovery after bariatric surgery: systematic review and meta-analysis. Obes Surg. 2017;27(1):226–35.

Magnetic Vascular Anastomosis

13

Michel Gagner

Introduction

The use of magnets for vascular anastomosis is interesting and dramatically different from that for GI anastomosis because the necrosis that occurs in the gastrointestinal tract causes the device to be expelled and passed in the stools per anus. In the cases of vascular anastomosis, such exit is not possible, and indeed would lead to embolization or vascular obstruction, with distal organ consequences. The necrosis in a side-to-side vascular anastomosis would lead to an anastomosis in device periphery just like sutures would have done; except in vascular anastomosis, permanent sutures are usually chosen as the wound healing and contraction are different. If non-healing occurs, a major haemorrhage or haematoma and/or pseudoaneurysm would ensue. The foreign body could also cause a partial vascular occlusion with clotting or vessel thrombosis. Hence, the vascular anastomosis would probably require a lumen to allow flow right away, a difference with the GI tract, and magnetic devices that approximate would have to become endothelialized and stay in the vessel walls permanently to become incorporated. There have been three groups of research efforts, the first is microvascular anastomosis (mostly by plastic surgeons and others using the microscope), the second is arterial anastomosis devices, and finally, venous. I will review the literature on these three subjects separately.

Microvascular

It is really Obora and colleagues Tamaki and Matsumoto from Kobe Japan (from the Department of Neurosurgery) who had the original idea of using compression/attraction for vascular anastomosis in their classic paper of 1978, *Nonsuture Microvascular Anastomosis Using Magnet Rings*. A new method of non-suture microvascular anastomosis was developed, using magnet rings and cogwheel-shaped hollow metal instruments with six spurs or oval hollow instruments (Fig. 13.1). With this method, both end-to-end and end-to-side anastomoses are possible. End-to-end anastomosis in experimental animals was possible for small vessels with outer diameters of up to 1 mm with an average patency rate of 90%, requiring 8 minutes on average to complete. In cases of end-to-side anastomosis, the patency rate was 84%, requiring 8.4 minutes on average. In end-to-end anastomosis, electromagnetic flowmeter measurement showed that there was no difference in blood flow and blood flow patterns between control and operated vessels, even 40 days after anastomosis. In end-to-side anastomosis, blood flow at the donor vessel and the total blood flow at the recipient vessel were the same after 40 days in cases of artery-to-artery

M. Gagner (✉)
Hôpital du Sacré-Cœur de Montréal, Montréal, QC, Canada

Chief of Surgery, Westmount Square Surgical Center, Westmount, QC, Canada

M. Gagner (ed.), *Magnetic Surgery*, https://doi.org/10.1007/978-3-030-73947-8_13

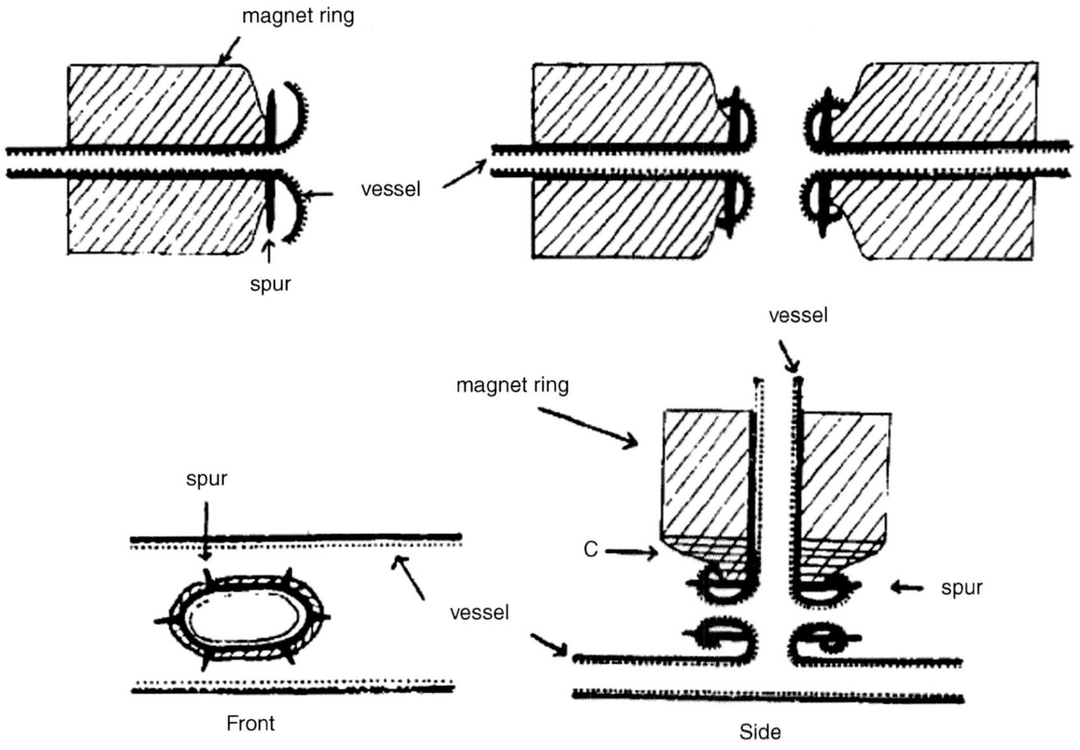

Fig. 13.1 Magnet rings and cogwheel-shaped hollow metal instruments with six spurs. Front and side views. (From Obora et al. [2]. Neurologia medico-chirurgica. Published by the Japan Neurosurgical Society (Open Access))

anastomosis. Histological assessment in experimental animals 20 days after anastomosis revealed a continuity of the media and the intima; at 180 days, no noticeable abnormal findings were documented. In a scanning electron microscope study, no disturbance and flattening of longitudinal endothelial folds on the inner surface of the vessels were detected. Histological examinations revealed that magnetic force did not alter blood vessel walls and adjacent tissues [1, 2].

Almost 25 years later, Erdman et al. revisited this experiment using their own novel device for a side-to-side arteriovenous anastomosis in a dog model. The femoral artery and vein were exposed unilaterally in three dogs and bilaterally in four dogs to create 11 anastomoses. A 4-mm arteriotomy was performed, and one oval magnet 0.5 mm thick was inserted into the lumen of the artery. A second magnet was applied external to the artery, compressing and stabilizing the arterial wall to create a magnetic port. An identical venous magnetic port was created with another pair of oval magnets. When the two devices were permitted to contact each other, they self-aligned and magnetically coupled to accomplish the arteriovenous anastomosis. All 11 anastomoses were patent under direct observation and palpation. Ten of 11 anastomoses were clearly patent on duplex scans, with hydrodynamic resistance averaged 0.73 ± 0.33 mm Hg min/mL (mean ± SEM). Arteriovenous vascular anastomoses performed with magnets were feasible with 100% patency after 10 weeks in a dog model. It did not present aneurysm or leaks, with a nice remodelling of the vessel wall after several weeks, which incorporated the magnets [3].

Arterial

I have been involved in the efforts to make coronary bypass with minimally invasive techniques. Indeed, at the Hotel-Dieu de Montreal in the early 1990s, my efforts with the interventional radiologist Gilles Soulez have been to try to perform a mammo-coronary anastomosis end-to-side with the use of catheter-guided anastomosis and glue to keep it in place [4]. Another has been with the use of the first robot called "Zeus" to assist and I performed a robotic sutured mammary-coronary anastomosis in a pig with 6-0 or 7-0 sutures. I was the first successful surgeon to perform in the lab of Computer Motion in Carpinteria California in the mid-1990s, with engineers James Wright and Moji Ghodoussi, amongst several [5]. This proof of concept prompted the race between Computer Motion and Intuitive Surgical about a robotics-assisted technique to make sutured coronary bypass anastomosis in the thorax.

While the handsewn anastomosis with sternotomy is considered the "gold standard" for performing coronary artery bypass grafts, they are still cumbersome, demanding, and time-consuming, especially on a beating heart. A device called Magnetic Vascular Positioner System was invented; it consists of four magnetic, gold-plated implants and two delivery devices that facilitate the creation of a functional end-to-side anastomosis (Fig. 13.2). The company Ventrica Inc., a Delaware Corporation, had several patents including the devices and methods for forming magnetic anastomoses between vessels in USA with a publication number: 20060282106, filed on November 18, 2002. The inventors, David Cole, Darin Gittings, Stephen Olson, Dean Carson, Michael Reo, Keke Lepulu, and A. Sharkawy, described "an anastomosis device with first and second components which each having first and second parts. The first and second components are magnetically attracted to one another. The device forms a through hole when in use. The first parts of the first and second components are positioned radially outward from the second parts relative to the longitudinal axis with the first parts of the first and second components contacting one another and being magnetically attracted to one another. The second parts of the first and second components also being magnetically attracted to one another and are separated by the vessel walls". Another patent was filed on 23 May 2003, and included components, systems and methods for forming anastomoses using magnetism or other coupling means, with publication number: 2004011694, Inventors A. Adam Sharkawy, J. Greg Stine, David H. Cole, Samuel Crews, Darin C. Gittings, Adam Kessler, and Mark J. Foley. By 5 May 2003, Ventrica, Inc. had announced that it has received CE Mark for its MVP(R) Distal Anastomosis System, allowing

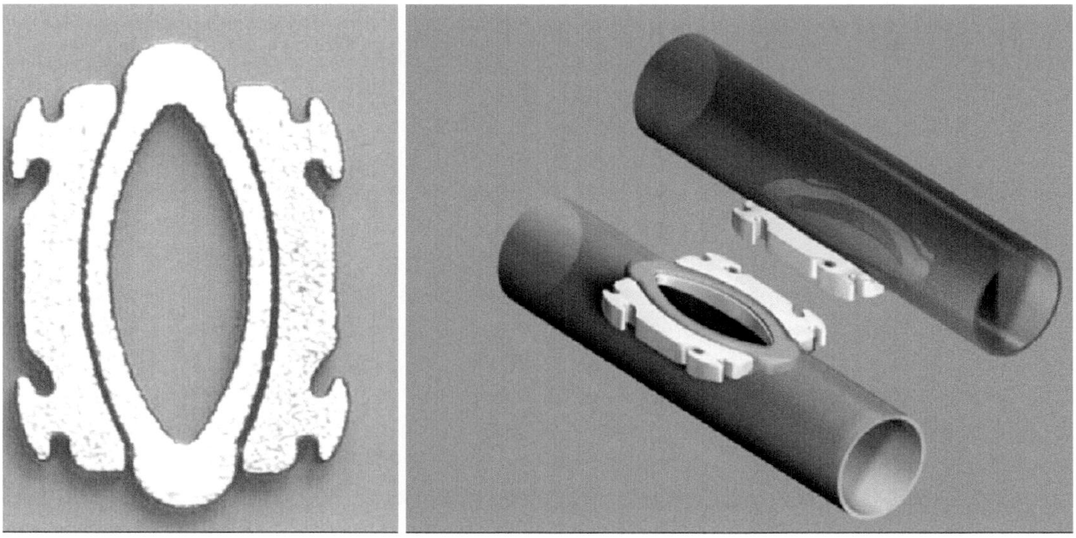

Fig. 13.2 Magnetic anastomotic device Ventrica MVP®. (From Morbiducci et al. [12]. Reprinted with permission (STM Signatory Agreement Springer/SAGE Publications)

the device to be sold in all countries of the European Union. Also, Medtronic, Inc. became the sole distributor of this new magnetic connector technology in Europe. However, in 2004, the company Ventrica Inc. was finally acquired totally by Medtronic, Inc.

The device was supported by prior animal work by Filsoufi et al. [6] In 40 pigs, a right internal thoracic artery to right coronary artery anastomoses and left internal thoracic artery to left anterior descending artery anastomoses were successfully performed and self-aligning properties of the implants permitted for immediate and secure approximation, with a total anastomotic time between 2 and 3 minutes. Five non-device-related deaths occurred postoperatively. At 1 week, angiography performed in 35 surviving animals showed a patent graft and anastomosis in all cases. The patency rate at 1 month was 97% (33/34). Histologic studies as late as 6 months displayed neointimal coverage of the magnets without any significant luminal hindrance. Histology also corroborated the existence of sustainable tissue between magnets. Others have published animals and early clinical experiences with the device [7–13]. This was followed by clinical experience by Klima et al., a multicentre trial which tested the device in 32 patients (mean age: 65 ± 9 years; 85% men) requiring multivessel coronary artery bypass surgery, in which one of the anastomoses was performed using this novel anastomotic technology. The application of the magnetic vascular positioner device was successful in 32 of 41 cases (78%). In five of the cases, the coronary artery was too small; one case had a posterior wall plaque in the target artery; and three patients had a non-haemostatic anastomosis after coupling of the port and were subsequently converted to hand-sewn anastomoses. The median total magnetic vascular positioner anastomotic time was 137 seconds, with a range from 65 to 370 seconds. Overall patency rate of the magnetic vascular positioner anastomosis was 93.5% versus 91.7% (non-significant) in hand-sewn grafts. One patient (3.1%) died due to low cardiac output but had patent grafts at autopsy. One myocardial infarction (3.1%) occurred the day after a percutaneous transluminal coronary angioplasty of a hand-sewn graft. It was concluded that the magnetic vascular coupling in coronary surgery is safe and effective and has acceptable early patency rates [14, 15]. They also reported a reoperation 8 months after minimally invasive direct coronary artery bypass grafting with magnetic vascular coupling due to a symptomatic subtotal obstruction at the anastomotic site [16].

Vicol et al. had a similar experience in a small number of patients, reporting a UK experience [16, 17]. According to Tossios, the 10-year review showed 150 patients implanted with good patency [18]. But less favourable mid-term results and no long-term patency outcomes of those recipients have been investigated. Tossios described excellent patency 10 years after the magnetic device, between a left internal thoracic artery to left anterior descending grafting, in a man who underwent coronary angiography prior to thymectomy [19].

Arterial coupling can be done with ring devices, magnetic or not. The non-magnetic ones show promising coupling and get incorporated in the walls, especially the non-metallic ones. Li et al. have shown reliable vessel anastomosis with a metal-free vascular coupling system that can be used for both arteries and veins. Mechanical testing results showed that vessels reconnected with these devices could withstand 12.7 ± 2.2 N tensile force and have superior leak profiles (0.049 ± 0.015, 0.078 ± 0.016, 0.089 ± 0.008 mL/s at 160, 260, 360 mmHg, respectively) compared to hand-sutured vessels (0.310 ± 0.014, 1.123 ± 0.033, 2.092 ± 0.072 mL/s at 160, 260, 360 mmHg, respectively). The anastomotic process was successfully demonstrated on both arteries and veins in cadaver pigs [20]. The system consists of an engaging ring made from high-density polyethylene using computer numerical control machining, and a back ring made from polymethylmethacrylate using laser cutting. A segment of expanded polytetrafluoroethylene (ePTFE) tubing was interposed into a transected carotid artery by anastomosis using two couplers, and end-to-end anastomoses were accomplished. MRI performed 2 weeks after the surgery evaluated vessel and ePTFE graft patency. This could facilitate vascular anastomosis procedures in trauma and reconstructive surgeries [21].

But the other elegant solution is a magnetic pinned-ring device, which consists of paired magnetic rings coated with titanium nitride and entrenched in a polypropylene casing; the rings are furnished with alternately spaced holes and titanium pins. The vascular anastomosis technique employing magnetic pinned-ring devices was achieved on 14 mongrel dogs and compared to hand-sewing anastomosis on 14 additional dogs, end-to-end anastomoses between the femoral artery and the inferior vena cava. The time required to perform the anastomosis was significantly briefer for the magnetic device. A continuity of re-endothelialization was confirmed in all anastomotic stomas after 24 weeks, and neither formation of aneurysms nor thickening of the vascular wall was recorded. The re-endothelialization was smooth at the anastomotic site of the device, whereas hand sewing occasioned rougher and uneven endothelialization and the presence of observable sutures. Application of the magnetic tool was accompanied by significantly lower deposition of fibrotic collagen compared with hand-sewing technique. Hence, the magnetic pinned-ring device offered a simple, fast, reliable and efficacious technique for non-suture vascular anastomosis, it shortened operation time and maintained a high patency rate [9, 22].

The same group investigated burst pressure of femoral artery anastomosis with magnets using adult mongrel dogs compared to hand-suturing (group B). At immediate, 4 weeks, and 12 weeks after operation, the vascular bursting pressure of anastomosis site in group A was more than 280 mm Hg (1 mm Hg = 0.133 kPa), and was (140.11 ± 15.23), (180.31 ± 24.55), and more than 280 mm Hg in group B, showing significant differences at immediate and 4 weeks ($P < 0.05$), but no significant difference at 12 weeks ($P > 0.05$) [23].

Cirillo et al. have proposed a new way to secure complex grafts for aortic dissection [24]. Connections can be made with catheters having magnetic tips, using neodymium iron boron (NdFeB) magnetic catheters to create transcatheter cavopulmonary and aortopulmonary shunts. "Target" catheters were placed in the pulmonary arteries (PAs), and radiofrequency "perforation" catheters were placed in either the descending aorta (DAo) for central shunts or the superior vena cava (SVC) for Glenn shunts. The magnet technique or "balloon target" method was used to pass wires from the DAo or the SVC into the PA. Aortopulmonary and cavopulmonary connections were then created using Atrium iCAST covered stents. Magnet catheters were used to perforate the left pulmonary artery from the DAo, thereby establishing a transcatheter central shunt. Given the orientation of the vasculature, magnetic catheters could not be used for SVC-to-PA connections; however, perforation from the SVC to the right pulmonary artery was accomplished with a trans-septal needle and balloon target. Transcatheter Glenn or central shunts were successfully created in four swine [25].

Venous

Wang HH et al. have proposed the use of a novel magnetic compression technique (magnamosis) for creating a portacaval shunt in a canine model of portal hypertension. After portal hypertension was induced in 18 dogs by partial ligation of the portal vein (baseline), half had 6 weeks later a magnetic anastomosis rings porto-caval shunt vs. the other half getting manual suturing ($n = 9$, each) [26]. Anastomotic leakage did not occur and the operative time for magnamosis (4.1 min) was significantly less than manual suture (24.5 min, $P < 0.01$). Histology uncovered better evenness and continuity of the vascular intima with magnamosis than sutures. Portocaval pressures were similar; therefore, magnetic venous anastomosis appeared superior to manual suture for the creation of a portacaval shunt for the treatment of portal hypertension [26]. Yan achieved something similar in dogs and cadavers [27, 28]. In Figs. 13.3, 13.4, 13.5, and 13.6, the parent and daughter magnets are attached to catheters: one in the vena cava and the other in the portal vein.

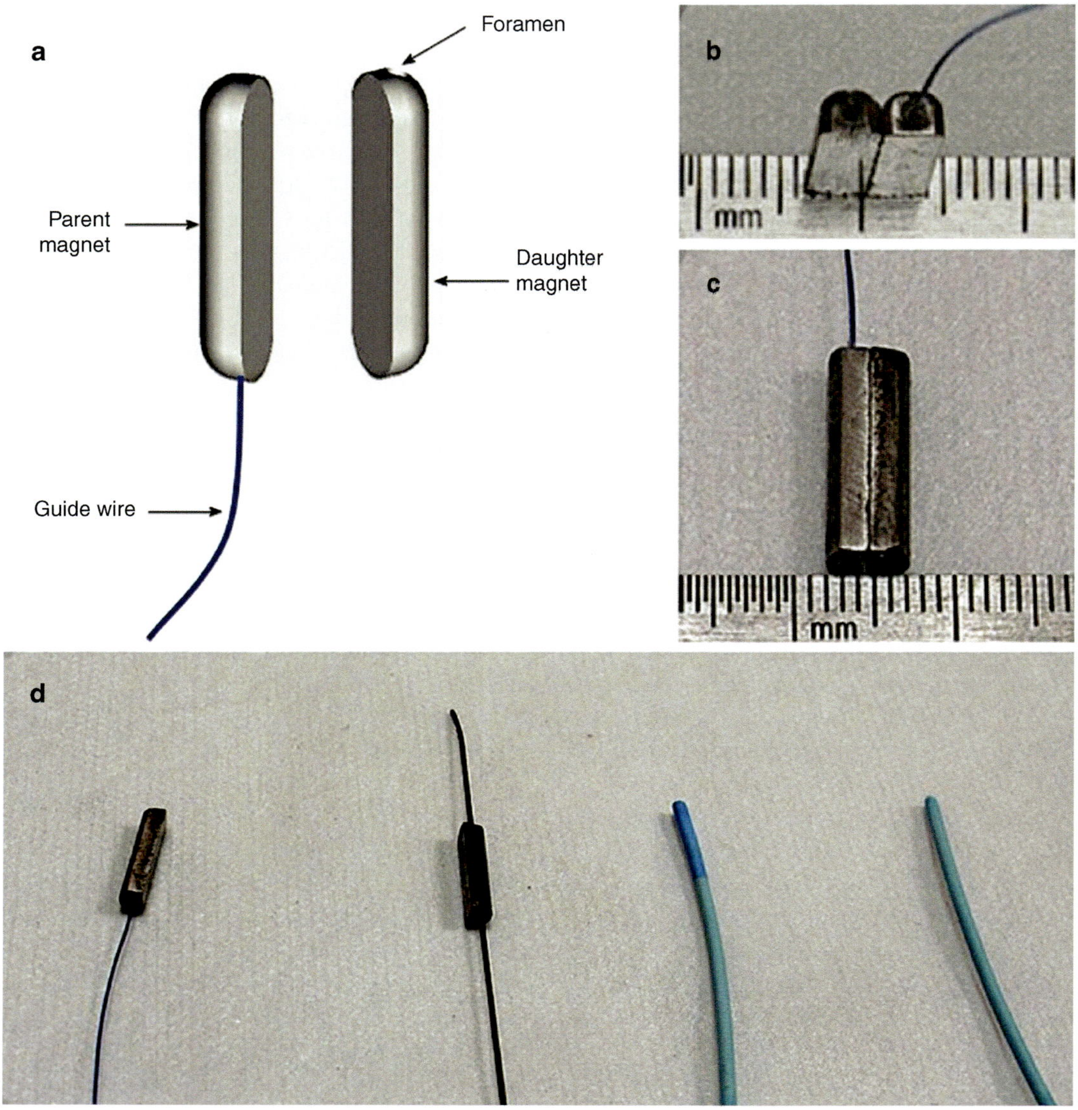

Fig. 13.3 Magnets for portocaval shunts. (**a**) Longitudinal parent and daughter magnets. (**b**, **c**) Sizes. (**d**) Catheter attachments. (From Yan et al. [28]. ©The Author(s) 2015. Published by Baishideng Publishing Group Inc. All rights reserved. Reprinted with permission)

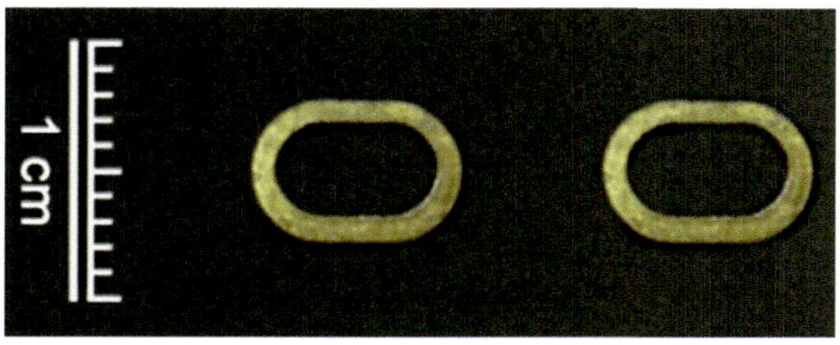

Fig. 13.4 Oval shape magnets. (Adapted with permission from Yang et al. [30])

Xue et al. pursued a similar concept for splenorenal shunts, explored in both a canine model and cadavers [29]. After manufacturing the devices based on CT image measurements from 30 patients with portal hypertension and in 20 adult cadavers, the magnetic splenorenal shunt procedure was performed in three dogs and five human cadavers. Follow-up at 7 days revealed necrotic tissues stuck between the two

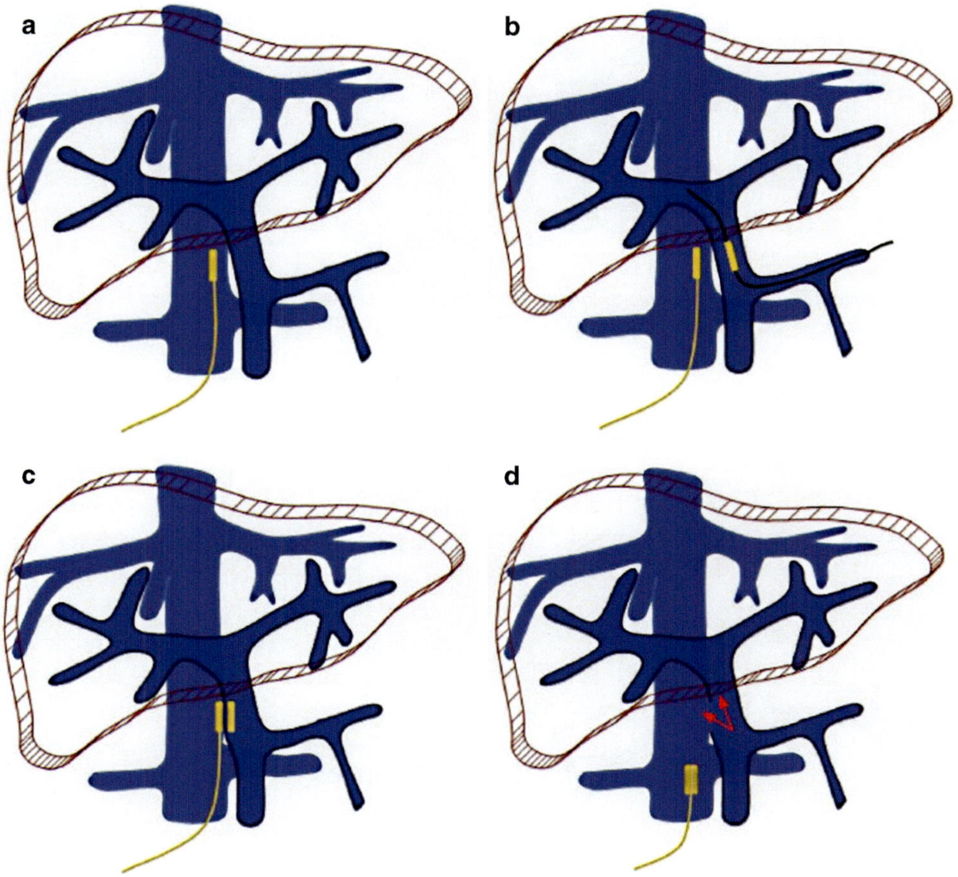

Fig. 13.5 Magnets in place in the portal vein and cava. (**a**) Parent magnet in venal cava. (**b**) Daughter magnet in portal vein. (**c**) Portal vein catheter removed, and attraction. (**d**) Patent anastomosis with retrieval from IVC. (From Yan et al. [28]. ©The Author(s) 2015. Published by Baishideng Publishing Group Inc. All rights reserved. Reprinted with permission)

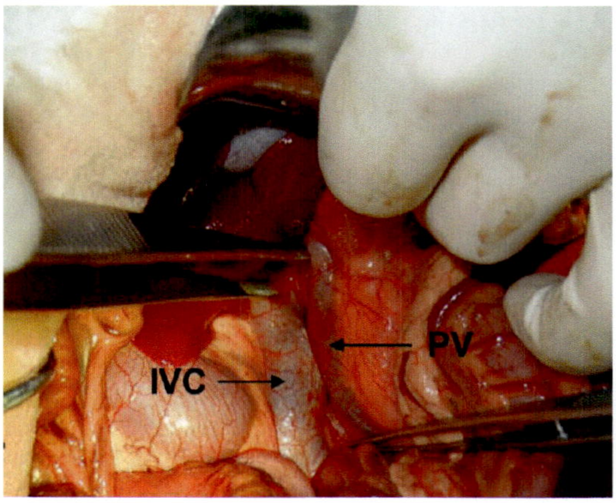

Fig. 13.6 Magnetic ring for vascular anastomosis in porto-cava shunt, intraoperative view. (From Yan et al. [27]. © 2013 Yan et al. Open-Access, distributed under the terms of the Creative Commons Attribution License)

magnets, which were shed, and the magnets were taken away with an anchor wire [29].

Apart from the portocaval shunt, the suprahepatic cava anastomosis to facilitate orthotopic liver transplantation has been explored. Using a rat model of orthotopic liver transplantation (OLT), Yang et al. used a magnetic anastomosis technique for connecting two vessels (Fig. 13.7) using the attractive force between two magnets (Fig. 13.8) and made the suprahepatic vena cava reconstruction much easier and significantly shortened [30]. Shi et al. confirmed those findings in their experiment [31, 32]. To improve the portal vein reconstructions, magnets were also used by Wang et al. [33].

Magnetic devices for anastomosing vein grafts to an artery have also been done in the

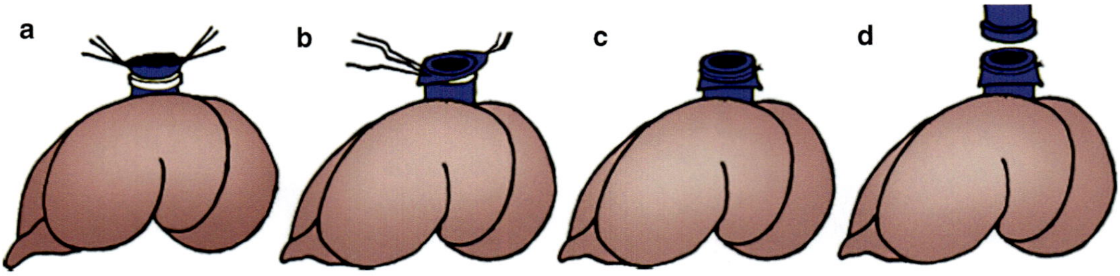

Fig. 13.7 Preparation and insertion of the rings for vascular anastomosis in suprahepatic venae cava. (**a**) Lowering (**b**) Eversion (**c**) Suture in place (**d**) Attraction. (Adapted with permission from Yang et al. [30])

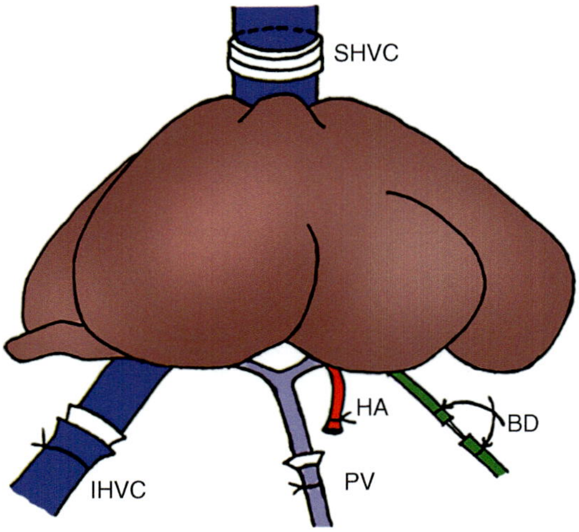

Fig. 13.8 Final results. (This is adapted with permission from Yang et al. [30])

laboratory. Indeed, Heitmann et al. looked at oval ring magnets using six male foxhounds. After femoral artery ligation, a femoral vein was harvested, reversed, and a magnet was inserted into each vessel lumen and a second magnet was placed outside the vessel but aligned directly over the intraluminal magnet, establishing a magnetic port in each vessel, creating a side-to-side anastomosis. After explant, there was no significant difference in flow resistance between the acute and 14-week grafts. Microscopic examination of 14-week anastomoses exhibited well-endothelialized vascular surfaces. It proved that oval ring magnets are useful for anastomosis of large and small vessels [34].

Conclusion

We must conclude that the field is fertile and should lead to clinical utilization of these magnetic devices for faster operating time and superior endothelialization that could lead to longer patency duration. It is unclear why such devices are not widely used clinically, is it conservatism in surgical practice?

References

1. Obora Y, Tamaki N, Matsumoto S. Nonsuture microvascular anastomosis using magnet rings: preliminary report. Surg Neurol. 1978;9(2):117–20.
2. Obora Y, Tamaki N, Matsumoto S. Nonsuture microvascular anastomosis using magnet rings (author's transl). Neurol Med Chir (Tokyo). 1980;20(5):497–505.
3. Erdmann D, Sweis R, Heitmann C, et al. Side-to-side sutureless vascular anastomosis with magnets. J Vasc Surg. 2004;40(3):505–11.
4. Soulez G, Gagner M, Therasse E, et al. Catheter-assisted totally thoracoscopic coronary artery bypass grafting: a feasibility study. Ann Thorac Surg. 1997;64(4):1036–40.
5. Garcia-Ruiz A, Smedira NG, Loop FD, et al. Robotic surgical instruments for dexterity enhancement in thoracoscopic coronary artery bypass graft. J Laparoendosc Adv Surg Tech A. 1997;7(5):277–83.
6. Filsoufi F, Farivar RS, Aklog L, et al. Automated distal coronary bypass with a novel magnetic coupler (MVP system). J Thorac Cardiovasc Surg. 2004;127(1):185–92.
7. Athanasiou T, Ashrafian H, Glenville B, Casula R. Coronary artery bypass with the use of a magnetic distal anastomotic device: surgical technique and preliminary experience. Heart Surg

Forum. 2004;7(6):356–9. https://doi.org/10.1532/HSF98.2004-1024.
8. Wong T, Mayet J, Casula RP. Minimal invasive direct revascularisation of the left anterior descending artery using a novel magnetic vascular anastomotic device. Heart. 2004;90(6):632. https://doi.org/10.1136/hrt.2003.023929. see attached paper
9. Liu S, Lei P, Lü Y, et al. Zhongguo Xiu Fu Chong Jian Wai Ke Za Zhi. 2014;28(7):885–90.
10. Falk V, Walther T, Jacobs S, Wolf RK, Mohr FW. Facilitated MIDCAB using a magnetic coupling device. Ann Thorac Surg. 2005;79(2):691–3.
11. Charitou A, Panesar SS, DeL Stanbridge R, Athanasiou T. Novel use of a magnetic coupling device to repair damage of the internal thoracic artery. J Card Surg. 2006;21(1):89–91.
12. Morbiducci U, Lemma M, Ponzini R, et al. Does the Ventrica magnetic vascular positioner (MVP) for coronary artery bypass grafting significantly alter local fluid dynamics? A numeric study. Int J Artif Organs. 2007;30(7):628–39.
13. Falk V, Walther T, Stein H, et al. Facilitated endoscopic beating heart coronary artery bypass grafting using a magnetic coupling device. J Thorac Cardiovasc Surg. 2003;126(5):1575–9.
14. Klima U, Falk V, Maringka M, et al. Magnetic vascular coupling for distal anastomosis in coronary artery bypass grafting: a multicenter trial. J Thorac Cardiovasc Surg. 2003;126(5):1568–74.
15. Klima U, Maringka M, Bagaev E, Kirschner S, Haverich A. Total magnetic vascular coupling for arterial revascularization. J Thorac Cardiovasc Surg. 2004;127(2):602–3.
16. Klima U, Kofidis T, Beilner J, Maringka M, Kirschner S, Haverich A. Anastomotic obstruction after magnetic vascular coupling after minimally invasive direct coronary artery bypass grafting. Ann Thorac Surg. 2006;81(2):728–9.
17. Vicol C, Eifert S, Oberhoffer M, et al. Early clinical results with a magnetic connector for distal coronary artery anastomoses. Ann Thorac Surg. 2005;79(5):1738–43.
18. Vicol C, Eifert S, Oberhoffer M, Boekstegers P, Reichart B. Mid-term patency after magnetic coupling for distal bypass anastomosis in coronary surgery. Ann Thorac Surg. 2006;82(4):1452–6.
19. Tossios P, Triantafillopoulou K, Sianos G, Karapanayiotides T, Foroulis CN. Magnetic connectors for coronary surgery: what do we know a decade later? Minim Invasive Ther Allied Technol. 2014;23(5):313–6.
20. Li H, Gale BK, Sant H, Shea J, David Bell E, Agarwal J. A novel vascular coupling system for end-to-end anastomosis. Cardiovasc Eng Technol. 2015;6(3):294–302.
21. Li H, Gale B, Shea J, Sant H, Terry CM, Agarwal J. Vascular coupling system for end-to-end anastomosis: an in vivo pilot case report. Cardiovasc Eng Technol. 2017;8(1):91–5.
22. Liu SQ, Lei P, Cao ZP, Lv Y, Li JH, Cui XH. Nonsuture anastomosis of arteries and veins using the magnetic pinned-ring device: a histologic and scanning electron microscopic study. Ann Vasc Surg. 2012;26(7):985–95.
23. Liu SQ, Lei P, Cui XH, et al. Sutureless anastomoses using magnetic rings in canine liver transplantation model. J Surg Res. 2013;185(2):923–33.
24. Cirillo M. A new concentric double prosthesis for sutureless, magnetic-assisted aortic arch inclusion. Med Hypotheses. 2016;89:89–95.
25. Levi DS, Danon S, Gordon B, et al. Creation of transcatheter aortopulmonary and cavopulmonary shunts using magnetic catheters: feasibility study in swine. Pediatr Cardiol. 2009;30(4):397–403.
26. Wang HH, Ma J, Wang SP, et al. Magnetic anastomosis rings to create portacaval shunt in a canine model of portal hypertension. J Gastrointest Surg. 2019;23(11):2184–92.
27. Yan X, Fan C, Ma J, et al. Portacaval shunt established in six dogs using magnetic compression technique. PLoS One. 2013;8(9):e76873. Published 2013 Sep 30.
28. Yan XP, Liu WY, Ma J, Li JP, Lv Y. Extrahepatic portacaval shunt via a magnetic compression technique: a cadaveric feasibility study. World J Gastroenterol. 2015;21(26):8073–80.
29. Xue F, Li J, Lu J, et al. Splenorenal shunt via magnetic compression technique: a feasibility study in canine and cadaver. Minim Invasive Ther Allied Technol. 2016;25(6):329–36.
30. Yang L, Lu J, Wang Y, et al. A rat model of orthotopic liver transplantation using a novel magnetic anastomosis technique for suprahepatic vena cava reconstruction. J Vis Exp. 2018;(133):56933. Published 2018 Mar 19.
31. Shi Y, Zhang W, Deng YL, et al. Magnetic ring anastomosis of suprahepatic vena cava: novel technique for liver transplantation in rat. Transpl Int. 2015;28(1):89–94. https://doi.org/10.1111/tri.12418.
32. Shi Y, Lv Y, Wang B, et al. Novel magnetic rings for rapid vascular reconstruction in canine liver transplantation model. Transplant Proc. 2006;38(9):3070–4. https://doi.org/10.1016/j.transproceed.2006.08.174.
33. Wang SP, Yan XP, Xue F, et al. Fast magnetic reconstruction of the portal vein with allogeneic blood vessels in canines. Hepatobiliary Pancreat Dis Int. 2015;14(3):293–9.
34. Heitmann C, Khan FN, Erdmann D, Olbrich KC, Adam Sharkawy A, Klitzman B. Vein graft anastomoses with magnets. J Plast Reconstr Aesthet Surg. 2007;60(12):1296–301. https://doi.org/10.1016/j.bjps.2006.10.017.

14 Laparoendoscopic Magnetic Gastrointestinal Anastomosis

Michel Gagner

Gastrointestinal, colic, and vascular anastomoses have been fashioned by the use of sutures, but accelerated with the study of Antoine Lembert, a surgeon at the Hotel-Dieu de Paris, on the use of serosal sutures for apposition in 1826 [1]. Results varied in degrees of healing capabilities with or without permanent scarring, depending on the suture size, force, and material (permanent or temporary, absorbable or non-absorbable, from cotton to silk and catgut, chromic, nylon, wires, polyglycolic acids). Stapling was introduced in the early 1900s and becoming popular in the last half of the twentieth century which continues to this day. However, compression anastomoses have had a parallel development, which is important to review here.

The Murphy button, invented in 1892 by Dr. Murphy, was one of the first attempts to mechanize and standardize gastrointestinal compression anastomosis (Fig. 14.1a) [2]. This button has two hollow nickel-plated brass pieces. The male piece has a spring-loaded center band which inserts into the female piece and a purse string is delivered to both intestinal ends, resulting in a fast anastomosis (Fig. 14.1b). Indeed, John Benjamin Murphy (1857–1916), an American surgeon who practiced as Professor of Surgery at Rush Medical College and Northwestern University Medical School in Chicago, was a pioneer in recognizing the symptoms of appendicitis and recommended immediate removal of the appendix when a certain symptomatic pattern appeared [3].

The Mayo brothers published a small series of cases of gastroenterostomy, cholecystoduodenostomy, and various colic resections or enteric bypasses done in 1894 and added several unpublished from other American surgeons [4]. Leveen published in 1949 on its use for vascular anastomosis and later Prioton reported on esophageal applications [5, 6].

And so after 100 years of the Murphy button [7], a biodegradable one made of polyglycolic acid was manufactured. The Valtrac™ is a biodegradable compression button that squeezes tissue to perform an endoluminal digestive anastomosis (Fig. 14.2). In the context of Continuous development in the area of anastomotic sutures lead to exceptional results in surgical practice, the biofragmentable anastomosis ring (BAR) described in 1985 by Hardy et al. represented a breakthrough in a 100-year search of a paradigm [8, 9].

It was Czerny, in 1896 who stated the following: "The task of technology is ... to create buttons with material that is entirely or partly dissolved in the intestinal lumen." Then, polyglycolic acid, developed in the 60s and used for resorbable surgical sutures, was the material needed to redesign the Murphy's button into a resorbable button for quick GI anastomosis. Indeed, the Biofragmentable Anastomotic Ring (BAR) (Valtrac, Davis & Geck, Inc.) was an

M. Gagner (✉)
Hôpital du Sacré-Cœur de Montréal, Montréal, QC, Canada

Chief of Surgery, Westmount Square Surgical Center, Westmount, QC, Canada

M. Gagner (ed.), *Magnetic Surgery*, https://doi.org/10.1007/978-3-030-73947-8_14

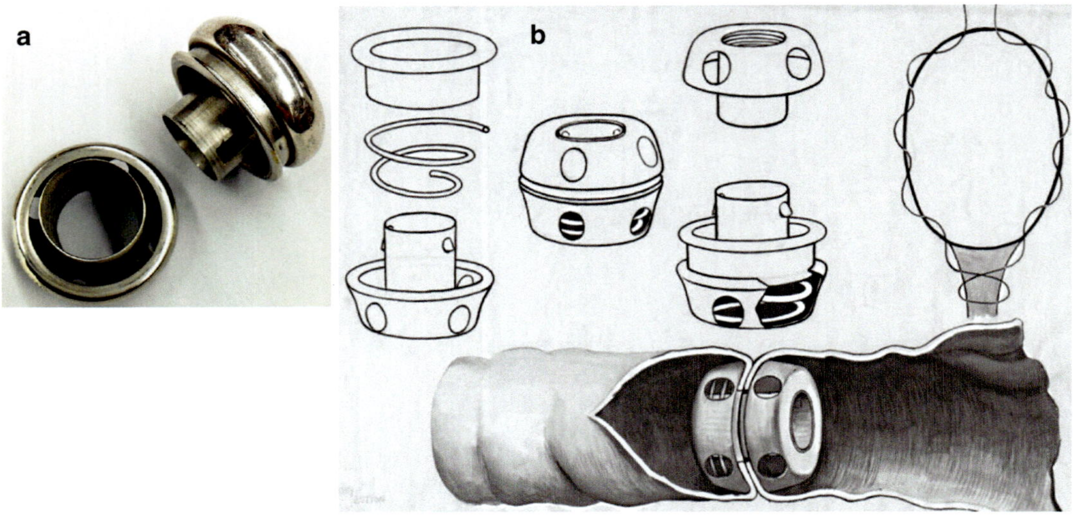

Fig. 14.1 (**a**) Murphy's button. Both metal ends separated. (**b**) Components, purse-stringing, and position in the bowel lumen

Fig. 14.2 (**a**) Biofragmentable Anastomotic Ring, Valtrac™ 1984 design. (**b**) Actual device mounted on a plastic delivery stick. (**c**) From open to closed positions

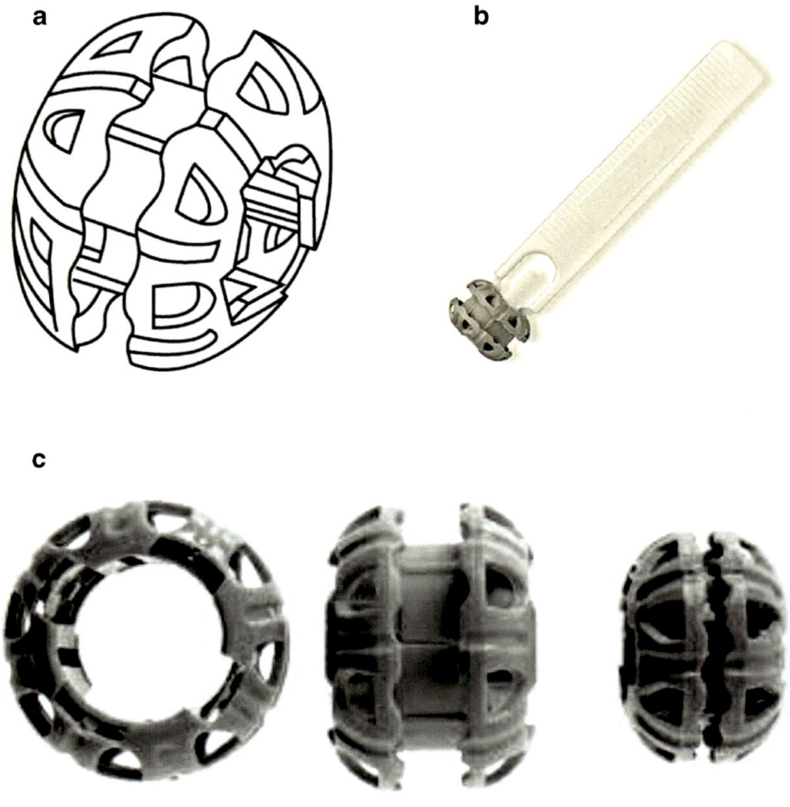

approved device intended for colonic anastomosis initially. Anastomosis is achieved by placing the two bowel lumens over the device, tying the purse-string sutures snugly, and after approximating both ends, the device closed with a click sound. The BAR fragments are passed in stools about 3 weeks postoperatively. Hardy animal experiments in 1985 and later a human series of 27 patients published in 1987 established the solid proof that biofragmentable bowel anastomosis rings (BAR) for sutureless intestinal anastomosis were safe [8, 10]. Those patients had bowel anastomoses with BAR without early complications, although one developed a stenosis perhaps caused by ischemia.

Hardy et al. did studies in dogs to look at the strengths of these anastomosis over time [11]. More specifically, wound healing, strength of the BAR, classic hand suturing, and metal staple colonic anastomoses were compared for intervals of up to 1 year. The BARs fragmented at a mean time of 15 days and passed per anus without incident. Gross healing evaluations at 21 days and beyond showed no differences from any anastomotic method. Microscopic evaluations suggested that residual granulation tissue was less with BAR than with regular sutures or metal staples at 1-year interval. This implies that wound healing is better with BAR than with standard methods of colon anastomosis, that when the wound scaffolding disappears between 14 and 21 days, it permits the return of a normal histology between the two merged ends [11].

Corman et al. published a randomized prospective study in 1989 of 438 patients, looking into the safety and efficacy of the Valtrac™ biofragmentable anastomotic ring compared with stapling and sutures [12]. It showed no significant difference in the morbidity, mortality, and clinical course of the patients. Further, it reestablished intestinal continuity more rapidly. Another one in 1991, essentially confirmed the latter [13]. It revealed no significant differences in wound complication, infections, bleeding, leaks, obstruction, or deaths. They were similar in return of bowel function, return to normal diet, or hospital stays. There were some concerns about intraoperative difficulties, which occurred in 17% of BAR patients, significantly higher (<0.001) than for sutured anastomoses, but these problems did not adversely affect the satisfactory outcome. In this series of 47 patients ranging from 14 to 82 years of age, various colonic resections and anastomosis with this absorbable device were successful with no anastomotic leaks and no complications [14].

I attempted to do this laparoscopically, colocolonic end-to-end anastomosis, in a series of canine experiments at Hotel-Dieu de Montreal in the early 1990s, but it required too much force laparoscopically [15]. A year later Sackier et al. found the same thing, that because of the need to have to "click" the device closed, BAR anastomosis after laparoscopic-assisted resection was rarely feasible intra-abdominally, perhaps when the anastomosis is exteriorized and hands can be used on the bowel itself [16]. Initially, the large diameter device precluded intestinal anastomosis, but eventually a smaller 25 mm and 21 mm diameters permitted small bowel anastomosis, including the smaller ileum in female patients as well as some parts of the duodenum.

It was quite popular in the 90s, I have seen it used for colic and intestinal anastomosis and it was used by Picard Marceau and Simon Biron from Quebec City in bariatric surgery to create the duodeno-ileal anastomosis during duodenal switches using a Valtrac™ 21 (21 mm circumference), creating a lumen of approximately 7 mm. It then slowly disappeared with the use of laparoscopic surgery, as the Valtrac™ required forceful hand closure and was causing dangerous lacerations on the bowel when laparoscopic instruments were used. Also, laparoscopic linear stapling technology appeared at the same time. The most recent publication in Chinese literature in 2017 attested that it is still in clinical use [17].

The literature then moved to the usage of compression anastomosis, using spring-loaded Nitinol Titanium rings (Fig. 14.3). Indeed, Stewart et al., with Dr. J. Fleshman as senior author, had looked at the use of an NITI Endoluminal Compression Anastomosis Ring (EndoCAR) to form compression anastomoses [18]. A total of 18 swine were utilized, using a 27-mm compression device and a 29-mm stapler, randomized to proximal and distal rectum. At 14 days, compression anastomoses had higher mean failure pressures than regular stapled anastomoses at the time the anastomosis was made (103 vs. 29.9 mm Hg). After 2 weeks, there was no difference between failure pressures (256 vs. 250 mm Hg). The mean anastomotic circumference of the compression anastomoses was narrower than the stapled anastomoses (9.6 vs. 11.3 cm, P = 0.001).

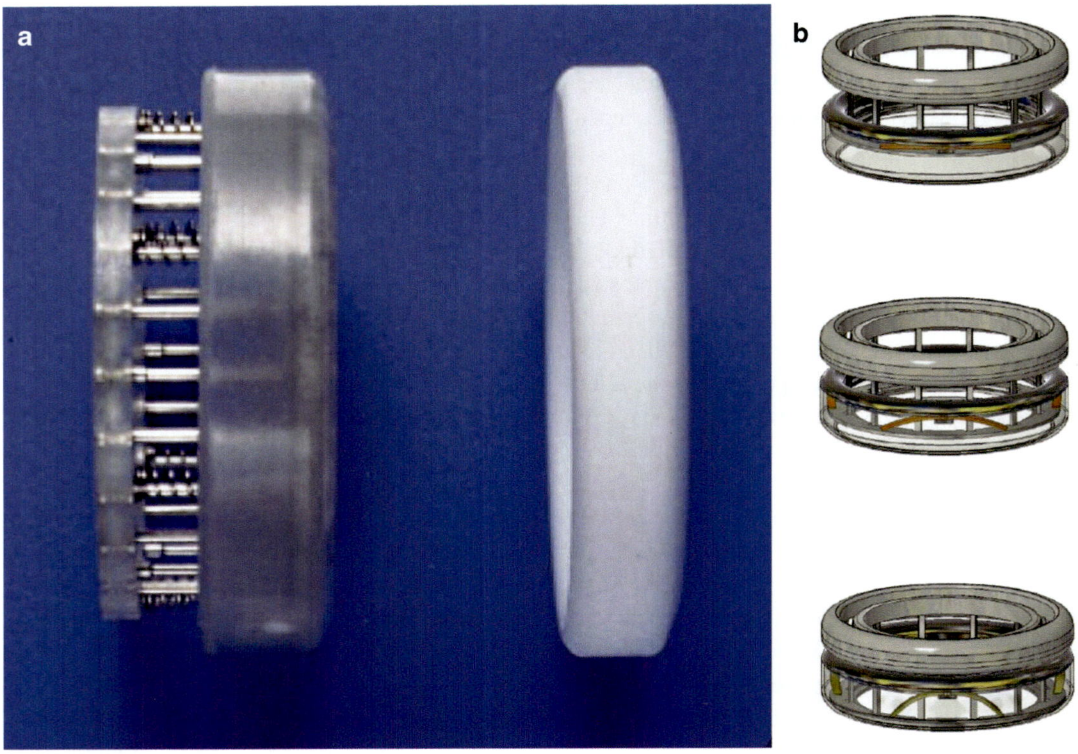

Fig. 14.3 NiTi™ Surgical Solutions (**a**) Components, side view. (**b**) From open to closed positions

There were no clinical leaks or radiographic leaks by barium enema at 2 weeks, no difference histologically. There were more dense adhesions to 7 of 12 (58.3%) of the stapled anastomoses, and only 1 of 12 flimsy adhesions (8.3%) from the NITI anastomoses. It was concluded that this new NITI Endoluminal Compression Anastomosis Ring might reduce leaks and eliminate foreign material, like titanium or permanent sutures, in the anastomosis [18].

Human clinical experiences followed. In a different early study on patients, Tulchinsky et al. exposed their clinical experience with the shape memory compression bowel anastomosis using a nickel and titanium alloy BioDynamix anastomosis with ColonRing™ for large-bowel end-to-end or side-to-end anastomosis. It was specifically compared to the standard double-stapled colorectal/colo-colonic anastomosis [19]. Ten study patients were compared to 13 matched controls, with a median anastomotic distance from the anal verge of 10 cm (6–20 cm). There were no anastomotic leaks and three minor complications in each group; however, two patients required transanal digital extraction of the ring, which was detached but not expelled. Therefore, the design of the closed rings was required to pass more easily and was modified with a smaller diameter for easiness of expulsion and travel in the bowel lumen [19].

The team of Dr. Stamos from the University of California in Irvine reported on the first human use in USA of the NiTi CAR™ 27, between March 2008 and August 2009 [20]. Used in 23 patients for a left-sided colectomy, the CAR™ 27 devices were positioned for a compression anastomosis. There were only minor morbidities, three of 23 (13%) patients, included one small postoperative abscess and two anastomotic strictures requiring balloon dilation. However, one patient required a surgical dismantling of the anastomosis and diversion for a partial anastomotic dehiscence/leak, concluding that larger series and multicenter studies are needed.

Certainly Hur et al. have moved to such multicenter prospective randomized trial to determine the clinical efficacy of the NiTi Hand CAC 30, a type of compression anastomosis clip (CAC), for jejunojejunostomy in gastric cancer surgery [21]. Forty-seven patients from six institutions who were diagnosed with gastric adenocarcinoma were enrolled. These patients were randomized to a CAC group and a hand-sewn (control) group. Of the 44 patients analyzed, 20 had the CAC and 24 had the hand-sewn anastomosis.

Anastomosis time was faster in the CAC group than in the control group ($P < 0.001$), but the complication rates of the two groups did not differ ($P = 0.908$). However, jejunojejunostomy leakage occurred in two patients in the CAC group. It is not clear from the manuscript why two leaks occurred, and it was concluded that the extended use of the NiTi Hand CAC™ 30 should be carefully applied.

Kim et al. also used the same device, the NiTi endoluminal Compression Anastomotic Clip (CAC™) 30 (NiTi CAC30) (NiTi Alloys Technologies, Ltd., Netanya, Israel), to investigate the safety and early surgical outcomes of intestinal anastomosis in patients with gastrointestinal malignancy [22]. No differences were noted with conventional group; the study provided additional information about migration and expulsion of the device. First, migration started in one patient between 3 and 5 days, 11 patients between 6 and 7 days, and 37 patients after 8 days. The expulsion of 31 cases occurred between post-op weeks 2 and 3. The NiTi CAC 30 was expulsed within 1 week in four patients and between 1 and 2 weeks in eight patients. An expulsion occurred in one case at over 4 weeks. No problems related to early migration and expulsion were observed, and no anastomotic leakage and bleeding occurred.

In a multinational (16 countries), multicenter (178 centers) data registry provided by NiTi Surgical Solutions (Netanya, Israel), we retrospectively examined clinical data of patients who underwent elective laparoscopic or open left-sided colectomy and anterior resection from January 2008 to June 2010 [23]. A total of 1180 patients underwent end-to-end anastomosis using the ColonRing device during the study period. The overall anastomotic leak rate was 3% and the median length of hospital stay was 6 days. The median ring expulsion time was 8 days, with earliest ring expulsion time at 6 days. However, in one patient, the ring did not expel. In four patients, the anastomosis had to be immediately recreated because of one misfiring and three incomplete anastomoses. The use of the ColonRing device was considered feasible and safe for end-to-end colorectal anastomosis.

In a single-center study, 157 consecutive patients who received an operation between March 2010 and December 2011 were retrospectively assessed. The Niti CAR 27 (CAR group, 63 patients) colorectal anastomoses were compared with the conventional double-stapled (CDS group, 94 patients) colorectal anastomoses [24]. Intraoperative, immediate postoperative, and 6-month follow-up data were recorded. There were no statistically significant differences between the two groups in terms of age, gender, tumor location, and other clinical characteristics. One patient (1.6%) in the CAR group and two patients (2.1%) in the CDS group experienced complications of anastomotic leakage ($P = 0.647$). These three patients underwent a diverting loop ileostomy. There were two cases (2.1%) of bleeding at the anastomosis site in the CDS group. All patients underwent a follow-up colonoscopy (median, 6 months). One patient in the CAR group experienced anastomotic stricture (1.6% vs. 0%; $P = 0.401$). This complication was resolved by using balloon dilatation. Anastomosis using the Niti CAR 27 device in a laparoscopic anterior resection for sigmoid colon cancer is safe and feasible. Its use is equivalent to that of the conventional double-stapler.

Most of these devices were from NiTi™ Surgical Solutions, and according to this company, the unique line of products utilized Nitinol-based elements to press together the ends of resected tissue, enabling seamless anastomosis of the intestine after removing a section. After it was cleared for use by the US Food and Drug Administration and CE-certified, NiTi's innovative devices were declared suitable for open, laparoscopic, and hand-assisted laparoscopic (HALS) surgeries.

NiTi Surgical Solutions Ltd. was founded in 1996 as a privately held, venture-backed company headquartered in Israel, with sales offices in the USA and representatives around the globe. In 2009, the company had raised $18.5 million in a financing round led by Dutch life sciences and biomedical venture capital fund Forbion Capital Partners. NiTi's investors included Israeli and European funds Alice Ventures, Evergreen Venture Partners, Israel Healthcare Ventures Ltd., Kreos Capital, Millennium Material Technologies Fund, and Vitalife Life Sciences Venture. NiTi is a graduate of Meytav Technological Enterprises Innovation Center Ltd., a technology incubator owned by Capital Point Ltd. NiTi was founded by its CSO, Dr. Leonid Monassevitch, formerly a senior researcher of shape memory alloys at the Siberian Institute of Physics and Technology. NiTi president and CEO Itay Itzhaky was CEO of ColBar, which was sold in 2016 to Johnson & Johnson for $159 million.

Thousands of BioDynamix™ Anastomosis cases have been completed in hundreds of medical centers around the world with both the ColonRing™ and the Hand CAC™ 30. The ColonRing™ has been successfully used in various regions of the colon and rectum (≤4 to >50 cm from the anal verge) regardless of age, gender, and BMI. Surgeons have confirmed ease of use and removal of the deployment device and the absence of disruption caused to the anastomosis due to the post-deployment anvil residing distal to the anastomosis. Eventually, Niti Surgical Solutions was renamed as novoGI. It was announced in June 1, 2012 that novoGI was now led by Gavriel Meron, the founding President and CEO of Given Imaging Ltd., which pioneered Capsule Endoscopy. By mid-2012, it had been used globally in more than 10,000 patients undergoing colorectal resection procedures. In December 2013, it was announced that 100% of Given Imaging's shares were purchased by Covidien for over 800 million, and then, in 2015, Covidien itself was purchased by Medtronic [25].

Strangely, in spite of these clinical successes, since the acquisitions, this technology has not reappeared on the markets nor in publications since, perhaps a business strategy by a stapling company to "kill" the concept before it gets too successful? This is unfortunate, as patients have not benefited from this and surgeons have fewer choices. We are left with the experience of endoluminal magnets.

The historical aspects of magnets have been reviewed in Chap. 3 and will not be repeated here, except to mention that in 2005, Chopita et al. published a series of patients treated for malignant obstruction of the upper digestive tract using a novel technique of endoscopic gastroenteric anastomosis using magnets (EGAM) [26, 27]. They treated 15 patients (13 men, 2 women; mean age 64.5 years) with EGAM for malignant obstructions and had monthly follow-ups between December 2001 and May 2003. The procedure was efficacious in 13 patients (89%) with a mean survival of 5 months. Four minor complications (31%) were encountered during the follow-up period. Their results demonstrated the feasibility, safety, and efficacy of creating a gastroenteric anastomosis endoscopically with magnets; it appeared to be safe in the short term as there was no mortality related to the procedure.

I always had a strong interest in developing this for the treatment of diabetes and severe obesity; hence, I had the idea of creating a short circuit with the GI tract, mainly between the proximal and distal gut, to create an incretins surge by the ileum and another from the colon. Those ideas permitted the creation and foundation of a company in Minneapolis called "Endometabolic Solutions Inc." in 2007, with the engineer David Blaeser, the late engineer Dale Spencer, and me as co-founder. By early 2009, venture capitalist firm McNerney and partners, also from Minneapolis, had provided $3.8 millions in round A of financing. One of several animal experiments that led to this endoluminal GI anastomosis was published [28, 29]. The first patent was deposed in July 15, 2009 and had the magnetic anastomosis incorporated between the proximal and distal GI tract (Fig. 14.4).

In the purest form of malabsorptive surgery for weight loss, the jejunoileal bypass (JIB), one of the earliest types of bariatric surgery, was introduced with its many variations more than five decades ago. The JIB was performed end-to-

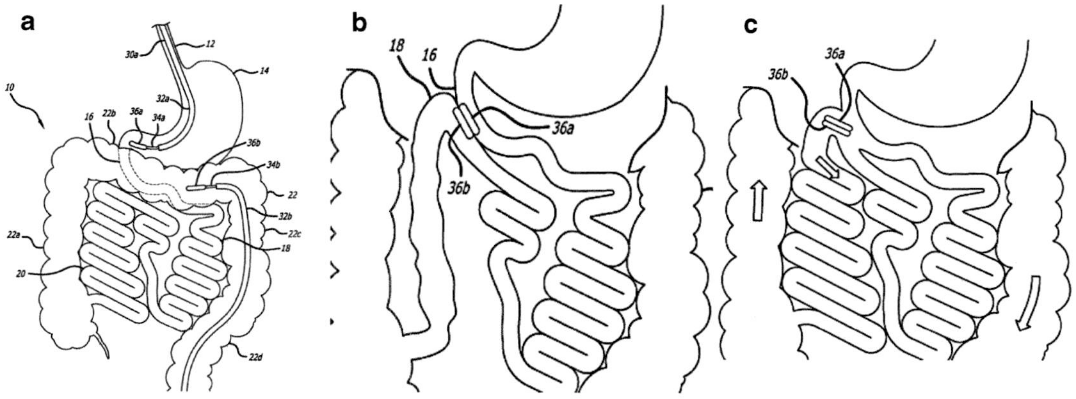

Fig. 14.4 (**a**) Linear magnetic anastomosis. Positioning the proximal piece in the duodenum by gastroscopy and the distal piece in the ileum, but with initial travel in the colon by colonoscopy. (**b**) Final position of the proximal and distal linear magnets for a duodeno-ileal anastomosis. (**c**) After tissue compression, passage of united linear magnets distally, for transanal natural evacuation

side, with the proximal 30 cm jejunum anastomosed to the distal 15 cm of ileum, or end-to-end, with bypassed small bowel derived end-to-side to the colon. In both instances, more than 90% of small intestine was bypassed, unexcised, excluding it from the alimentary channel leaving a blind end, causing bacterial overgrowth.

Excellent weight loss and complete resolution of type-2 diabetes mellitus were reported after JIB [30, 31]. However, a variety of serious complications related to JIB were reported including hypoalbuminemia, hypokalemia, hypocalcemia, hyperbilirubinemia, migratory polyarthralgias, calcium oxalate urinary calculi, and elevated liver enzymes levels and deaths due to liver failure [32, 33]. Diarrhea and flatulence were common. The excluded intestinal segment was associated with various problems including intussusceptions, bypass enteritis, and colonic pseudo-obstruction. Other authors reported that the risk of progressive liver disease existed indefinitely, and that ongoing careful follow-up was necessary [34, 35].

However, when a 90% small bowel resection in germ-free rats is compared to a 90% small bowel bypass, the resected animals have retained normal liver histology after a prolonged period. This means that any blind limb promoting bacterial overgrowth is possibly responsible for liver insufficiency. Therefore, the development of a new surgical malabsorptive procedure should not involve any blind segment [36]. A model of partial malabsorptive bypass is constructed with a side-to-side anastomosis between the second and third portions of the duodenum and last 50 cm of the ileum (anatomically in close proximity), allowing a partial flow of nutrients to move in the proximal jejunum for normal mineral absorption and caloric intake, while a portion is bypassed into the distal ileum, causing a decreased absorption resulting in weight loss. Since both limbs have flow, bacterial overgrowth is of a lesser concern, theoretically comparable to Roux-en-Y gastric bypass. To perform this anastomosis, a compression anastomotic device was used for its simplicity.

Compression anastomotic devices for the performance of gastrointestinal anastomosis have been available for more than a century and used extensively in colon surgery in its resorbable form, more recently simulating a commercial end-to-end anastomotic device [4, 12, 18].

The animal protocol was approved by the Institutional Animal Care and Use Committee (IACUC) of American Preclinical Services, LLC (APS), a facility licensed with the United States Department of Agriculture. We used seven Yorkshire pigs, >2 months old, weighing approximately 40–60 kg, and housed individually. The porcine diet consisted of a fixed formula certified by the manufacturer to be free of environmental contaminants; tap water was given ad libitum. Blood samples were taken for minimal hematology parameters (red blood cell count, hemoglobin, hematocrit, platelet count, white blood cell count, and differential), minimal serum biochemistry parameters (urea nitrogen (BUN), creatinine, total protein, albumin, aspartate aminotransferase (AST), gamma-glutamyl transferase (GGT), glucose, sodium, potassium, chloride, calcium, phosphorus, bicarbonate). Prior to surgery, animals were administered a 3-day bowel prep with 2 l per day of Golitely (PEG-3350, Braintree Laboratories, Inc., Braintree, MA) and Ensure (Abbott Nutrition, Columbus, OH) to cleanse the colon, and were fasted the night before except for water. Preoperative medication included Telazol 2–8 mg/kg for anesthesia induction (Tiletamine HCL and Zolazepram HCL, Animal Healthcare, Wyeth (now Pfizer, Inc.), Fort Dodge, IA), Xylazine 2–8 mg/kg (Bayer Healthcare, Leverkusen, Germany) for anesthesia induction, Buprenorphine 0.01–0.05 mg/kg for pain management (Buprenex, Reckitt & Colman Pharmaceuticals, Inc., Richmond, VA), and Oxytetracycline (long acting) 20 mg/kg (Hebei New Century Pharmaceutical Co., Ltd., Hebei, China) for infection prophylaxis.

Four animals were allocated to a side-to-side duodenoileostomy with the compression anastomotic device, 3 to a control group. After endotracheal intubation, anesthesia was maintained with isoflurane in 100% O2 and propofol at 2–8 mg/kg, with an intravenous Ringers' lactate solution at 2–10 ml/kg/hr. After laparotomy with a 25-cm upper midline incision, a duodenotomy of approximately 2.5 cm was created anterior to admit the proximal part of the compression anastomotic device, and an ileotomy approximately 50 cm from the ileocecal valve was made to insert the distal part compression anastomotic device. The anastomosis was performed by compression of both parts away from the duodenotomy and ileotomy. Both openings of the small bowel were closed with a running suture of 3-0 Vicryl (Polyglactin-910, Ethicon, Cincinnati, OH). The control group had both enterotomies closed with a running suture only. A liver biopsy was also performed by a wedge. The abdominal wound is closed with Vicryl 1-0 for fascia and 3-0 for skin.

During recovery in the pen and postoperative period, the animals received Buprenorphine 0.01–0.05 mg/kg IM as needed, ketoprofen 1.8–2.2 mg/kg IM daily for the first 3 days (Ketofen, Fort Dodge Animal Health, Fort Dodge, IA), Prilosec 20 mg once daily (Omeprazole, AstraZeneca, Wilmington, DE), and Oxytetracycline (long acting) 18–25 mg/kg IM on day 3. During the first 24 hours, the animals could drink water; afterward, soft food was introduced to gradually progress to a normal solid diet over 10 days. Elimination of the device was recorded, including signs of infection. Blood samples were taken at days 0, 3, and 56.

On Day 28, a gastroscopy (Olympus, GIF-2 T20, 11.2 mm diameter) was performed under general anesthesia using a similar protocol, and photographs were obtained of the anastomosis and nearby intraluminal organs to assess patency, diameter, and degree of inflammation and presence of macroscopic abnormalities. An attempt was made to measure the intestinal shunting from the procedure by introducing approximately 25 radiopaque doughnut-type markers (Sitzmark, Konsyl Pharmaceutis, Inc., TX) in the proximal stomach for a gastrointestinal transit study, by taking abdominal x-rays every 2 hours for 6 hours.

At 8 weeks, euthanasia and necropsy of the abdominal cavity were performed. Samples of the liver were taken at the time of the anastomotic procedure (pre-sample) and at necropsy (left medial liver lobe, post-sample) and immersion-fixed in 10% neutral buffered formalin (NBF). The gastrointestinal tract was rinsed with water to remove food content and images were taken of each excised anastomotic site. Additionally, a sample of the right gluteus maximus was procured from each animal. All tissue samples were immersion-fixed in 10% NBF. Two sections from each anastomotic site were trimmed, sections of pre- and post-anastomosis lever samples and a section of right gluteus maximus skeletal muscle were taken for histological processing. The sections were placed in labeled cassettes and tissues

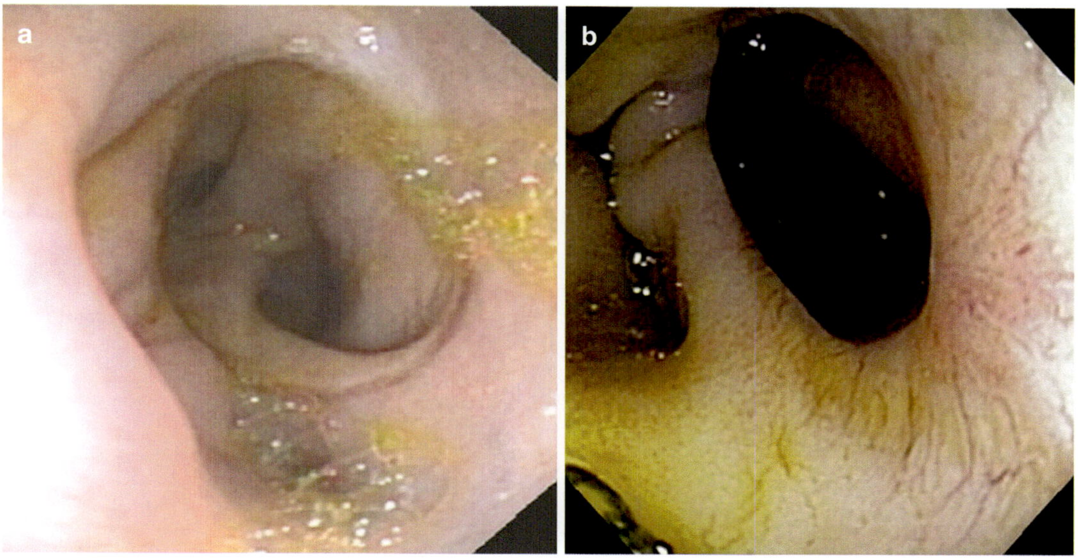

Fig. 14.5 (**a**) Duodenoscopy of the third portion of the duodenum, showing a healed side-to-side duodeno-ileal anastomosis, with proximal ileum on the right and distal ileum on the left of the figure. (**b**) Duodenoscopy of the third portion of the duodenum from a different subject, showing a healed side-to-side duodeno-ileal anastomosis, with distal duodenum on the far right of the figure

were processed through a graded series of alcohols, embedded in paraffin, cut with a rotary microtome to approximately 5 μm in thickness, mounted on microscopic slides, and stained with hematoxylin and eosin (H & E) and Masson's trichrome stains. American Preclinical Services (APS) sent the digital images taken at necropsy, completed gross pathology forms, trim sheets, and microscopic slides to a board-certified veterinary pathologist for independent interpretation. The sections of the anastomotic sites were evaluated for healing response and the presence of inflammation, infection, or dehiscence at the site of apposition.

At 28 days post-surgery, all pigs were healthy, with good appetite, eating the proposed diet with normal feces. However, one pig had developed a small, external incisional hernia, which had to be corrected. At 28 days, duodenoscopy of all animals showed a widely patent healed side-to-side duodeno-ileal anastomosis, with proximal ileum on the right and distal ileum on the left (Fig. 14.5). The gastroscope was able to pass through the anastomosis in all limbs. There was no evidence of gross ulcerations in all parts of the duodenum nor in the ileum. There was no visible inflammation either. The anastomosis itself revealed a smooth transition between both mucosae. Since the pigs had been fasting, mostly bilious fluids with saponification from the air insufflations were visible. We were not successful in determining various gastrointestinal transit times from both limbs, as the transit of markers was too slow (the majority remained in the stomach during the study period).

Weight progression in both the DI animals and controls was recorded weekly and plotted for comparison. In fact, for better understanding of the progression, the mean percentage of weight change from baseline in animals that had a side-to-side duodeno-ileal anastomosis (study group) versus sham controls, over time in days was projected (Fig. 14.6). At 56 days, control animals had gained 33.2% of weight, while study animals had lost 6.8% of weight. Figure 14.7 shows the weight loss in kilograms from duodenocolic anastomosis, not reported in this chapter.

Mean values for hematological profiles at baseline, day 3, and day 56 show a decline in RBC count (−21%), hemoglobin (−15%), hema-

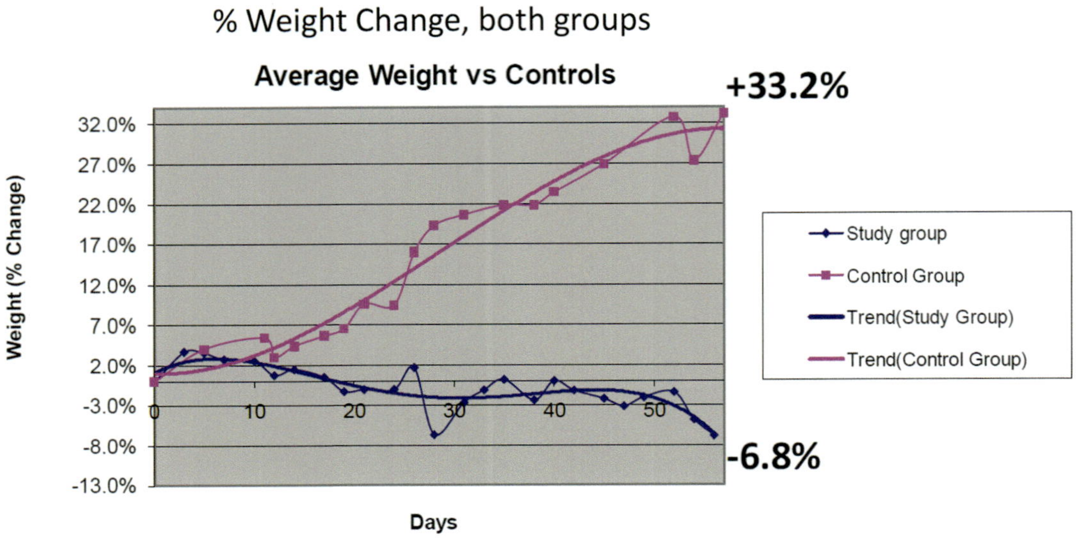

Fig. 14.6 Graph of % of weight change in animals that had a side-to-side duodeno-ileal anastomosis (study group) versus sham controls, over time in days. At 56 days, control animals had gained 33.2% of weight, while study animals had lost 6.8% of weight

Fig. 14.7 Graph of weight change in animals that had a side-to-side duodeno-colic anastomosis

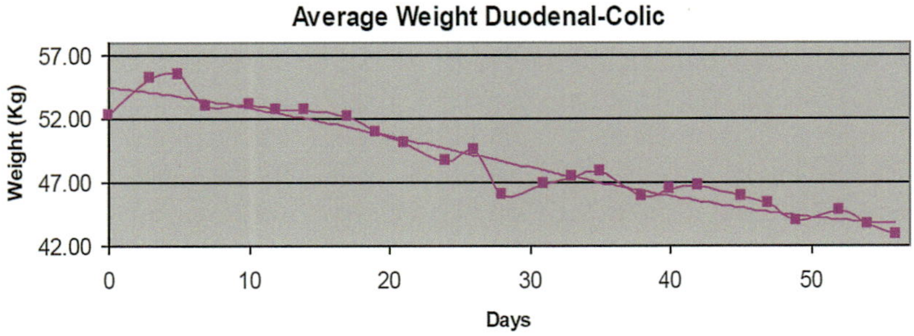

tocrit (−19%) and increases in platelet counts (+60%) and WBC counts (+16%) at 56 days, compared to baseline. Equally, mean values of serum biochemical profiles at baseline, days 3 and 36. After a slight increase (+33%) in serum glucose at day 3, presumably from stress response after surgery, the mean value returns within normal range at 56 days. There is a notable decrease in serum total protein and albumin at 56 days by 23% and 25%, attributable to a fixed diet. Equally, the BUN has increased threefold at 56 days. Nitrogen loss maybe attributable to inadequate intake of calories from a restricted diet and decreased absorption from bypass of the GI tract. A slight and subtle change of serum calcium (−11%) and phosphorus (−17%) is observed at 56 days, but within normal range, and may parallel the decrease in serum proteins. The serum potassium, sodium, chloride, and bicarbonate remained within normal range. The only serum liver enzyme measured remained constantly normal.

At necropsy, general flimsy adhesions were encountered near the anastomosis; the liver had a normal macroscopic appearance. Each gastroduodenal area was harvested for measurements and histological sampling. Macroscopic external view of a side-to-side duodeno-ileal anastomosis revealed a smooth surface serosal apposition, and inside the anastomosis could admit the index finger. Once this duodeno-ileal anastomosis was opened along its longitudinal axis, a smooth sur-

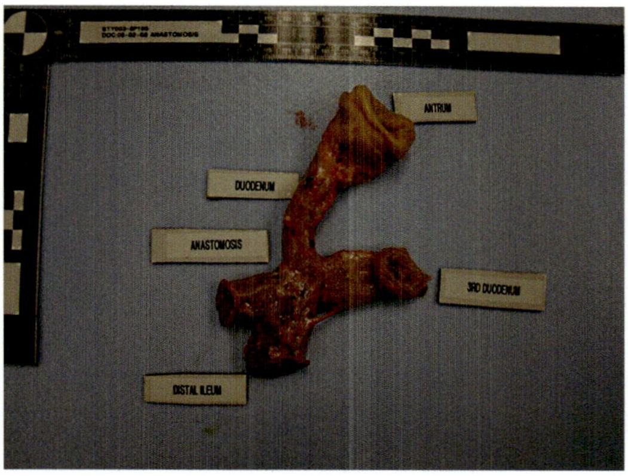

Fig. 14.8 Macroscopic external view of a side-to-side duodeno-colic anastomosis at 56 days

face was revealed. Figure 14.8 shows the macroscopic external view of a side-to-side duodeno-colic anastomosis, revealing a smooth surface serosal apposition.

All layers of the intestine were well healed with good apposition of the mucosa and muscular layers of the duodenum and ileum. A variable amount of fibrous connective tissue was noted in the muscular layers of the two apposed edges of the intestine which extended into the surrounding muscle bundles. The muscle layers at the anastomotic site appeared to align. The vasculature throughout the intestinal sections appeared normal with no evidence of thrombus formation or occlusion. Mild serosal edema was seen, and serosa vessels appeared prominent with some perivascular edema noted. No evidence of infection, inflammation, or dehiscence was noted at any of the anastomotic sites. Two of the four post-liver samples taken were considered within normal limits (WNL). The other two samples showed subtle changes of hepatocellular swelling with glycogen accumulation. Similar microscopic changes of glycogen accumulation can also be seen during various stages of fasting in animals. No evidence of muscle fiber vacuolization, loss, inflammation, fatty infiltration, or increased fibrous connective tissue deposition was seen in any of muscle sections examined.

The use of a new compressive device for GI anastomosis allowed a safe and effective creation of an anastomosis between two portions of the small bowel. The anastomosis created was robust, healthy, and permanent, which facilitated a partial diversion of nutrient flow and thus altered nutrients absorption, causing effective weight loss in this porcine model with short follow-up. A side-to-side duodeno-ileal anastomosis provided excellent weight loss without diarrhea or grossly aberrant histological changes, especially in the liver. However, a notable decline in serum total protein and albumin levels (and elevated BUN) may indicate inadequate protein/calorie absorption. In the absence of proper nitrogen balance measurements, resting energy expenditure, one cannot conclude that inadequate intake resulted in this early phenomenon, especially considering the energetic and protein needs to heal a midline laparotomy and two enterotomies. It is also possible that if the animal had access to an ad libitum diet that serum protein and albumin levels would have been maintained.

In the real clinical world, humans have free access to nutrients and are provided with protein supplementation and nutritional counseling after surgery. It is expected that any malabsorptive procedure must include these components and serial serum levels of protein, albumin, minerals, fat soluble vitamins, and liver enzymes, similarly to gastric bypass, biliopancreatic diversion with or without duodenal switch must be carried out at regular intervals. Equally remarkable is that the bypassed intestine in the pig is greater with (97% bypass, 50 cm from 18 m) a ratio of 1:36 when compared to humans (90% bypass, 50 cm from 5 m) with a ratio of 1:10 [37]. Therefore, this phenomenon may be seen less in humans.

Recent literature still appears on jejunoileal bypass and its modifications. Recently, Fazel et al. have reported a successful consecutive series of 43 patients who underwent a modified jejunoileal bypass, where the defunctionalized limb was anastomosed to the gall bladder and cecum, resulting in a loss of 43 kg (or 15 kg/m^2 of BMI) at 5 years, without changes in liver histology [38]. One of the main reasons why jejunoileal bypass was abandoned was reports of deaths from liver failure. Meinhardt and colleagues have carefully followed 50 consecutive patients who underwent JIB, in which liver biopsies were performed intraoperatively in 41 patients and in follow-up of 31 patients. With good weight loss at a mean of 67 months, no deaths occurred from liver failures and liver histology was stable [34].

Rosina's team [39] extensively studied bacterial overgrowth on 49 patients. Only 45% of patients had some colonic micro flora in the excluded limb of jejunoileal bypass. The colonization appeared to correlate with clinical symptoms of bloating, migratory arthralgia, and rashes and skin lesions. Conversely, the positive cultures were not always associated with symptoms. No specific bacteriology was associated with this phenomenon. According to Rosina, the "success of an intestinal bypass may depend not only on anatomic and functional adaptation to the new, surgically created conditions, but also to the attainment of microbiological equilibrium in the intestinal ecosystem" [39]. Riordan et al. reported that bacterial overgrowth does not necessarily correlate with liver damage or increased intestinal permeability in human subjects [40].

The main advantage of a duodeno-ileostomy would be the fast ileal stimulation, causing an early incretin release and offering a potential tool for the resolution of type-2 diabetes. Recent hypothesis concerning the resolution of type-2 diabetes after weight loss surgery seems to point out that distal bowel stimulation may promote the production of glucagon-like peptide-1 (GLP-1) from the ileal and colonic L cells. There has been some evidence of this phenomenon when ileal transposition has been performed in Goto-Kakizaki type-2 diabetic rats [41]. Mason had proposed an ileal transposition to promote the early release of GLP-1 for the cure of type-2 diabetes [42]. Although we did not measure this hormone in pigs after duodeno-ileostomy, we postulate that an early release of GLP-1 will be a main endocrine feature of this operation.

Peptide YY (PYY) is also released from the distal small bowel endocrine cells in the circulation after a fatty meal, and PYY seemed to appear in the ileal lumen at greater concentration when glucose is used predominantly in the diet [43]. In fact, when oleic acid is infused into the duodenum, PYY is released approximately 10–30 minutes after. The site of production of circulating PYY appears to be the ileum, colon, and rectum. If an ileocolectomy is performed, an abolished production of PYY to intraduodenal stimulation of oleic acid is observed. This release is not mediated by neural pathway, but solely from endocrine nature [44]. In turn, the increasing concentration of intravenous infusion of PYY reduces the glucose-stimulated insulin release. This suggests that PYY affects the beta-cell function by a possible autonomic regulation [45]. Similarly, we are postulating that an early ileal release of PYY will occur after a side-to-side duodeno-ileostomy and could be one hypothesis behind the effective weight loss seen in these animals. In this porcine model with short follow-up, a side-to-side duodeno-ileal anastomosis provided excellent weight loss without apparent nutritional or grossly aberrant histological changes. This intervention is likely to cause weight loss by numerous mechanisms including decreased food absorption and decreased satiety from endocrine stimulation [46, 47].

Lately efforts have been made using stents to create GI anastomoses. It appears from my perspective, to be convoluted, labor intensive, and requiring more skills than magnets. This may not be suitable after all; nevertheless, it is sensible to pay attention. It is used mainly in terminal malignant patients because gastric outlet obstruction, afferent or efferent limb obstruction, and biliary obstruction will often require surgical intervention, which is associated with significant morbidity and mortality. These self-expandable metal stents are currently in use for strictures and malignant etiologies, but the tumor in-growth eventually re-occludes them; hence, lumen apposing metal stents placed endoscopically, creating de novo anastomosis, and bypassing the obstruction.

In this study cohort of 79 patients, the technical success rate and clinical success was 91% [48]. Various techniques were employed: 43% underwent a balloon-assisted method, 28% undertook endoscopic ultrasound-guided balloon occluded gastrojejunostomy bypass, 20% a direct technique, 6% a rendezvous technique, and 3% went through a natural orifice transluminal endoscopic surgery (NOTES)-assisted procedure. All techniques required an echo endoscope, except the NOTES cases. In all, 53% had non-cautery enhanced Axios stent, 44% had hot Axios stent, and 3% had Niti-S spaxus stent. Only 6% had a complication (bleeding, abdominal pain, or peritonitis). Currently, the AXIOS™ Stent and Electrocautery Enhanced Delivery System from Boston Scientific is the only stent indicated for transgastric or transduodenal endoscopic drainage of symptomatic pancreatic pseudocysts and walled-off necrosis under EUS imaging guidance. These techniques require the help and availability of adequate surgical backup, in case of perforation and/or peritonitis post-intervention.

In conclusion, compression anastomosis has been popular in the past and a resurgence is possible, if the method is simple, fast, reproducible, cost-effective and results in the lowest complication rates.

References

1. Lembert A. Memoire sur l'enterorraphie avec description d'un procede nouveau pour pratiquer cette operation chirurgicale. Rep Gen D'Anat Physiol Pathol Clin Chir. 1826;2:100–7.
2. Murphy JB. Cholecysto-intestinal, gastro-intestinal, entero-intestinal anastomosis, and approximation without sutures. Med Rec, New York. 1892;42:665–76.
3. Gordon RC, John B. Murphy: unique among American surgeons. Invest Surg. 2006;19(5):279–81.
4. Mayo WJ, Mayo CH. V. Clinical report. I. Complete section of the vas deferens, end-to-end union; II. Acute suppuration of knee-joint: open treatment; III. Gastroenterostomy by the Murphy button: anastomoses by this method. Ann Surg. 1895;21(1):35–44.
5. LeVEEN HH. Nonsuture method for vascular anastomosis utilizing the Murphy button principle. Arch Surg. 1949;58(4):504–10.
6. Prioton JB. Ligation of the esophagus on the Murphy button in hemorrhages caused by rupture of esophageal varices. [article in French]. Ann Chir. 1973;27(3):343–9.
7. Weisser C. 100 years Murphy button: development, dissemination and further development. [article in German]. Chirurg. 1993;64(4):359–63.
8. Hardy TG Jr, Pace WG, Maney JW, Katz AR, Kaganov AL. A biofragmentable ring for sutureless bowel anastomosis. An experimental study. Dis Colon Rectum. 1985;28(7):484–90.
9. Dietz UA, Debus ES, Hirt AL, Czeczko NG, Malafaia O, Geiger D, Thiede A. From Murphy's button to the Valtrac ring. 100 years in search of a paradigm. [article in German]. Zentralbl Chir. 1999;124(7):653–6.
10. Hardy TG Jr, Aguilar PS, Stewart WR, Katz AR, Maney JW, Costanzo JT, Pace WG. Initial clinical experience with a biofragmentable ring for sutureless bowel anastomosis. Dis Colon Rectum. 1987;30(1):55–61.
11. Maney JW, Katz AR, Li LK, Pace WG, Hardy TG. Biofragmentable bowel anastomosis ring: comparative efficacy studies in dogs. Surgery. 1988;103(1):56–62.
12. Corman ML, Prager ED, Hardy TG Jr, Bubrick MP. Comparison of the Valtrac biofragmentable anastomosis ring with conventional suture and stapled anastomosis in colon surgery. Results of a prospective, randomized clinical trial. Dis Colon Rectum. 1989;32(3):183–7.
13. Bubrick MP, Corman ML, Cahill CJ, Hardy TG Jr, Nance FC, Shatney CH. Prospective, randomized trial of the biofragmentable anastomosis ring. The BAR Investigational Group. Am J Surg. 1991;161(1):136–42. discussion 142-3
14. Wood JS, Frost DB. Results using the biofragmentable anastomotic ring for colon anastomosis. Am Surg. 1993;59(10):642–4.
15. Gagner M, Heppell J, Lamarre L, Carioto S. L'anastomose colique par laparoscopie avec l'anneau biodégradable valtrac: Une étude comparative dans un modèle canin. Ann Chir. 1993;46(9):875.
16. Sackier JM, Jessup G, Krenz H, Allen W, Ahari F. Biofragmentable anastomosis ring for laparoscopic bowel surgery. Surg Endosc. 1994;8(10):1190–4.
17. Huang Q, Cao F, Zhou J, Liu L, Ge B. Clinical application of compound anastomotic device in protective terminal ileostomy during rectal cancer operation [article in Chinese]. Zhonghua Wei Chang Wai Ke Za Zhi. 2017;20(12):1375–80.
18. Stewart D, Hunt S, Pierce R, Mao D, Frisella M, Cook K, Starcher B, Fleshman J. Validation of the NITI Endoluminal Compression Anastomosis Ring (EndoCAR) device and comparison to the traditional circular stapled colorectal anastomosis in a porcine model. Surg Innov. 2007;14(4):252–60.
19. Tulchinsky H, Kashtan H, Rabau M, Wasserberg N. Evaluation of the NiTi Shape Memory BioDynamix ColonRing™ in colorectal anastomosis: first in human multi-center study. Int J Color Dis. 2010;25(12):1453–8.
20. Buchberg BS, Masoomi H, Bergman H, Mills SD, Stamos MJ. The use of a compression device as an alternative to hand-sewn and stapled colorectal anastomoses: is three a crowd? J Gastrointest Surg. 2011;15(2):304–10.
21. Hur H, Kim HH, Hyung WJ, Cho GS, Kim W, Ryo SW, Han SU. Efficacy of NiTi Hand CAC 30 for jejunojejunostomy in gastric cancer surgery: results from a multicenter prospective randomized trial. Gastric Cancer. 2011;14(2):124–9.
22. Kim HR, Lee WY, Jung KU, Yun HR, Cho YB, Yun SH, Kim HC, Chun HK. Early surgical outcomes

of NiTi endoluminal compression anastomotic clip (NiTi CAC 30) use in patients with gastrointestinal malignancy. J Laparoendosc Adv Surg Tech A. 2012;22(5):472–8.
23. Masoomi H, Luo R, Mills S, Carmichael JC, Senagore AJ, Stamos MJ. Compression anastomosis ring device in colorectal anastomosis: a review of 1,180 patients. Am J Surg. 2013;205(4):447–51.
24. Kwag SJ, Kim JG, Kang WK, Lee JK, Oh ST. Niti CAR 27 versus a conventional end-to-end anastomosis Stapler in a laparoscopic anterior resection for sigmoid colon cancer. Ann Coloproctol. 2014;30(2):77–82. 25.
25. Kaidar-Person O, Rosenthal RJ, Wexner SD, Szomstein S, Person B. Compression anastomosis: history and clinical considerations. Am J Surg. 2008;195(6):818–26.
26. Chopita N, Vaillaverde A, Cope C, Bernedo A, Martinez H, Landoni N, Jmelnitzky A, Burgos H. Endoscopic gastroenteric anastomosis using magnets. Endoscopy. 2005;37(4):313–7.
27. Chopita N, Landoni N, Ross A, Villaverde A. Malignant gastroenteric obstruction: therapeutic options. Gastrointest Endosc Clin N Am. 2007;17(3):533–44.
28. Gagner M. Safety and efficacy of a side-to-side duodeno-ileal anastomosis for weight loss and type-2 diabetes: duodenal bipartition, a novel metabolic surgery procedure. Ann Surg Innov Res. 2015;9:6.
29. Gagner M. Side-to-side duodeno-colic anastomosis provides dramatic weight loss. A potentially strong anti-diabetic operation for type-2 diabetes. Minerva Chir. 2017;72(3):169–77.
30. Våge V, Solhaug JH, Berstad A, Svanes K, Viste A. Jejunoileal bypass in the treatment of morbid obesity: a 25-year follow-up study of 36 patients. Obes Surg. 2002;12(3):312–8.
31. Näslund E, Backman L, Holst JJ, Theodorsson E, Hellström PM. Importance of small bowel peptides for the improved glucose metabolism 20 years after jejunoileal bypass for obesity. Obes Surg. 1998;8(3):253–60.
32. Singh D, Laya AS, Clarkston WK, Allen MJ. Jejunoileal bypass: a surgery of the past and a review of its complications. World J Gastroenterol. 2009;15(18):2277–9.
33. Vyberg M, Ravn V, Andersen B. Pattern of progression in liver injury following jejunoileal bypass for morbid obesity. Liver. 1987;7(5):271–6.
34. Meinhardt NG, Souto KE, Ulbrich-Kulczynski JM, Stein AT. Hepatic outcomes after jejunoileal bypass: is there a publication bias? Obes Surg. 2006;16(9):1171–8.
35. Wills CE. Long-term follow-up of jejunoileal bypass patients with preoperative cirrhosis of the liver. Obes Surg. 1994;4(1):37–9.
36. Viddal KO, Midtvedt T, Nygaard K. Comparison of bypass and resection of the small intestine in germfree rats. Eur Surg Res. 1984;16(suppl 2):147–53.
37. Kararli TT. Review article: comparison of the gastrointestinal anatomy, physiology, and biochemistry of humans and commonly used laboratory animals. Biopharm Drug Dispos. 1995;16:351–80.
38. Fazel I, Pourshams A, Merat S, Hemayati R, Sotoudeh M, Malekzadeh R. Modified jejunoileal bypass surgery with biliary diversion for morbid obesity and changes in liver histology during follow-up. J Gastrointest Surg. 2007;11(8):1033–8.
39. Rosina M, Micheletto G, Vita PM, Restelli A, Caspani P, Ferla G, Doldi SB. Intestinal microflora settlement in patients with jejunoileal bypass for morbid obesity. Obes Surg. 1993;3(3):239–45.
40. Riordan SM, McIver CJ, Williams R. Liver damage in human small intestinal bacterial overgrowth. Am J Gastroenterol. 1998;93(2):234–7.
41. Patriti A, Aisa MC, Annetti C, Sidoni A, Galli F, Ferri I, Gullà N, Donini A. How the hindgut can cure type 2 diabetes. Ileal transposition improves glucose metabolism and beta-cell function in Goto-kakizaki rats through an enhanced Proglucagon gene expression and L-cell number. Surgery. 2007;142(1):74–85.
42. Mason EE. Ileal [correction of ilial] transposition and enteroglucagon/GLP-1 in obesity (and diabetic?) surgery. Obes Surg. 1999;9(3):223–8.
43. McFadden DW, Rudnicki M, Nussbaum MS, Balasubramaniam A, Fischer JE. Independent release of peptide YY (PYY) into the circulation and ileal lumen of the awake dog. J Surg Res. 1989;46(4):380–5.
44. Greeley GH, Jeng YJ, Gomez G, Hashimoto T, Hill FL, Kern K, Kurosky T, Chuo HF, Thompson JC. Evidence for regulation of peptide-YY release by the proximal gut. Endocrinology. 1989;124(3):1438–43.
45. Greeley GH Jr, Lluis F, Gomez G, Ishizuka J, Holland B, Thompson JC. Peptide YY antagonizes beta-adrenergic-stimulated release of insulin in dogs. Am J Phys. 1988;254(4 Pt 1):E513–7.
46. Sclafani A, Koopmans HS, Vasselli JR, Reichman M. Effects of intestinal bypass surgery on appetite, food intake, and body weight in obese and lean rats. Am J Phys. 1978;234(4):E389–98.
47. Näslund E, Melin I, Gryböck P, Hägg A, Hellström PM, Jacobsson H, Theodorsson E, Rössner S, Backman L. Reduced food intake after jejunoileal bypass: a possible association with prolonged gastric emptying and altered gut hormone patterns. Am J Clin Nutr. 1997;66(1):26–32.
48. Jain D, Chhoda A, Sharma A, Singhal S. De-novo gastrointestinal anastomosis with lumen apposing metal stent. Clin Endosc. 2018;51(5):439–49.

15 Endoscopic Magnetic Bowel Anastomosis

Vitor Ottoboni Brunaldi and Manoel Galvão Neto

Introduction

Magnets are intriguing components since they may exert long-lasting force over a distance. The application of the magnetic force in clinical surgery remotes to a report published in 1957 describing the retrieval of ingested foreign bodies by using magnets [1]. Since then, several studies, animal and clinical, have investigated different types of magnets to address a wide variety of GI disorders. More recently, the emerging GI endoscopy field embraced it as a potential point of interest, especially in performing sutureless and incisionless anastomoses which could preclude a more aggressive surgical approach. This chapter summarizes available data regarding the use of a magnetic force in creating endoscopic bowel anastomoses to treat different types of GI disorders.

V. O. Brunaldi (✉)
Gastrointestinal Endoscopy Unit, Gastroenterology Department, University of São Paulo Medical School, São Paulo, Brazil
e-mail: vitor.brunaldi@usp.br

M. Galvão Neto
Surgery Department, Florida International University, Miami, FL, USA

Gastrojejunal Anastomosis

The gastric outlet obstruction (GOO) syndrome may be caused by neoplasms from the stomach, duodenum, or periampullary [2]. Nausea, vomiting, dysphagia, weight loss, and severe malnutrition are the main symptoms [3]. Usually, in a palliative setting, the prognosis is dismal, and the focus of the best supportive care is to address obstruction along with bleeding, nausea/vomiting, and pain [4]. The gastrojejunostomy is the standard surgical technique employed in the context of a gastric outlet obstruction. If it functions, the patient normally experiences long-term relief of dysphagia [5]. However, some individuals are unfit for surgery since it carries non-negligible morbidity and mortality rates [6, 7]. Therefore, less invasive approaches like the endoluminal magnet-assisted gastrojejunostomy are particularly opportune.

Several studies evaluated different devices, deployment, and assembling techniques in performing this incisionless gastrojejunal anastomosis (GJA). We are going to discuss them chronologically.

Initially, Cope reported the feasibility of the rationale in an animal study in 1995 [8]. In 1999, Cope et al. published a second animal study in which the authors deployed rare earth magnets perorally in 15 dogs and managed them to assemble across the gastric and jejunal wall. Different sizes and types of magnets were employed, and their excretion occurred within a week of the

M. Gagner (ed.), *Magnetic Surgery*, https://doi.org/10.1007/978-3-030-73947-8_15

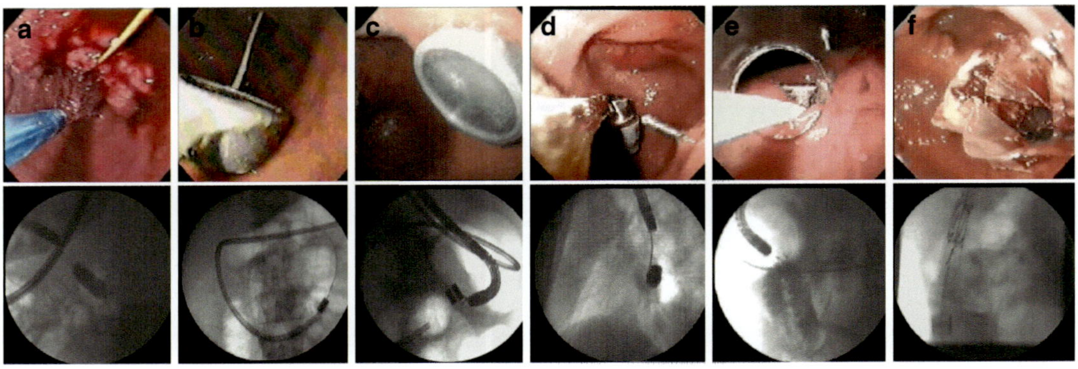

Fig. 15.1 Magnetic gastrojejunostomy procedure as reported by Chopita et al. (**a**) Dilation of the duodenal malignant stricture. (**b**) Distal magnet delivery using a specific catheter. (**c**) Gastric magnet deployment and coupling. (**d**) Magnets retrieval. (**e, f**) Dilation and stenting of the magnetic gastrojejunostomy. (From Chopita et al. [11]. Reprinted with permission from Georg Thieme Verlag KG)

procedure. The GJA was then assessed endoscopically and stenting was attempted aiming at increasing its patency time. The results, however, were somewhat disappointing: 6 out of the 15 anastomoses presented early closure; 2 could not be located; 1 animal suffered from a pancreatic abscess and another from a perforation with peritonitis. Among the remaining GJAs, the patency was 19 days after balloon dilation alone, 40–64 days with uncovered stents, and 58–147 days (mean, 90 days) with partially covered stents [9]. Two years later, the same group published a similar study testing a new "yo-yo"-shaped covered stent after the magnetic GJA was accomplished. The authors showed 6-month patency in four out of five dogs with no reported morbidity or mortality related to the procedure [10].

These results encouraged a pilot first-in-human study conducted in Argentina in cooperation with one of the authors from the aforementioned animal reports. Chopita et al. enrolled 15 patients diagnosed with malignant GOO who were unfit for surgery due to poor clinical status and advanced disease. The gastric and duodenal magnets were 14 mm and 12 mm wide, respectively. After dilating the duodenal stricture, the distal magnet was placed using a wire-guided catheter under fluoroscopic control. Then, the gastroscope directed the gastric magnet against its mate and across the gastric and duodenal wall. The coupled magnet buttons were withdrawn 7–10 days later and the "yo-yo"-shaped stent was deployed through the gastroduodenostomy (Fig. 15.1). The technical success was 86% (13/15). The first failure was due to a perforation that required surgical intervention and the second because the duodenal obstruction could not be dilated. Of the 13 successfully treated patients, 12 died from the underlying disease. All of them were able to eat solid food until their deaths. There were three cases of uneventful stent migration and one stent obstruction by food [11]. Based on these results, the authors concluded that the endoscopic magnetic gastrojejunostomy could be a third option to address GOO aside surgery and sole stenting.

Then, van Hooft et al. published a multicenter study investigating the safety and efficacy of the endoluminal gastrojejunostomy with similar technique and accessories (magnets and "yo-yo"-shaped stents) in patients with malignant GOO. The enrollment goal was 40, but the study was prematurely terminated with 18 patients due to serious adverse events. Initially, there were two stent migrations out of twelve procedures. The Ethics Committee placed the trial on hold but eventually allowed continuation with a different stent. Ultimately, a free peritoneal perforation of the second type of stent led to enrollment suspension by the data safety monitoring board.

Among the 18 patients, the magnets could be aligned in 15, but 2 patients died within 10 days of the procedure from unrelated causes. Stenting was successful in 12 out of the 13 remaining. Seven patients died from the underlying disease with a functional anastomosis and another one was followed up to 180 days and still had a functional stoma. This study mistrusted the efficacy and safety of technique and the types of magnet employed so far. Since all adverse events were related to the stent, most groups went back to the animal lab aiming at developing a magnetic gastrojejunostomy that waived stenting [12].

Within a few years, novel articles investigating the ideal features of a magnet became available. In 2009, Jamshidi et al. compared four types of anastomoses: hand-sutured, stapled, magnetic with uniform compression, and magnetic with gradient compression. The authors hypothesized that the ideal magnet should be ring-shaped to avoid necrosis in the actual site of the anastomosis. Moreover, it should exert the greater pressure in the central border of the ring, while the lower in the external edge. This property would lead to a wide anastomosis and would grant time for the stoma to mature centripetally, ultimately preventing leaks (Fig. 15.2). Although the differences among the types of anastomoses were not statistically significant, the researchers found a trend toward greater mechanical strength favoring the magnetic anastomoses. Also, the gradient compression trended toward greater strength and patency at 1 week compared to the uniform compression. The authors criticized previous publications employing round and uniform magnets and supposed they had created a chronic fistula rather than an anastomosis. According to them, that would explain the high rates of early closure and the need for stenting [13]. Similarly, Myers et al. reported another animal study 1 year later evaluating the combination of a thick and a thin magnet in performing GJAs. They employed external magnetic forces to guide the internal assembling of the magnets across the stomach and the jejunum. The success of the procedure was 85% (6/7), also confirmed through gross and histological analysis [14].

In 2011, the same group that studied the ideal features of these magnets published a new version of the gradual force device, the so-called "Magnamosis II." This new animal study assessed the histological changes of the gastrojejunostomy in time. At 1 week, they found necrosis at the compression point between the mated magnets with a simultaneous necrotic central plug. At 2 weeks, the patent anastomoses presented marked fibrosis between the bowel wall of the stoma. At 6 weeks, there was re-epithelialization permeating the fibrosis. Again, the burst pressure

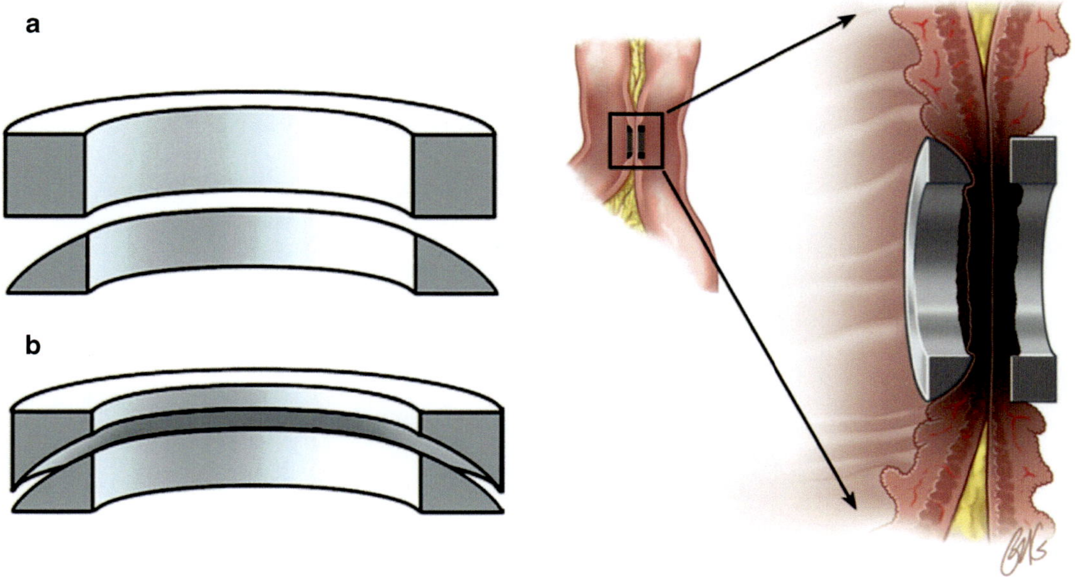

Fig. 15.2 Schematics of the gradient (**a**) and uniform (**b**) compression magnets. (From Jamshidi et al. [13]. Reprinted with permission from Elsevier)

of the magnamosis was similar to either stapled or hand-sewn anastomoses [15].

The major shortcomings of the technique employed so far were the waiting time for the anastomosis to form and its small diameter. Aiming to address those issues, a group from Boston, USA, developed magnets that automatically assembled in a predetermined 2.25 cm × 2.25 cm window-shape after deployment and might be pushed through the working channel of the endoscope. Once both jejunal and gastric magnets had been released, they would mate together across the GI wall. Initially, the group performed the gastrojejunostomy in six cadaveric pigs and one human cadaver to improve the technique. The final technique consisted of a transgastric full-thickness incision followed by placement of a specific overtube armed with graspers that stabilized the proximal jejunum. Then, they created a jejunostomy and introduced the jejunal magnet. Finally, the gastric magnet was released and managed to couple to the distal one (Fig. 15.3). Live animal procedures were then undertaken in five Yorkshire pigs and succeeded with an average procedure time of 1.75 hours. There were no immediate contrast leakages or hemorrhage. After euthanasia, a necropsy found adequate coupling of the magnets and no perforation or peritoneal perforations [16].

Since this last article was released in 2011, no other relevant report was published concerning magnetic anastomoses to treat GOO. Of note, the knowledge and technology derived from all aforementioned research allowed further studies on obesity treatment using the magnetic jejunal bypass, which will be discussed ahead.

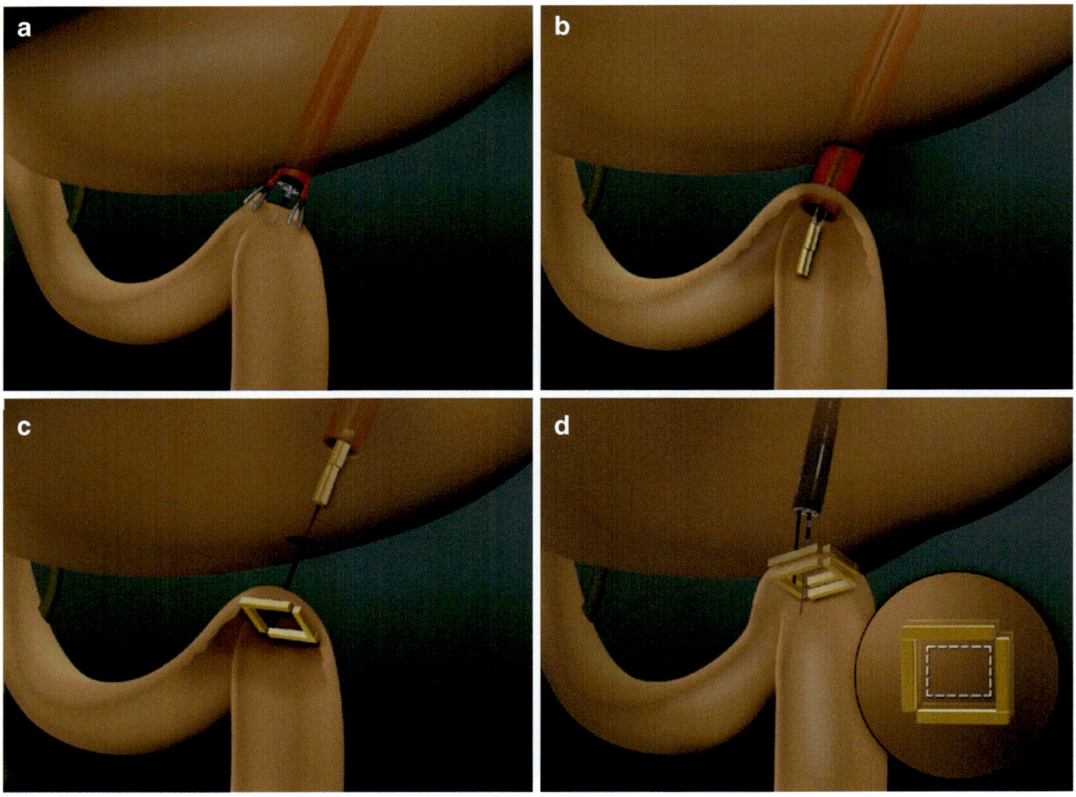

Fig. 15.3 Schematics of the immediate magnetic gastrojejunostomy procedure using the self-assembling magnets (SAMSEN ®). (**a**) Gastrotomy using a specific overtube equipped with two graspers that secure the proximal jejunum. (**b**) Deployment of the jejunal magnet. (**c**) Assembling and positioning of the jejunal magnet. (**d**) Deployment and assembling of the gastric magnet followed by coupling. (From Ryou et al. [16]. Reprinted with permission from Elsevier)

Jejunoileal Anastomosis (Enteric Diversion)

Obesity is a rising pandemic. While bariatric surgery is the standard-of-care to address grades II and III (BMI $\geq$ 35 kg/m^2), there is still no consensus on how to treat grade I obesity and the overweight [17]. Since surgery is not exempt from complications, the benefit must be carefully weighed on a case-by-case basis for high-risk patients or borderline indications. Moreover, less than 2% of patients who have an indication for a bariatric procedure actually undergoes surgery [18]. As a consequence, several obese patients remain aside medical care. In this situation, a less invasive approach such as the endoluminal treatment is particularly attractive since it could reach a greater number of patients in need. In recent years, studies have reported employment of magnets to create bowel anastomoses aiming to bypass different segments of the intestine.

The abandoned traditional surgical jejunoileal bypass was aggressive and posed a high risk of metabolic disorders including liver failure [19, 20]. That fact was related to the excessive malabsorption due to the creation of a blind defunctionalized segment of small intestine. Unlike them, recent studies aim at creating a partial jejunal diversion, that is, the original path remains intact and only a fraction of food bolus bypass the jejunum into the ileum (Fig. 15.4).

This procedure is based on the hindgut hypothesis also seen in the duodenal switch, ileum transposition, and biliopancreatic diversion surgery. This theory advocates that the early passage of food and enzymes into the distal small bowel stimulates the release of glucagon-like peptide 1 (GLP-1), peptide YY (PYY), and other gut hormones from enteric cells in terminal ileum and colon. These hormones, besides the inherent malabsorption, downregulate serum glucose and help promote weight loss [21].

The same group that developed the self-assembling magnets for gastrojejunostomy improved the device into an updated version. Instead of being square-shaped, the new one was a large self-assembling octagon coated with a biosafe exoskeleton. It could be delivered through the working channel of a colonoscope allowing a fully endoluminal approach (Fig. 15.5) [22].

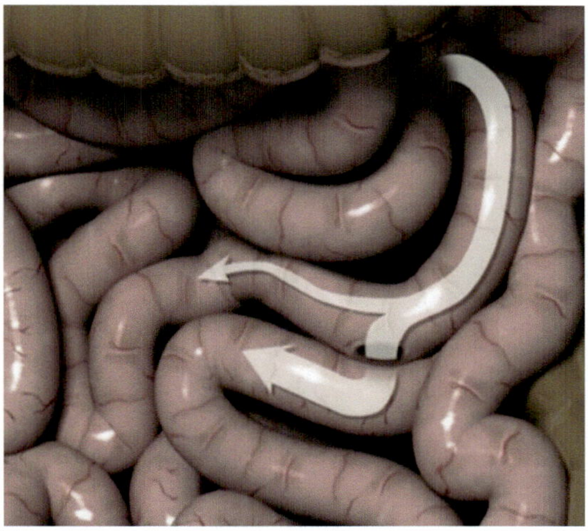

Fig. 15.4 Schematics of a side-to-side jejunoileal anastomosis creating partial jejunal diversion. (From Machytka et al. [24]. Reprinted with permission from Elsevier)

The first related report was a proof-of-concept feasibility animal study published in 2016. Five pigs underwent the endoscopic partial jejunal diversion procedure. Initially, simultaneous colonoscopy and antegrade enteroscopy were performed. Jejunal and colon magnets were deployed through the enteroscope and colonoscope, respectively. After self-assembling, they were managed to couple using magnet-tipped catheters under endoscopic and fluoroscopic guidance (Fig. 15.6).

After the procedure, all animals were kept alive with daily assessment for food intake and general appearance. Every 3–5 days, an upper endoscopy evaluated the status of the enteral anastomosis. At 3 months, the pigs were euthanized, and a necropsy was performed. The researchers resected the anastomosis and assessed the burst pressure, besides a standard histological evaluation.

All five pigs underwent successful deployment, assembling, and coupling of the magnets. Due to the porcine anatomy, the only feasible anastomosis was jejunocolostomy. The mean duration of the procedure was 14.7 minutes. The endoscopic examination showed central tissue necrosis with a patent bypass within the coupled magnets by day 4. At 12 days, there was a wide

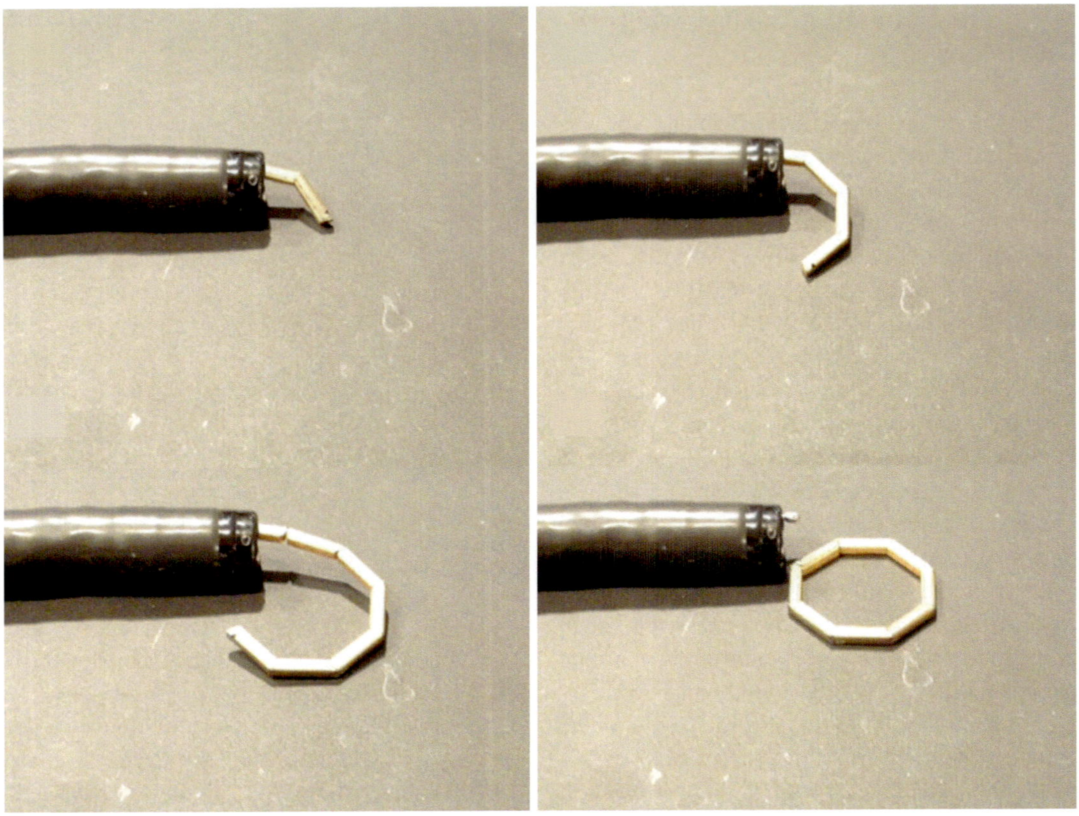

Fig. 15.5 Self-assembling octagon magnet being deployed through the working channel of a standard colonoscope. (From Ryou et al. [22]. Reprinted with permission from Elsevier)

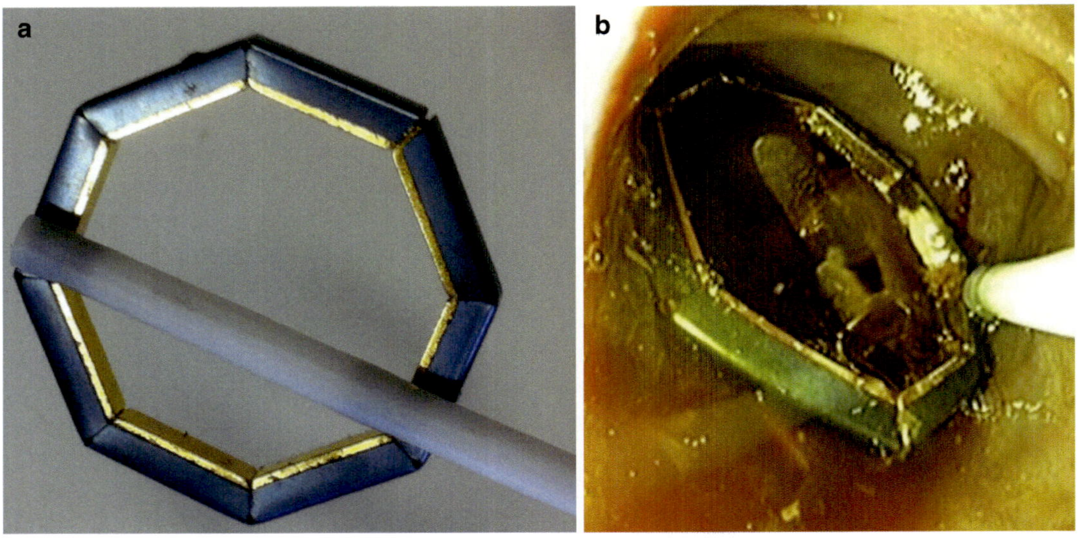

Fig. 15.6 Magnets after assembling and attached to the magnet-tipped catheter used to manage the coupling. (**a**) Bench demonstration of the self-assembling magnets from Cummings DE, et al. [21]. Reprinted with permission from Elsevier. (**b**) In vivo demonstration of the self-assembling magnets. (From Ryou et al. [23]. Reprinted with permission from Springer Nature)

dual-path anastomosis and all magnet couples had already been expelled. At 3 months, they found a completely re-epithelized 3.5 cm wide anastomosis. The postmortem analysis revealed no signs of adhesions, hemorrhage, or abscess. Histology demonstrated the absence of active inflammation, minimal fibrosis, and scar formation—typical findings of a well-healed anastomotic site. Of note, the intervention animals had weight stabilization compared to control litter-matched pigs [22].

The next study of this timeline aimed to confirm the feasibility of a jejunoileal magnetic anastomosis. The particular corkscrew-like anatomy of the porcine ileum precludes the trans-anal endoluminal delivery of the distal magnet. Therefore, all animals underwent laparotomy followed by an ileotomy that allowed the colonoscope to access and deploy the magnet into the distal ileum.

In total, eight survival studies were successfully performed. All animals recovered uneventfully from the procedure. The last three pigs had their anastomosis resected at month 3 and were kept alive for 15 days to confirm reversibility of the procedure. Of note, these last animals recovered from the reversal surgery and resumed the preprocedural growth rates. The endoscopic follow-up showed patent stomas at 10 days, and epithelized anastomosis by day 90 (Fig. 15.7). All magnets sloughed off and were naturally expelled. The necropsy at 3 months demonstrated a clean and fully healed anastomosis with no adhesions (Fig. 15.8). No leaks or hemorrhage have been reported [23].

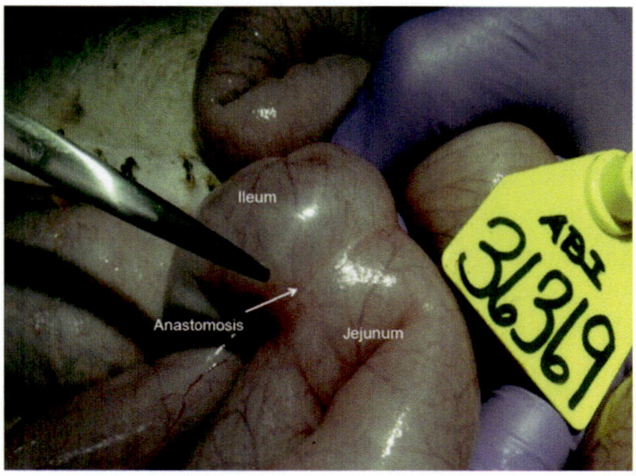

Fig. 15.8 Gross assessment of the porcine magnetic jejunoileal anastomosis during a necropsy at 3 months. (From Ryou et al. [23]. Reprinted with permission from Springer Nature)

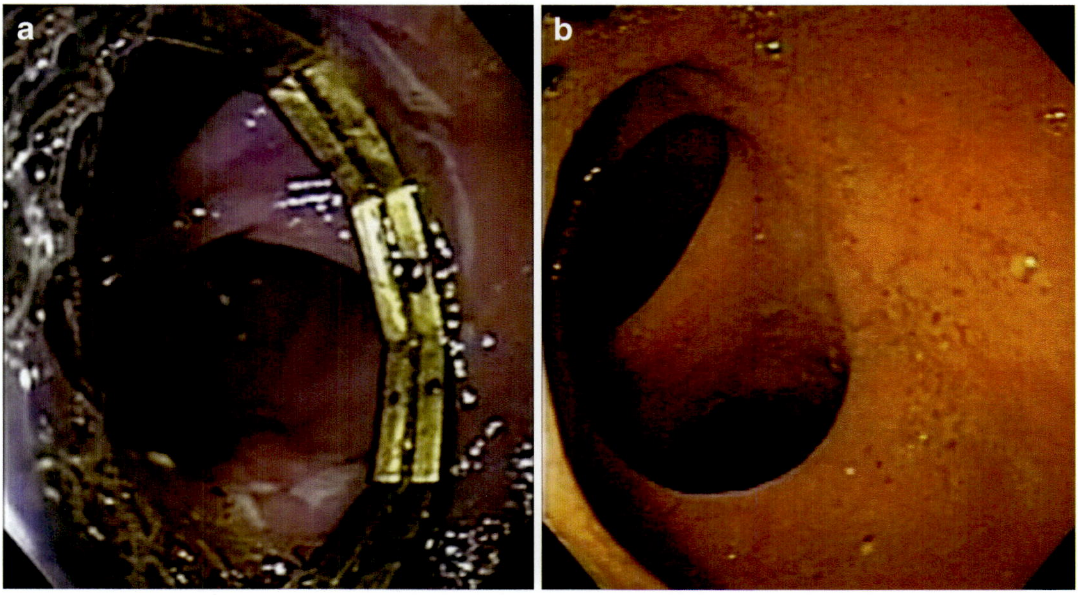

Fig. 15.7 Endoscopic follow-up of the magnetic jejunoileal anastomosis. (**a**) Appearance after 10 days. (**b**) Appearance after 90 days. (From Ryou et al. [23]. Reprinted with permission from Springer Nature)

The exciting results encouraged this group to perform a first-in-human, single-center, pilot study in the Czech Republic assessing feasibility, safety, and clinical performance of the endoluminal magnetic partial jejunal diversion (EMPJD). Inclusion criteria were participants with moderate or severe obesity (BMI of 35–50 kg/m^2); mild obesity (BMI = 30–35 kg/m^2) if associated at least one clinically significant obesity-related comorbidity; and adults (18–65 years). Exclusion criteria were BMI higher than 50 kg/m^2; type 1 diabetes; use of more than two oral antidiabetic medications, dipeptidyl peptidase 4 inhibitor, insulin, or a GLP-1 agonist; previous abdominal surgery; and hypersensitivity to nickel.

Fourteen individuals met eligibility criteria and were enrolled between October 2014 and March 2015. Two patients later withdrew consent, and another was diagnosed with an exclusory lung disease. Thus, the EMPJD was attempted in 11 patients. The first two cases failed because of an inability to approximate the adequate loops of bowel. The researchers hypothesized it was due to excessive air insufflation. Further procedures were executed with CO_2 insufflation only, which allowed the adequate magnet coupling in 10 cases, including one of the previously failed. As this was a first-in-human study, all procedures were laparoscopically monitored. Per protocol, if attempting to couple magnets was still unsuccessful after 40 minutes, laparoscopic graspers were employed to guarantee the coupling.

All magnets were successfully deployed through the working channel of the colonoscope. Coupling required laparoscopic assistance in 8 out of 10 cases because of the predetermined time limit. Of note, the two completely endoluminal couplings occurred among the four last cases, suggesting that greater experience could eventually exempt laparoscopy. The average duration of the procedure was 115 minutes (131 minutes for the first five procedures and 98 minutes for the last five ones). The magnets were targeted at 50–100 cm proximal to the ileocecal valve in the ileum and 50–100 cm distal to the ligament of Treitz in the jejunum in a fully anti-mesenteric position (Fig. 15.9). All patients expelled the magnets within 13 days, except for the first case that underwent uneventful endoscopic removal. They resumed normal daily activities after a mean of 1.7 days (1–3 days). Upper GI endoscopy confirmed wide and patent anastomoses at 2, 6, and 12 months (Fig. 15.10).

Patients presented progressive weight loss throughout follow-up. The mean total weight loss was 8.2%, 10.6%, and 14.6% at 3, 6, and 12 months, respectively. The mean excess weight loss was 21.7%, 28.3%, and 40.2%. Among the diabetic patients, the HbA1c dropped from 7.8 (baseline) to 5.9 at 12 months. Accordingly, the fasting blood glucose fell from 177 (baseline) to 116 at 1 month and kept stable until 1 year of follow-up. Regarding gut hormones, there were significant reductions in postprandial insulin and glucose levels at 2 and 6 months, and a significant increase in PYY at 2 months.

Concerning adverse events, all patients reported postoperative nausea and abdominal pain. The first was considered an anesthetic side effects while the latter was mostly related to trocar site pain. Moreover, all patients presented short-term diarrhea and four had recurrent diarrhea. Nutritional counseling, dietary changes, and a short course of loperamide fully resolved all cases. As to metabolic disorders, two of the three patients with preprocedural iron deficiency, three of ten with previous vitamin D deficiency, and one of two with baseline vitamin B12 deficiency still had serum levels below normal values at 12 months. Additionally, two patients presented magnesium deficiency, both of whom had preoperative subnormal values [24].

These results were extremely exciting and triggered an ongoing clinical trial settled in Argentina assessing the effectiveness of the EMPJD procedure with a strict methodological design [25]. If the results are favorable, EMPJD may turn into another weapon in the armamentarium against obesity and diabetes.

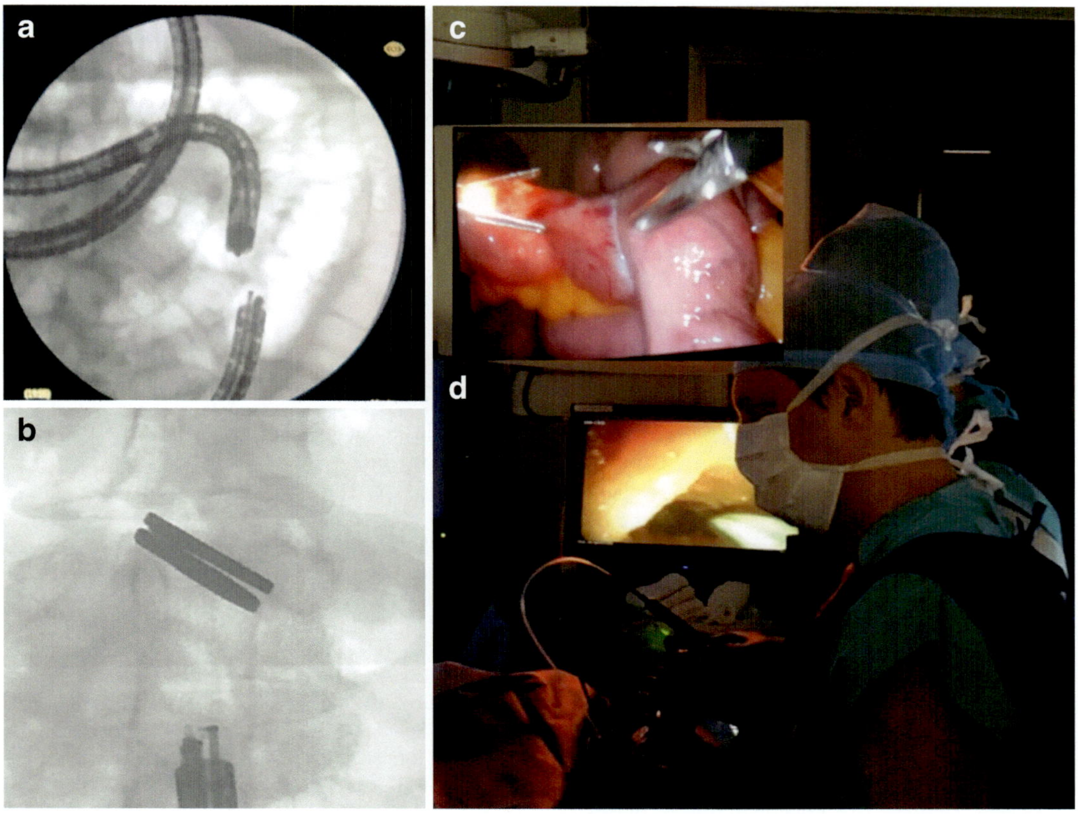

Fig. 15.9 In-human trial showing the endoluminal magnetic partial jejunal diversion procedure. (**a**) Colonoscopes from the bottom and from the top meeting at the "drop zone." (**b**) Magnets deployed and coupled. (**c**) Laparoscopic control of the magnets coupling across the jejunum and the ileum. (**d**) Endoscopic control of the delivery of the upper magnet

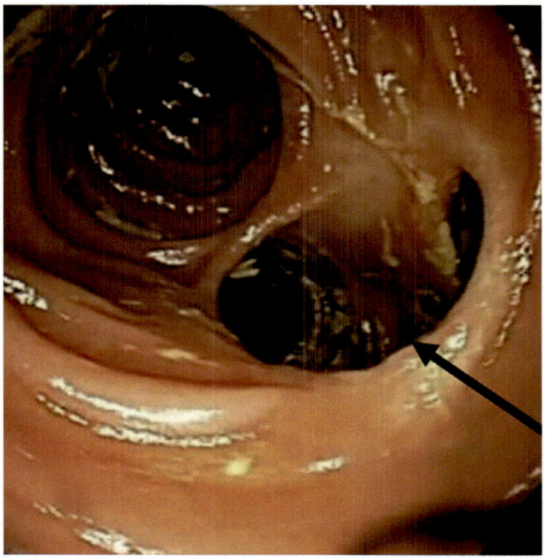

Fig. 15.10 The endoscopic appearance of the jejunoileal anastomosis of a human patient 12 months after the endoluminal partial jejunal diversion procedure. (From Machytka et al. [24]. Reprinted with permission from Elsevier)

Conclusion

Magnetic endoscopic bowel anastomoses are interesting alternatives to address different gastrointestinal diseases. Gastric outlet obstruction and obesity are their main targets currently. The magnets and accessories improved over time, allowing more safe and reproducible procedures. Still, further improvement and research are needed to guarantee safety and effectiveness.

References

1. Equen M, Roach G, Brown R, Bennett T. Magnetic removal of foreign bodies from the esophagus, stomach and duodenum. AMA Arch Otolaryngol. 1957;66(6):698–706.
2. Dormann A, Meisner S, Verin N, Wenk LA. Self-expanding metal stents for gastroduodenal malignan-

cies: systematic review of their clinical effectiveness. Endoscopy. 2004;36(6):543–50.
3. Jaka H, Mchembe MD, Rambau PF, Chalya PL. Gastric outlet obstruction at Bugando Medical Centre in Northwestern Tanzania: a prospective review of 184 cases. BMC Surg. 2013;13:41.
4. Network NCC. NCCN clinical practice guidelines in oncology (NCCN Guidelines) – gastric cancer, Version 2.2018 [Internet]. 2018. Available from https://www.nccn.org/professionals/physician_gls/pdf/gastric.pdf.
5. Jeurnink SM, van Eijck CHJ, Steyerberg EW, Kuipers EJ, Siersema PD. Stent versus gastrojejunostomy for the palliation of gastric outlet obstruction: a systematic review. BMC Gastroenterol. 2007;7:18.
6. Lo NN, Kee SG, Nambiar R. Palliative gastrojejunostomy for advanced carcinoma of the stomach. Ann Acad Med Singap. 1991;20(3):356–8.
7. Minata MK, Bernardo WM, Rocha RS de P, Morita FHA, Aquino JCM, Cheng S, et al. Stents and surgical interventions in the palliation of gastric outlet obstruction: a systematic review. Endosc Int open. 2016;4(11):E1158–70.
8. Cope C. Creation of compression gastroenterostomy by means of the oral, percutaneous, or surgical introduction of magnets: feasibility study in swine. J Vasc Interv Radiol. 1995;6(4):539–45.
9. Cope C, Clark TW, Ginsberg G, Habecker P. Stent placement of gastroenteric anastomoses formed by magnetic compression. J Vasc Interv Radiol. 1999;10(10):1379–86.
10. Cope C, Ginsberg GG. Long-term patency of experimental magnetic compression gastroenteric anastomoses achieved with covered stents. Gastrointest Endosc. 2001;53(7):780–4.
11. Chopita N, Vaillaverde A, Cope C, Bernedo A, Martinez H, Landoni N, et al. Endoscopic gastroenteric anastomosis using magnets. Endoscopy. 2005;37(4):313–7.
12. van Hooft JE, Vleggaar FP, Le Moine O, Bizzotto A, Voermans RP, Costamagna G, et al. Endoscopic magnetic gastroenteric anastomosis for palliation of malignant gastric outlet obstruction: a prospective multicenter study. Gastrointest Endosc. 2010;72(3):530–5.
13. Jamshidi R, Stephenson JT, Clay JG, Pichakron KO, Harrison MR. Magnamosis: magnetic compression anastomosis with comparison to suture and staple techniques. J Pediatr Surg. 2009;44(1):222–8.
14. Myers C, Yellen B, Evans J, DeMaria E, Pryor A. Using external magnet guidance and endoscopically placed magnets to create suture-free gastro-enteral anastomoses. Surg Endosc. 2010;24(5):1104–9.
15. Pichakron KO, Jelin EB, Hirose S, Curran PF, Jamshidi R, Stephenson JT, et al. Magnamosis II: magnetic compression anastomosis for minimally invasive gastrojejunostomy and jejunojejunostomy. J Am Coll Surg. 2011;212(1):42–9.
16. Ryou M, Cantillon-Murphy P, Azagury D, Shaikh SN, Ha G, Greenwalt I, et al. Smart Self-Assembling MagnetS for ENdoscopy (SAMSEN) for transoral endoscopic creation of immediate gastrojejunostomy (with video). Gastrointest Endosc. 2011;73(2):353–9.
17. Kim J, Eisenberg D, Azagury D, Rogers A, Campos GM. American Society for Metabolic and Bariatric Surgery position statement on long-term survival benefit after metabolic and bariatric surgery. Surg Obes Relat Dis. 2016;12(3):453–9.
18. Kumbhari V, Hill C, Sullivan S. Bariatric endoscopy: state-of-the-art. Curr Opin Gastroenterol. 2017;33(5):358–65.
19. DeWind LT, Payne JH. Intestinal bypass surgery for morbid obesity. Long-term results. JAMA. 1976;236(20):2298–301.
20. Complications of intestinal bypass for obesity. JAMA. 1967;200(7):638.
21. Cummings DE, Overduin J, Ph D, Shannon MH, Foster-Schubert KE. Hormonal mechanisms of weight loss and diabetes resolution after bariatric surgery. Surg Obes Relat Dis. 2005;1:358–68.
22. Ryou M, Agoston AT, Thompson CC. Endoscopic intestinal bypass creation by using self-assembling magnets in a porcine model. Gastrointest Endosc. 2016;83(4):821–5.
23. Ryou M, Aihara H, Thompson CC. Minimally invasive entero-enteral dual-path bypass using self-assembling magnets. Surg Endosc. 2016;30(10):4533–8.
24. Machytka E, Buzga M, Zonca P, Lautz DB, Ryou M, Simonson DC, et al. Partial jejunal diversion using an incisionless magnetic anastomosis system: 1-year interim results in patients with obesity and diabetes. Gastrointest Endosc. 2017;86(5):904–12.
25. ClinicalTrials.gov [Internet]. Bethesda (MD): National Library of Medicine (US). 2000 Feb 29 – Identifier NCT03130244, Endoscopic Procedure for Jejunal to Ileal Diversion to Treat Type 2 Diabetes; April 26, 2017 [cited 2018 Dec 17]; [about 5 screens]. Available from: https://clinicaltrials.gov/ct2/show/NCT03130244?term=gi+windows&rank=1.

16 Magnetic Compression Anastomosis and Magnetic Compression Revision for Stenosis

Eigoro Yamanouchi, Reiko Kumano, Hironori Ohdaira, and Yutaka Suzuki

Introduction

In 1989, we hit on this idea of magnetic compression anastomosis (MCA) from an accidental case of a 2-year-old girl who had swallowed small magnets that are sold and generally used to relieve shoulder stiffness in Japan. She was brought to the emergency room at our university hospital complaining of abdominal pain. It was revealed that she had swallowed 13 small magnets because "she was hungry" (Fig. 16.1). An abdominal computed tomography (CT) study showed complete obstruction of the bowel loops. A barium enema study showed that 3 magnets were in the cecum and the remaining 10 were outside of the colon, probably in the ileum (Fig. 16.2). The decision was made to perform open abdominal surgery to relieve the obstruction. During surgery, it was found that the terminal ileum was adhered to the cecum and the magnets had created an anastomosis between these two anatomical structures. The remanence of each small magnet was only 1200 gauss (Fig. 16.3). It was then that we realized that we could create such an anastomosis between organs if we could keep each organ in contact for a sufficient period of time using strong magnets (Fig. 16.4).

The concept of mechanical anastomosis was first proposed by Denan in 1821 and refined by Murphy in 1892 [1] at a time when lengthy abdominal surgery was still considered dangerous. Later, their mechanical anastomosis method was superseded by suturing devices because abdominal surgery became safer. Magnetic compression anastomosis (MCA) was also proposed, but was not used clinically due to many difficulties such as the lack of confirmation of magnet safety, no convenient method for delivery of the magnet to the stenosis site, and a high rate of acute restenosis [2–4]. In fact, clinical use did not occur until we applied this method without surgery and general anesthesia in 1997 and presented the results in 1998 [5, 6]. Since then, more than 400 MCA procedures have been performed in Japan. Yamanouchi have been involved in almost all cases [7–24].

In this chapter, we describe the results of basic experiments, the materials and methods used, results, typical clinical cases, and problems encountered during the many MCA procedures that have been performed since the report in 1998.

E. Yamanouchi (✉)
Department of Radiology, International University of Health and Welfare Hospital,
Nasushiobara-shi, Tochigi-ken, Japan
e-mail: doctor@nn.iij4u.or.jp

R. Kumano
Department of Radiology, St. Marianna University Yokohama Seibu Hospital,
Yokohama City, Kanagawa-ken, Japan

H. Ohdaira · Y. Suzuki
Department of Surgery, International University of Health and Welfare Hospital,
Nasushiobara-shi, Tochigi-ken, Japan

M. Gagner (ed.), *Magnetic Surgery*, https://doi.org/10.1007/978-3-030-73947-8_16

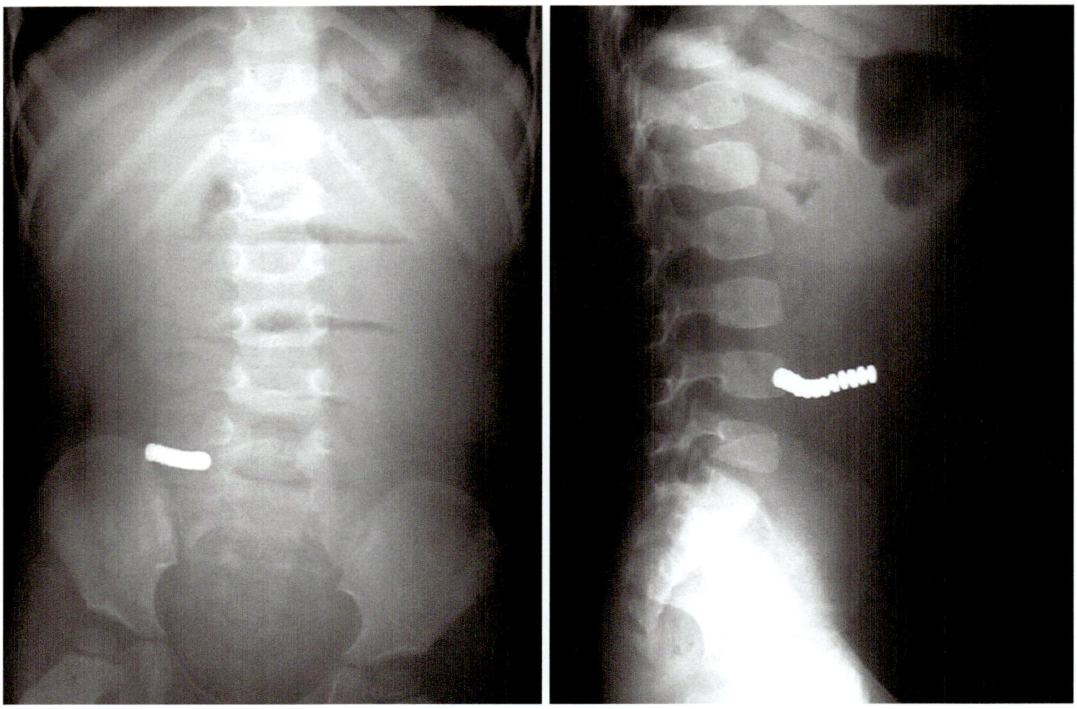

Fig. 16.1 A memorable case of accidental swallowing of magnets. Plain upright abdominal radiographs show foreign bodies (linearly mated small magnets) in the lower right quadrant of the abdomen. Fluid-filled dilated bowel loops are also noted, probably as a result of complete obstruction

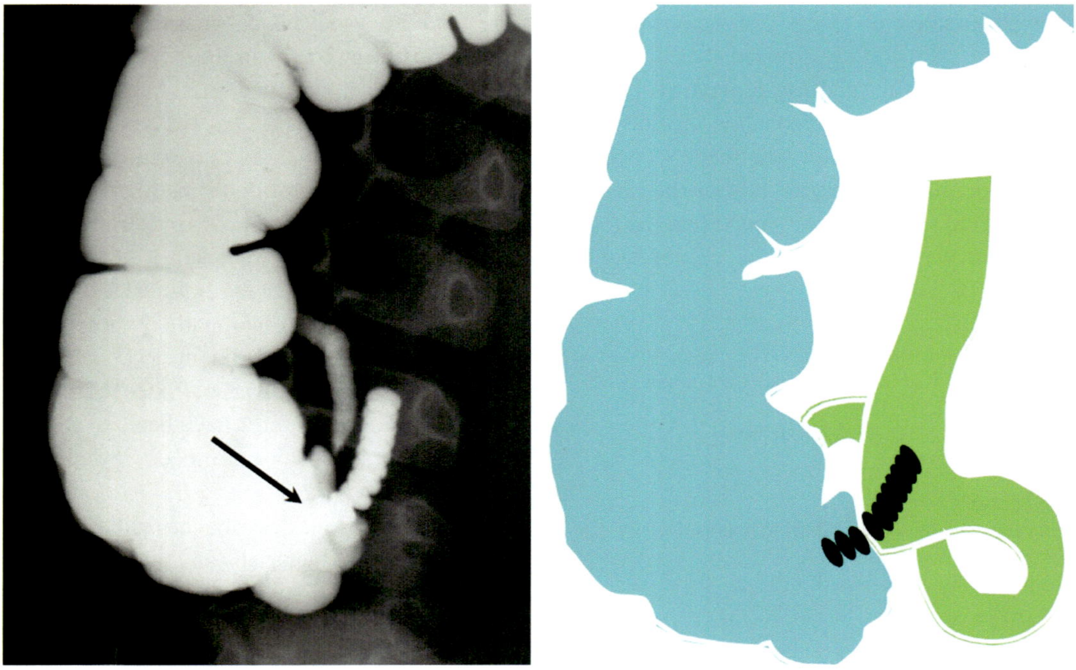

Fig. 16.2 A barium enema study showing three magnets in the cecum (*arrow*) and others in small bowel loops. A fistulous tract was found between the cecum and terminal ileum at the time of surgery

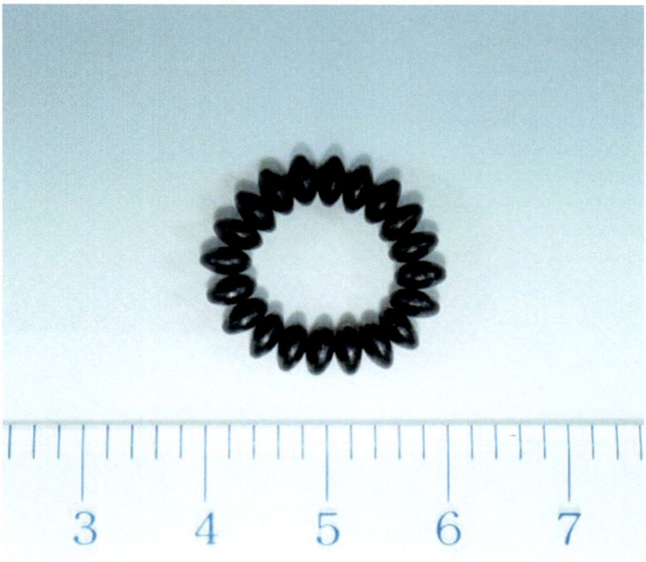

Fig. 16.3 Small magnets, similar to those accidentally swallowed, that have moderate remanence (1200 gauss) if mated (unit of measurement: centimeters)

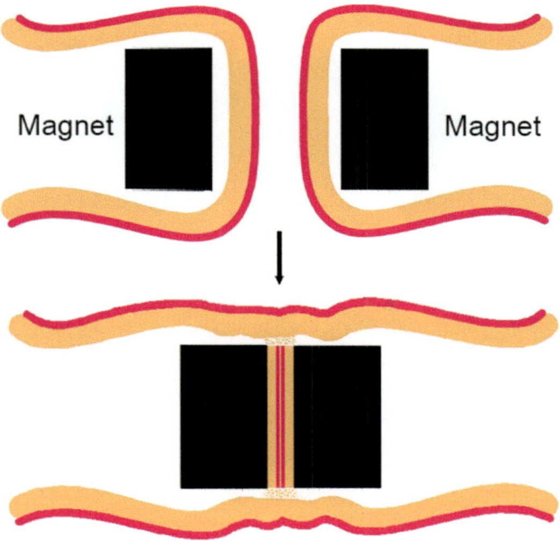

Fig. 16.4 Diagram illustrating magnetic compression anastomosis. If the magnetic grip is strong enough, a fistulous tract can be produced

Magnetic Compression Anastomosis

Basic Experimental Results

Multiple experiments were performed in rat and mongrel canine models to confirm the feasibility of MCA. In order to create an anastomosis, two rare-earth magnets (samarium-cobalt compound, 4 mm in diameter and 1.8 mm in thickness, with a remanence of 2300 gauss) were placed in each rat, one in the cecum and the other in the transverse colon (Fig. 16.5). The magnets in the cecum and transverse colon mated and subsequently created a fistulous anastomosis. The anastomosis was confirmed radiologically by a barium enema study (Fig. 16.6). Our experimental studies in rats confirmed that this method was safe and economical. Unlike with anastomoses created surgically, no white linear ischemic scar or inflammatory change was found at the site of the anastomosis after sacrifice (Fig. 16.7). Hematoxylin-eosin-stained pathological specimens obtained from the anastomotic site postmortem were checked for infiltration of inflammatory cells. The specimens were also stained with Masson's trichrome dye to check the state of the anastomosis layer by layer. Hardly any inflammatory change was found at the anastomotic site. Some multinucleated giant cells were found but without infiltration of inflammatory cells, suggesting that apoptosis may be involved in the process of forming an MCA. Furthermore, the site of the anastomosis was found to have an intact layer-by-layer structure, which cannot be obtained by surgical suturing (Fig. 16.8). Thus, we were finally able to create an MCA successfully. We determined that the optimal magnet strength was between 2000

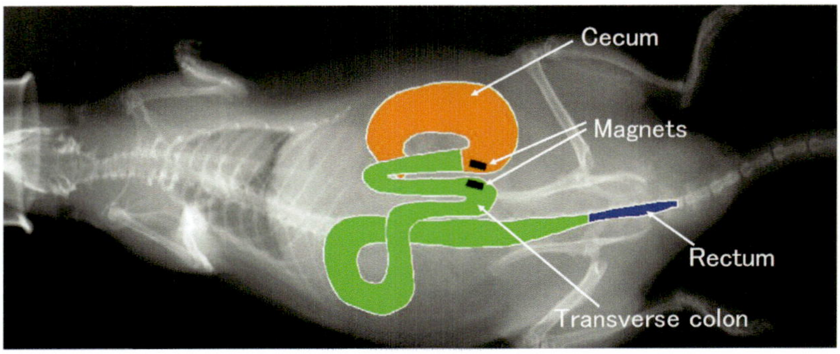

Fig. 16.5 Diagram of bowel loops in rats showing a magnet placed in the cecum and another in the transverse colon. Successful magnetic compression anastomosis was created between these two anatomical structures

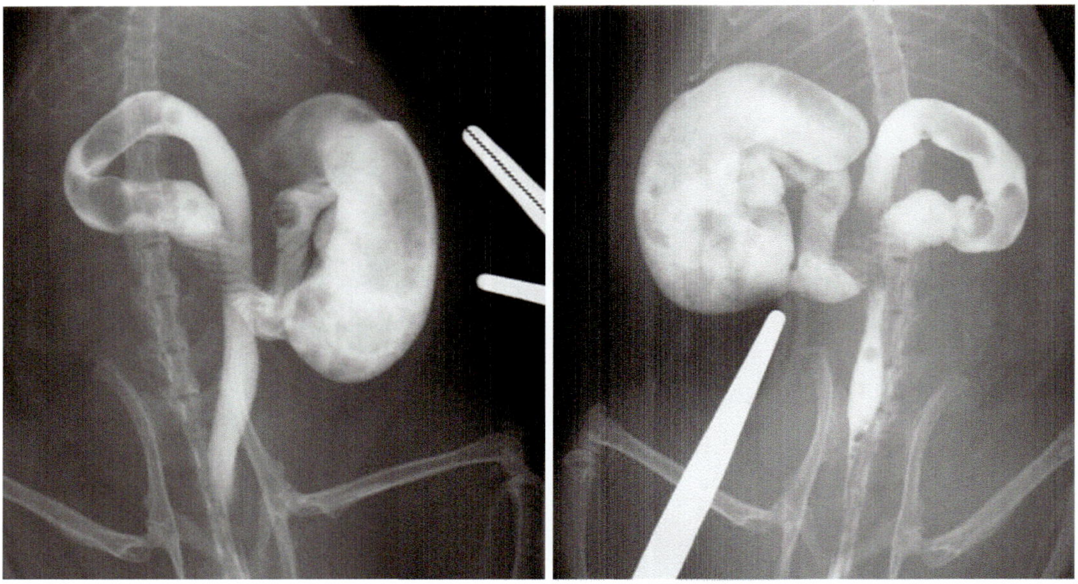

Fig. 16.6 A barium enema study in a rat showing a fistulous tract created by magnetic compression anastomosis (at the tip of the forceps)

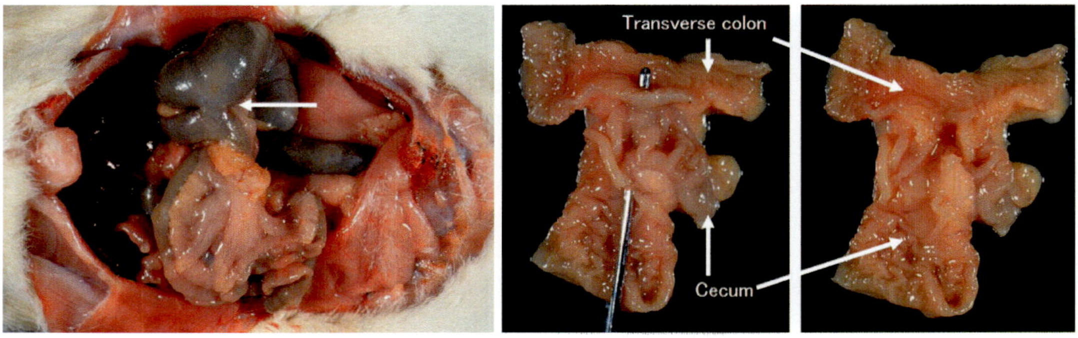

Fig. 16.7 A rat specimen obtained after sacrifice shows a fistulous tract (*arrow*) with no inflammatory change (*left*). A magnified view of the anastomotic site does not show the linear ischemic scar usually found in surgical cases. The surgical sonde is placed in the fistulous tract (*right*)

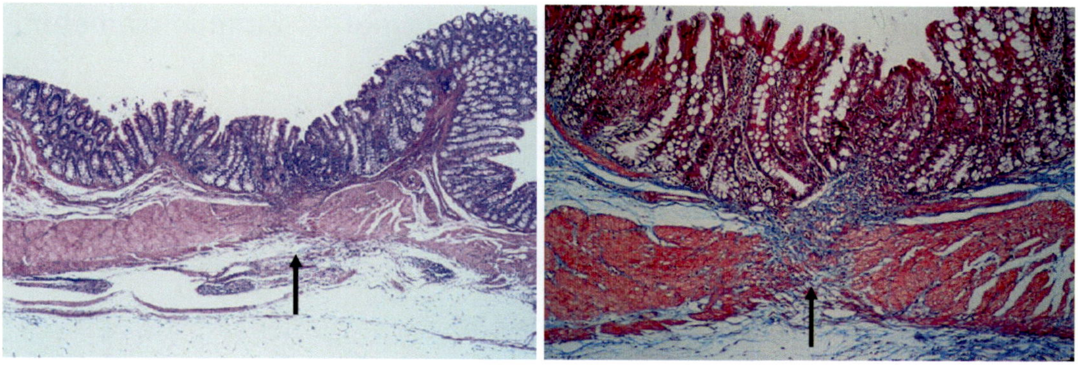

Fig. 16.8 Infiltration of inflammatory cells, which is usually seen in surgical specimens, is not noted at the anastomotic site on hematoxylin-eosin staining. Some multinucleated giant cells were found not to show infiltration of inflammatory cells. This finding suggests that apoptosis may participate in magnetic compression anastomosis (*left*). The anastomotic site shows wonderful layer-to-layer structure on Masson's trichrome staining (*right*)

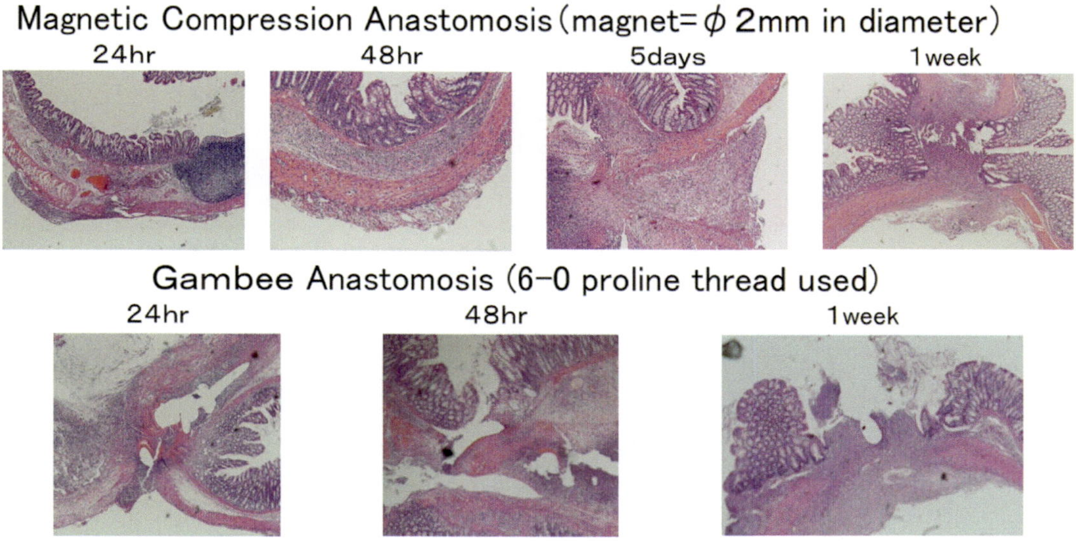

Fig. 16.9 The time course (24 hours to 1 week) of magnetic compression anastomosis and Gambee anastomosis. The main difference between the two methods is that a fibrin net appears around the site of the magnetic compression anastomosis within a few days but not around the site of the Gambee anastomosis until 1–3 weeks later

and 4500 gauss. Magnets weaker than 2000 gauss failed to create an anastomosis and there was a risk of anastomotic leak with magnets stronger than 4500 gauss.

We conducted further experiments to identify the key to maintaining the anastomosis. Studies in rat models confirmed that the main difference between the MCA and Gambee methods is that a fibrin net appears around an MCA within a few days but not around a Gambee anastomosis until 1–3 weeks (Figs. 16.9 and 16.10). Next, we investigated how the layer-by-layer structure was formed. TUNEL staining of specimens showed that many cells were in an apoptotic state, suggesting that apoptosis has an important role in structural remodeling at the site of the anastomosis (Fig. 16.11). Our experiments in rats also suggested that the MCA method could be used in humans if the magnets used were strong enough (see Fig. 16.4).

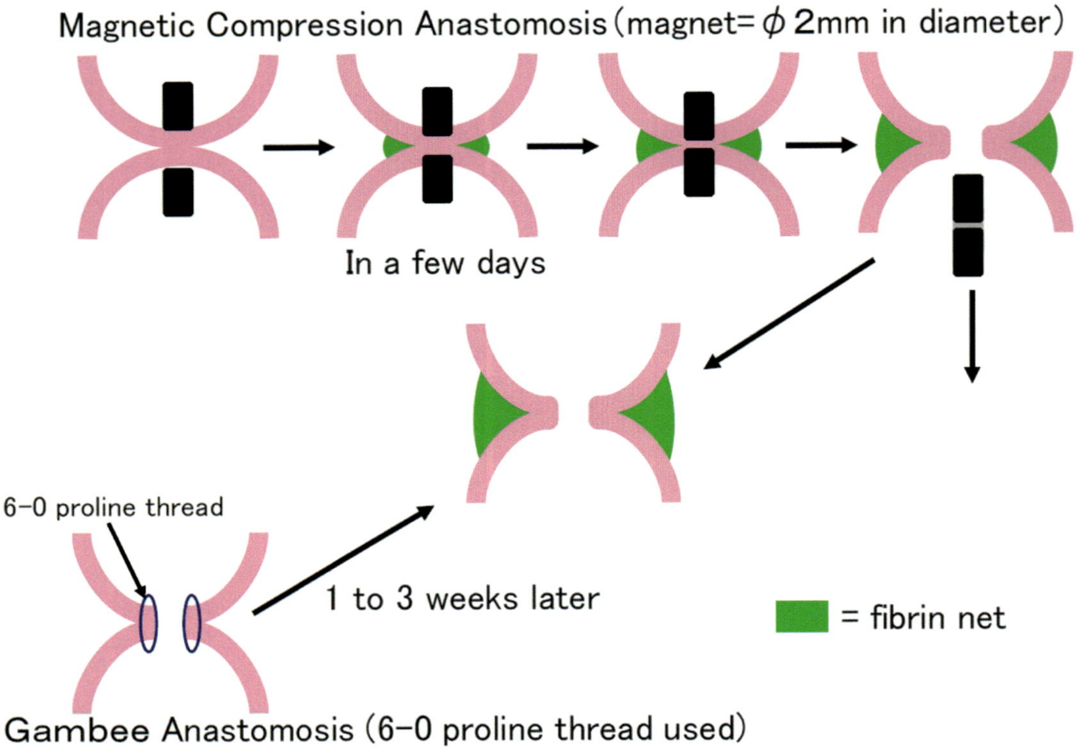

Fig. 16.10 Diagram showing magnetic compression anastomosis and Gambee anastomosis. The major difference between the two anastomosis methods is that fibrin net appears around the magnetic compression anastomosis site in a few days, but it does not appear around the Gambee anastomosis site until 1–3 weeks later

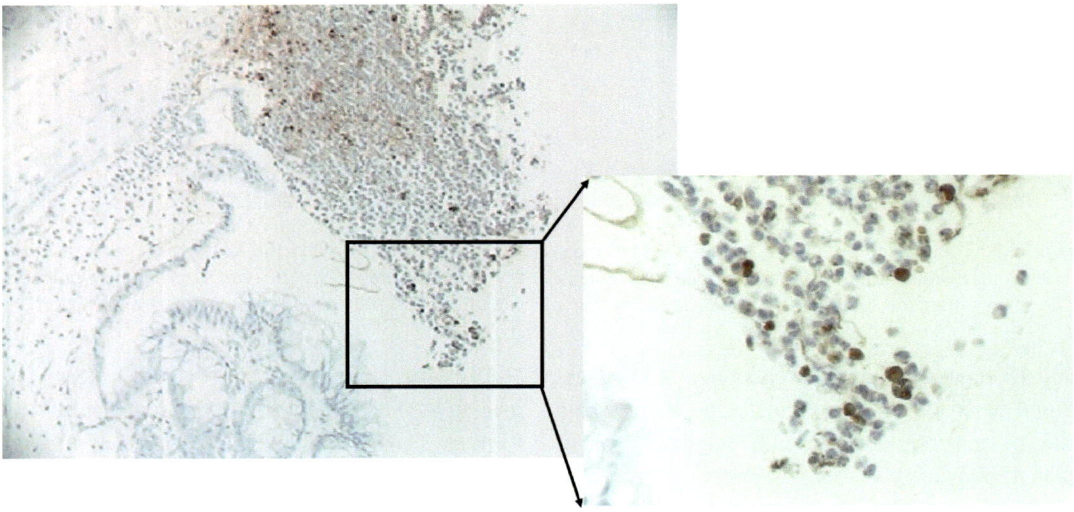

Fig. 16.11 The layers between the magnets remain as withered structures. Many apoptotic cells are apparent at the rim edge on TUNEL staining, suggesting that apoptosis may be involved in remodeling

Materials and Methods

Types of Magnets

Rare-earth magnets were already known to be strong magnets at the time we first started performing these procedures. There are two main types of rare-earth magnets, namely, samarium-cobalt magnet and neodymium-iron-boron magnet. Samarium-cobalt magnets (Magna Co., Ltd. Tokyo, Japan) were used for enteroenteric, bilioenteric, and biliobiliary anastomoses because neodymium magnets are usually nickel plated to prevent oxidation and thus are corrosive and biologically toxic. The two disk magnets were placed separately in the organs to be anastomosed and the joined magnets were excreted mainly in the feces after mating, usually within 1–2 weeks after an enteroenteric anastomosis. We designated the magnet placed at the distal site as the parent magnet and that placed at the proximal site as the daughter magnet (Fig. 16.12). However, two cylindrical magnets are usually used for a bilioenteric or biliobiliary MCA. The parent magnet is placed in the ascending jejunal limb, duodenum, or common bile duct (CBD) and the daughter magnet is placed in an intrahepatic bile duct (Fig. 16.13).

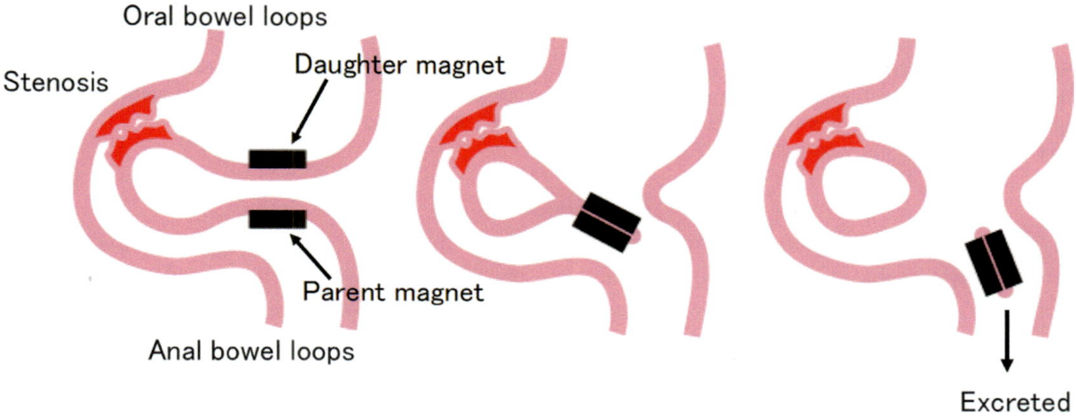

Fig. 16.12 Diagram showing the process of enteroenteric magnetic compression anastomosis. First, the parent magnet in most cases is transported across the stenosis, which is temporarily dilated by a balloon catheter. In other cases, the parent magnet is transported from the anal side. The daughter magnet is then positioned, and the magnets are mated. The soft tissue compressed by the magnets is finally removed from the anastomotic site and the new lumen provides an adequate tract

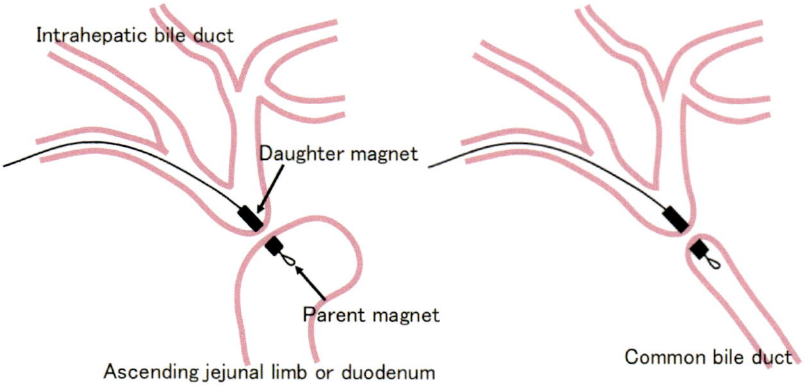

Fig. 16.13 Diagrams showing the process of bilioenteric and biliobiliary magnetic compression anastomosis. The figure on the left shows an anastomosis between the intrahepatic bile duct and the ascending jejunal limb or duodenum. The figure on the right shows an anastomosis between the intrahepatic bile duct and common bile duct. In some cases, the intrahepatic bile ducts may include the common bile duct

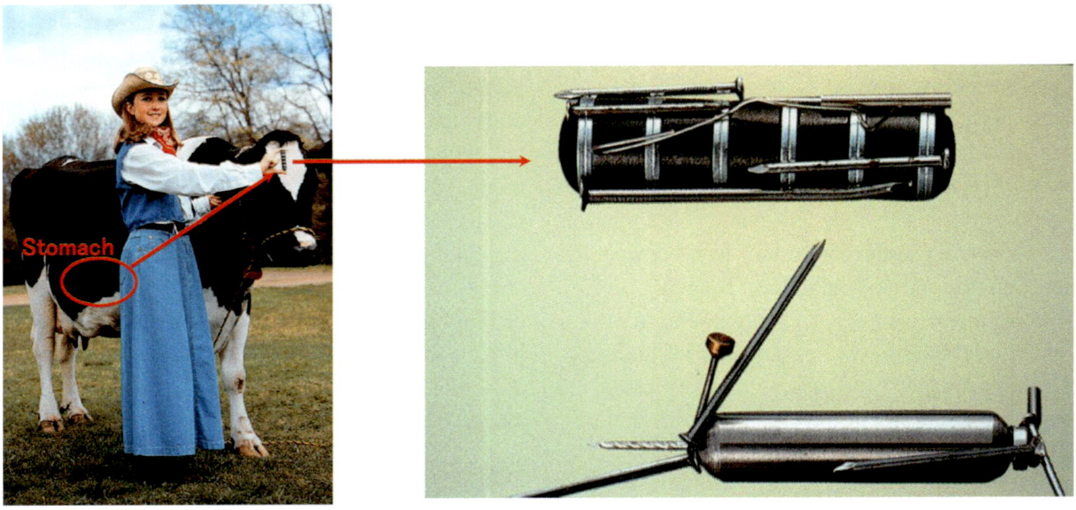

Fig. 16.14 Cows are known to accidentally swallow iron nails that can puncture the stomach. Farmers in Japan and the United States insert a cow magnet into the fourth stomach to prevent injury by iron nails. The magnets are left in the stomach for the cow's entire lifetime. The upper magnet is a new model to prevent iron nails from flaring. The lower magnet is an older model

The safety of the magnetic force and of a magnet itself when placed in the digestive tract is thought to be confirmed by the following observation. Cattle are known to like the taste of iron and often accidentally swallow iron nails that can puncture the wall of the stomach. To combat this problem, cattle are often fed magnets that enter the fourth stomach where they can attract an ingested iron nail and prevent its tip from piercing the stomach wall (Fig. 16.14). There are no problems with the milk and meat produced by cattle, which have these magnets in place lifelong.

Samarium-cobalt magnets were used to create enteroenteric and bilioenteric or biliobiliary MCA. Two disk magnets are used in enteroenteric MCA. The size of each magnet depends on the intended site of the anastomosis. For example, in the case of a gastroduodenal or gastrojejunal anastomosis, two disk magnets of the same size are used because when mated they can be removed from the stomach easily via an endoscope or are excreted uneventfully. However, in the case of ileus it is recommended that the parent magnet should not enter the dead-end loop, so the parent magnetic has a diameter that is 5 mm larger than that of the daughter magnet. If the mated magnet was to enter the dead-end bowel loop, it would be almost impossible to remove nonsurgically. Four types of disk magnets are commonly used in enteroenteric MCA (Fig. 16.15). These magnets are 15–22.5 mm in diameter, 5 mm in thickness, and have total remanence (magnetic strength) values in the range of 3200–2000 gauss. A small disk magnet is stronger than a large magnet if the thickness is the same. In children with esophageal atresia, smaller magnets with a diameter of 10–12.5 mm and a thickness of 5 mm are used. There are two holes in each disk magnet. The hole on the side of the magnet is called the side hole for the guidewire to transport. The hole on the top is called the top hole for lifting with a thread to perform magnetic compression revision of stenosis.

Two types of cylindrical magnet are used in bilioenteric or biliobiliary MCA. The parent magnet is 5 mm in diameter and 5 or 6 mm in length with a nylon snare for the forceps of the endoscope. The daughter magnet is 4 mm in diameter and 9 mm in length with a guidewire for manipulation (Fig. 16.16).

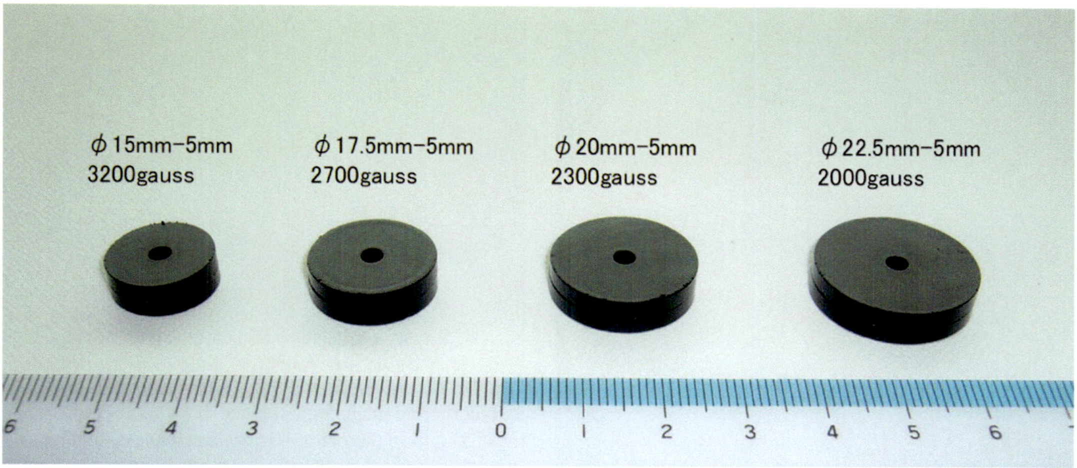
ϕ15mm-5mm
3200gauss
ϕ17.5mm-5mm
2700gauss
ϕ20mm-5mm
2300gauss
ϕ22.5mm-5mm
2000gauss

Fig. 16.15 Four types of disk magnets commonly used in enteroenteric magnetic compression anastomosis. They range in diameter from 15 mm to 22.5 mm and have a thickness of 5 mm. The remanence is shown beside the photograph of each magnet. Each disk magnet has two holes, namely a "side hole" for the guidewire and a "top hole" for lifting with a thread to perform the magnetic compression revision for stenosis procedure

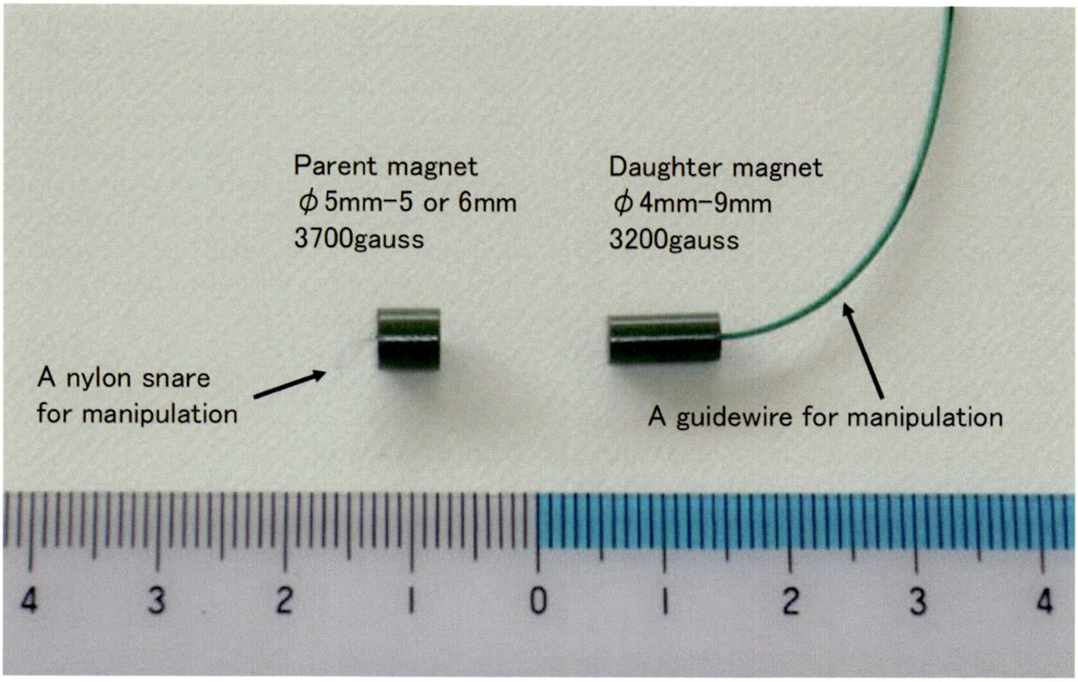

Fig. 16.16 In bilioenteric or biliobiliary magnetic anastomosis, the parent magnet is 5 mm in diameter and 5 or 6 mm in length with a nylon snare for the endoscopic forceps. The daughter magnet is 4 mm in diameter and 9 mm in length with a guidewire for manipulation

How to Transport and Remove the Magnet

We initially considered that an endoscope could be used to transport the magnet, but found that pushing the magnet over the guidewire was more effective than using the endoscope in enteroenteric MCA procedures. However, the endoscope is useful as a base when pushing the magnet over

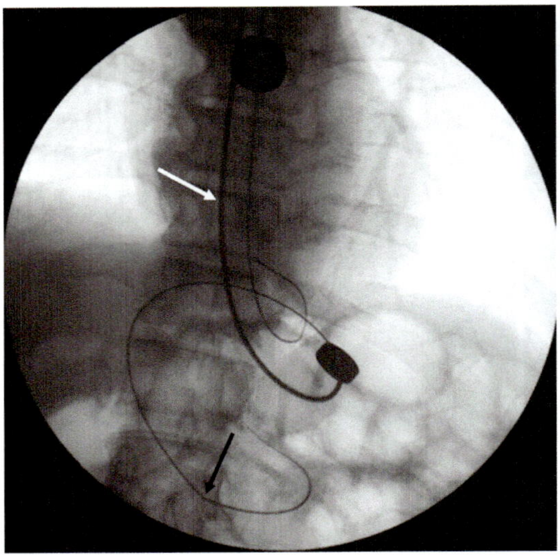

Fig. 16.17 Radiographic image of magnetic compression anastomosis performed to create a ρ-anastomosis between the jejunum and the blind end of the jejunum. The parent magnet, which was transported over the guidewire and bent 30 degrees at 5 cm from the tip (*black arrow*), is placed in the jejunal. The thick line over the guidewire is the pusher (*white arrow*), which is used to push and release the magnet

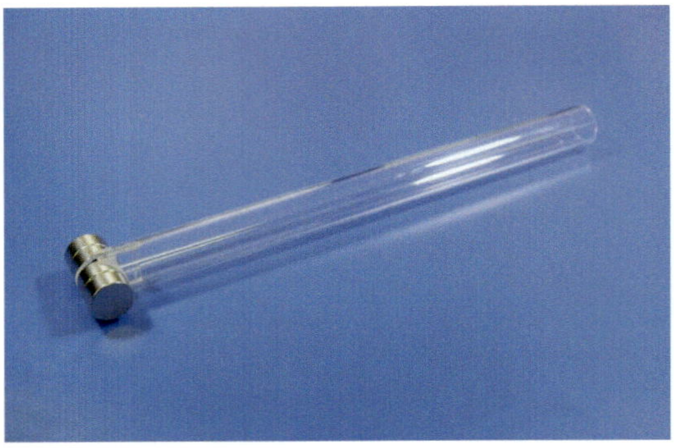

Fig. 16.18 Photograph showing the apparatus used for extracorporeal magnetic guidance. Four neodymium magnets (20 mm in diameter, 10 mm in thickness, 8000 gauss in total) are attached at the head of the handle. This apparatus is used to move or hold the magnet in the bowel loops

the guidewire. The guidewire is also useful for holding the magnet temporarily when bent to 30 degrees at 5 cm from the tip (Fig. 16.17). In some cases, extracorporeal magnetic guidance is very effective when holding and moving the magnet (Fig. 16.18). Extracorporeal magnetic guidance is also necessary when placing the magnet deeper within the bowel loops; an endoscope cannot reach deep within the jejunum or ileum and there was no endoscope that could enter the small intestine when we initially started performing MCA procedures. Insertion of an ileus tube made guidance easier than expected (see Fig. 16.20, left). However, this method cannot be used in obese patients because the extracorporeal magnetic force cannot reach the target depth in the body. The mated magnets are usually excreted via the bowel loop in which the parent magnet was placed. The mated magnets are heavier, and thus sometimes taking more time than expected to pass through the bowel loops.

In bilioenteric or biliobiliary MCA, an endoscope is required to transport the parent magnet into the ascending jejunal limb, duodenum, or CBD through the ampulla of Vater. The daughter magnet is attached to the guidewire, which is placed with deflection to create a pushing force. Using this pushing force, the mated magnets are moved into the ascending jejunal limb or CBD. The mated magnets are endoscopically removed in bilioenteric or biliobiliary cases. In some cases, the mated magnets can be released from the guidewire attached to the daughter magnet by pushing hard over the guidewire because the portion to which the guidewire is attached is designed to be released by strong external force. The mated magnets are excreted via the fecal route.

A Clinical Study

We performed a study involving 422 patients who had a stenosis in the intestine or CBD with a gap between the organs to be anastomosed of <3 cm on fluoroscopy using Gastrografin or abdominal CT. The patients (266 males, 156 females) had a mean age of 65.5 (range, aged 1–91) years. Four patients who underwent enteroenteric anastomosis required two procedures because of acute stenosis and one patient required bilioenteric anastomosis twice because of restenosis after 6 months. Therefore, a total of 427 procedures (206 enteroenteric anastomoses, 189 bilioenteric or biliobiliary anastomoses, and 32 magnetic compression revision for stenosis [MCRS]; described later) were performed. The most common cause of stenosis was postoperative complications in the enteroenteric, bilioenteric, or biliobiliary MCA cases. Informed consent was obtained from all patients or their guardians after they had received a detailed explanation of the procedure. Various representative clinical cases are described in the next section.

Representative Clinical Cases

A Case of Ileocolostomy

The patient was a woman in her 80s with chronic postoperative adhesive ileus. Surgery was contraindicated because of severe cardiac dysfunction, so an ileus tube had been placed percutaneously after gastrostomy a number of years earlier. Follow-through and barium enema studies were performed simultaneously to assess the possibility of MCA. The ileum and descending colon were next to one another (Fig. 16.19) with no other bowel loop in between, suggesting that the patient was a suitable candidate for MCA. The swallowed daughter magnet was moved along the ileus tube under extracorporeal magnetic guidance. The parent magnet was placed endoscopically, after which the two magnets were mated (Fig. 16.20). Endoscopic observation 10 days later showed passage of feces through the anastomosis. The endoscopic view showed a better anastomosis than we had ever seen with surgery. It would be impossible to create such a smooth anastomosis surgically. No inflammatory changes were noted around the anastomotic site (Fig. 16.21). A pathological specimen obtained from the area between the magnets showed each layer of the two bowel loops to be well preserved (Fig. 16.22). This was the first case of enteroenteric MCA performed in humans.

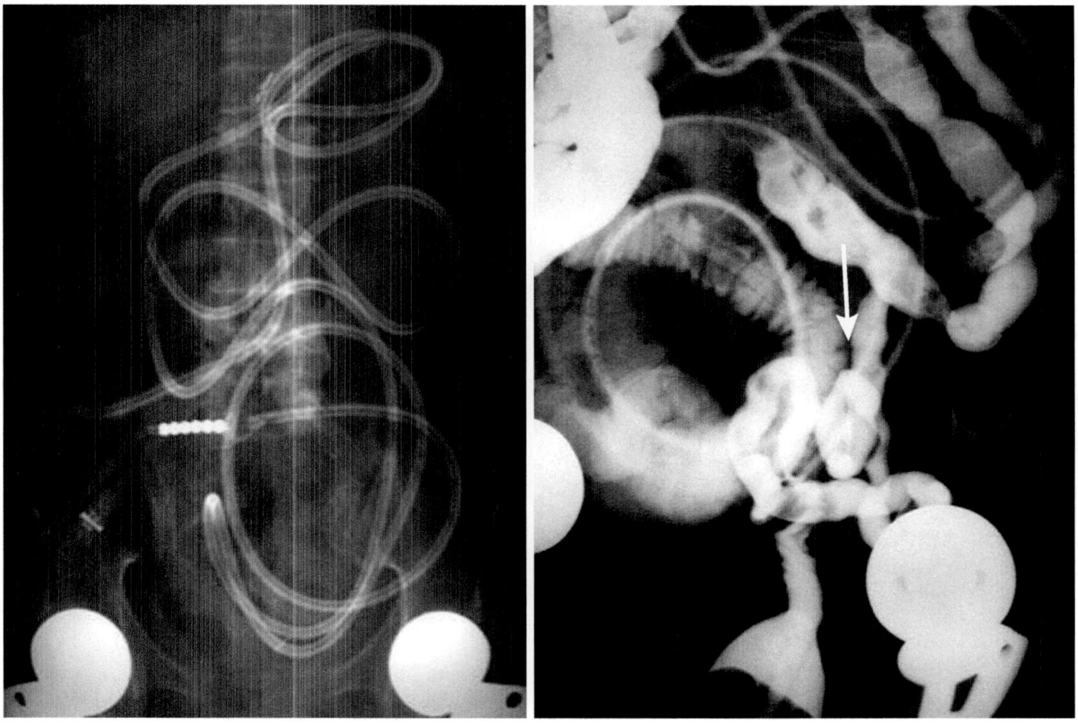

Fig. 16.19 Radiographic images showing an ileus tube that was placed percutaneously after gastrostomy many years earlier. Follow-through and barium enema studies were performed simultaneously. Microcolon due to no passage of fecal material can be identified. The ileum and descending colon are next to each other (*arrow*), and there is no other bowel loop between the two structures

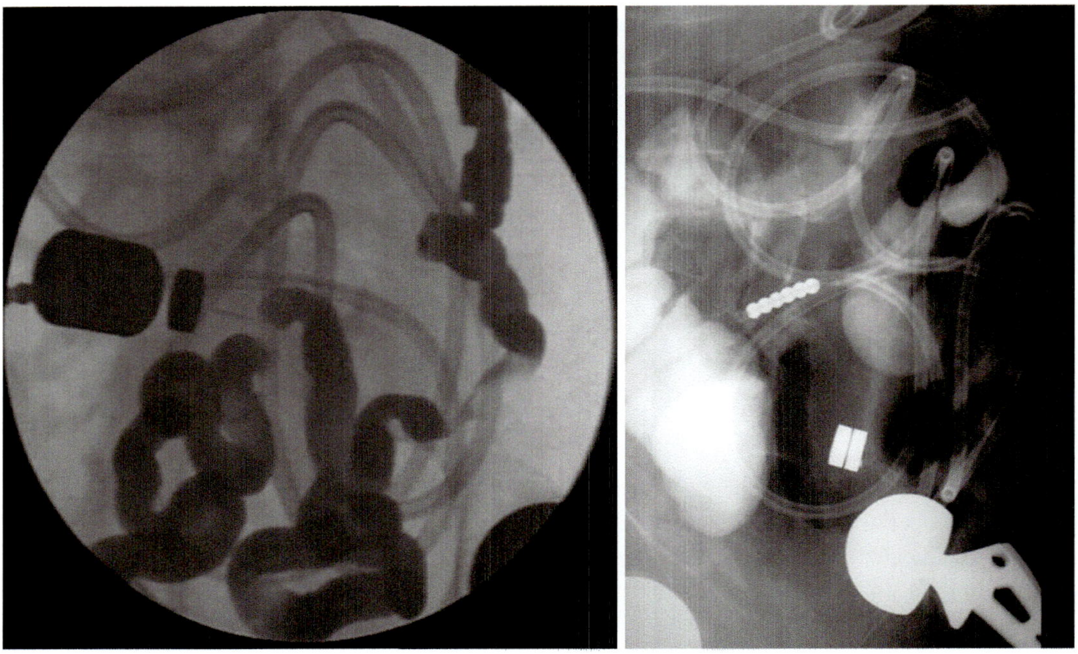

Fig. 16.20 Radiographic images showing that the swallowed daughter magnet is moved along the ileus tube under extracorporeal magnetic guidance. The parent magnet was placed endoscopically, and the two magnets were then mated

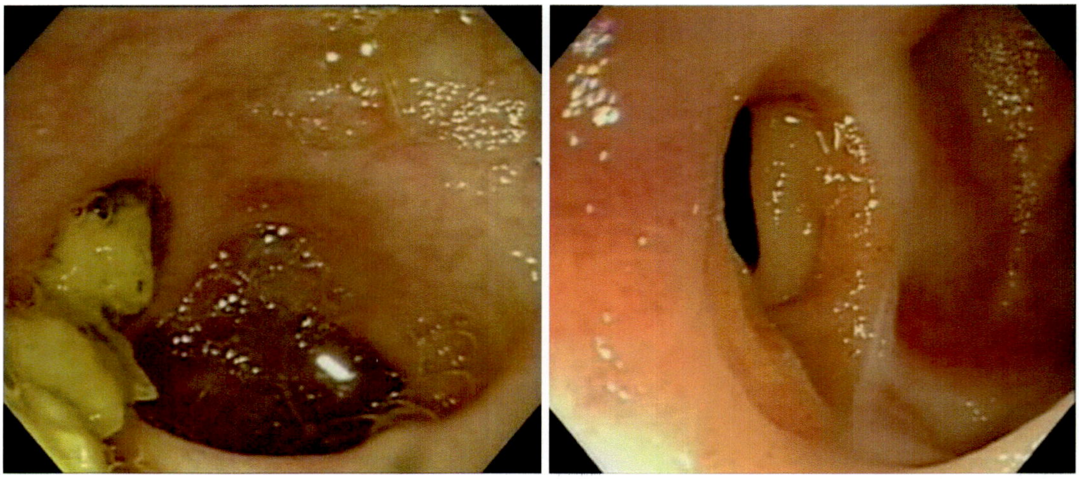

Fig. 16.21 After 10 days, endoscopic observation showed feces passing through the anastomosis. This endoscopic view showed a much better anastomosis than we had ever seen with surgery. It is impossible to create such a smooth anastomosis surgically. No inflammatory changes were noted around the anastomosis site

A Case of Gastroduodenal Anastomosis

The patient was a man in his 40s. Intake of solids was difficult because of scarring from a duodenal ulcer, and he had been on a liquid diet for approximately 6 months. He did not want to undergo distal gastrectomy because both his parents had died during surgery, so he chose MCA for gastroduodenal anastomosis. It was hard to transport the parent magnet across the pyloric stenosis,

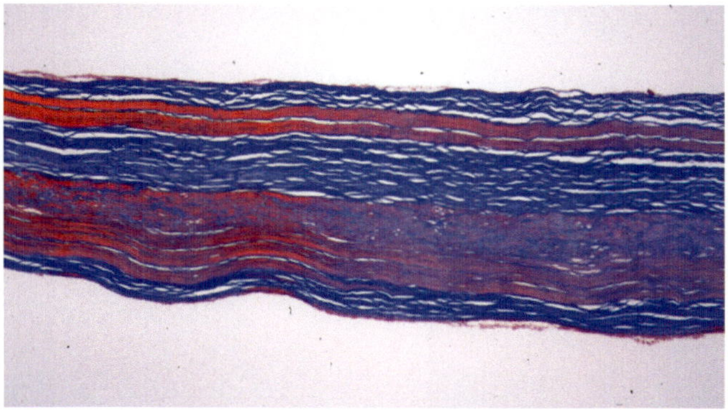

Fig. 16.22 A pathological specimen between the magnets showed each layer of the two bowel loops were well preserved without deterioration (Masson's trichrome staining). The lower thick zone is the muscular layer of the small intestine, and the upper thin zone is that of the large intestine. Note that the basic structure of the two intestinal walls is well preserved, although cells have disappeared, probably due to ischemic necrosis

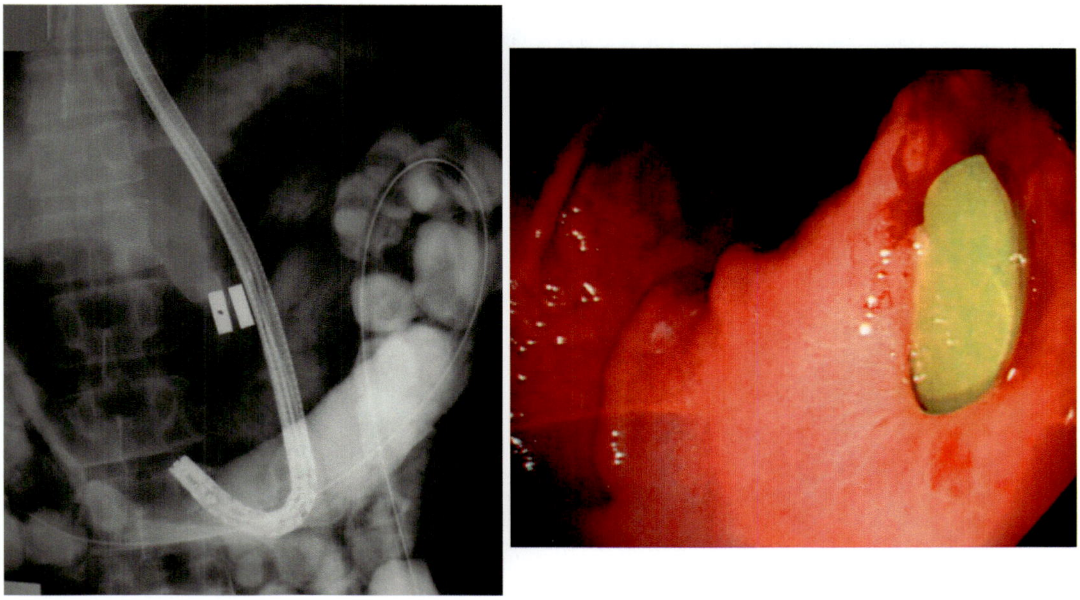

Fig. 16.23 The parent magnet (15 mm in diameter, 5 mm in thickness) placed in the fourth part of the duodenum after difficult passage across a pyloric stenosis, which was temporarily dilated by a balloon catheter. The 15-mm parent magnet was at the limit of the size able to enter through a pyloric stenosis. The daughter magnet (15 mm in diameter, 5 mm in thickness) was endoscopically placed in the body of the stomach. The magnets were finally mated and excreted after 14 days

which was temporarily dilated by a balloon catheter. Disk magnets measuring 17.5 mm are often used in this type of anastomosis, but 15-mm disk magnets were the limit in this case because of the severe stenosis. Transport of the daughter magnet was easier, and the two magnets mated immediately (Fig. 16.23). Two weeks later, the mated magnets had been released and were excreted. Acute stenosis is often noted after gastroduodenal MCA, but is easily controlled by frequent balloon dilatation (FBD), which is necessary once or twice weekly for several weeks (Fig. 16.24). At the 3-year follow-up, the anastomotic site showed good patency with smooth mucosal union. Now that he could have enough food, the patient was fat enough to misunderstand (Fig. 16.25).

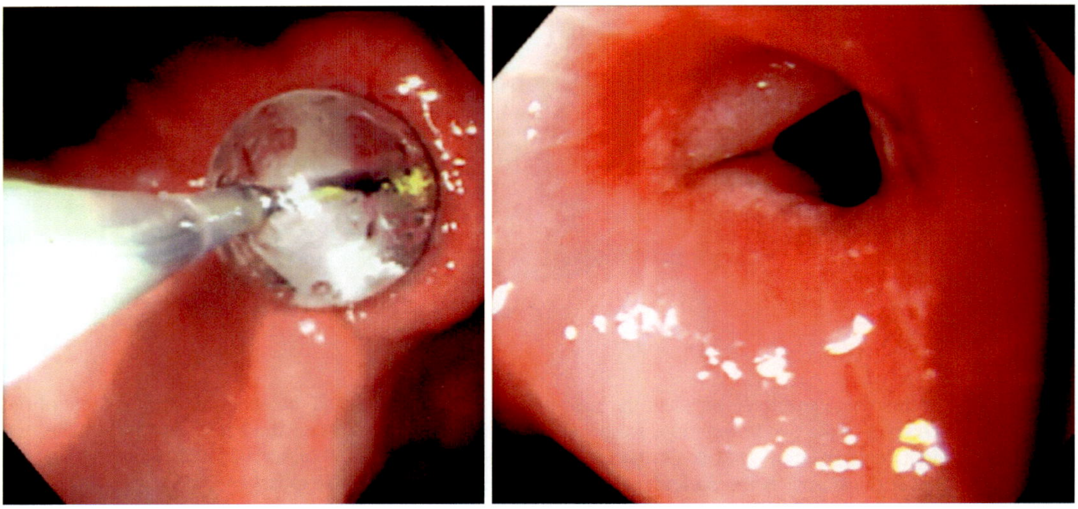

Fig. 16.24 Acute stenosis is often noted after gastroduodenal magnetic compression anastomosis but is easily controlled by frequent balloon dilatation (*left*). Smooth anastomosis may be noted on endoscopic examination at discharge (*right*)

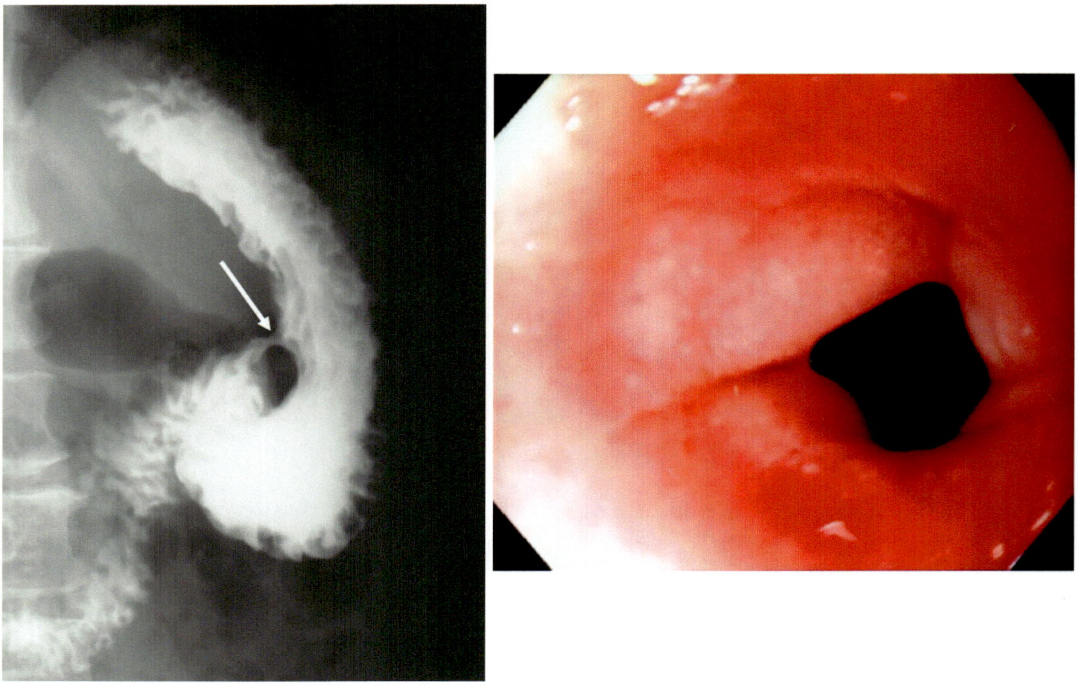

Fig. 16.25 Good passage of Gastrografin across an anastomosis (*white arrow*). No residual food material is visualized in the stomach (*left*). The anastomotic site showed good patency with smooth mucosal union between the stomach and duodenum on endoscopy at follow-up 3 years later (*right*)

A Case of Postoperative Occlusion After Low Anterior Resection

The patient was a man in his 70s who had undergone a low anterior resection 5 years earlier with stoma closure 3 years earlier and suddenly developed ileus because of complete obstruction of the anastomotic site (Fig. 16.26). Reoperation was predicted to be difficult because the site of the obstruction was located deep within the small

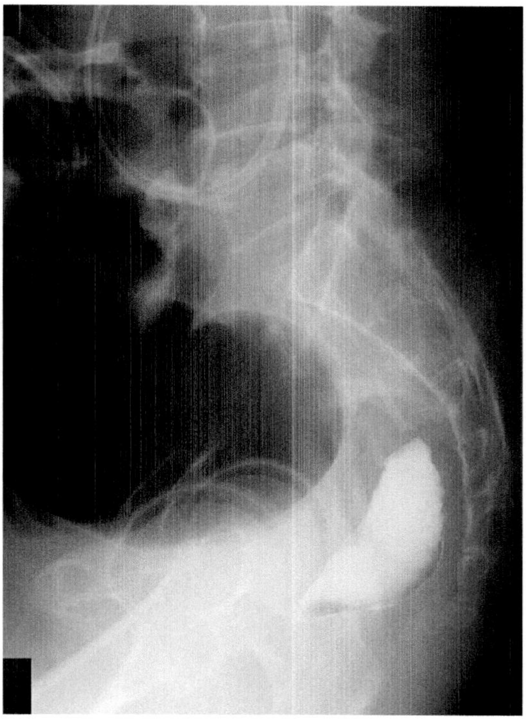

Fig. 16.26 This patient had undergone low anterior resection of the rectum for rectal cancer 5 years earlier and stoma closure 3 years earlier. Ileus developed suddenly. A barium enema study showed complete obstruction at the anastomotic site

pelvic cavity. Therefore, MCA was planned by swallowing the daughter magnet. The daughter magnet reached the blind end of the descending colon within a few days. The parent magnet was placed in the rectum by digital manipulation. The two magnets were mated in position uneventfully (Fig. 16.27) and excreted 10 days later. The created fistulous tract was not fully covered by normal mucosa, so balloon dilatation was applied several times to prevent stenosis. Fecal passage was also thought to work as good dilatation force in this case (Fig. 16.28). Good patency of the tract was observed at discharge, and the patient has had no problems since (Fig. 16.29).

A Case of Postoperative Occlusion After Low Anterior Resection

The patient was a man in his 60s who had developed a leak-related anastomotic occlusion after a low anterior resection, which was treated by creating a colostomy in the transverse colon. The surgeons were reluctant to perform repeat surgery because the site of obstruction was deep within the small pelvic cavity and there was con-

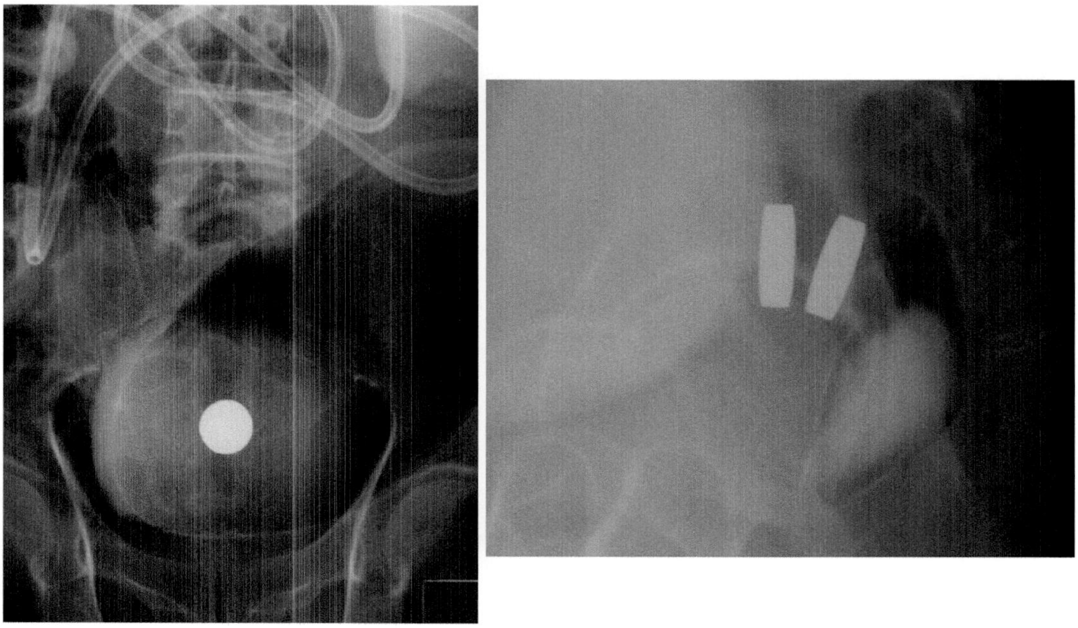

Fig. 16.27 The daughter magnet (17.5 mm in diameter, 5 mm in thickness) was swallowed and reached the blind end of the descending colon within a few days. The parent magnet (the same size as the daughter magnet) was carried into the rectum by digital manipulation. The two magnets were mated in position uneventfully

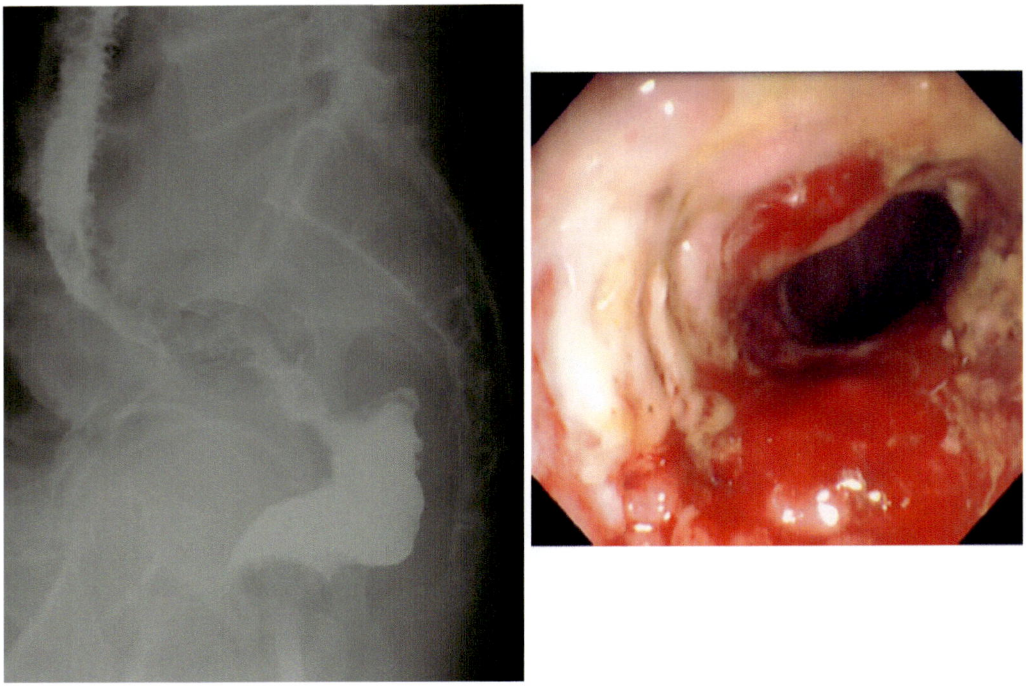

Fig. 16.28 A barium enema study and an endoscopic view showing a patent fistulous tract that was not fully covered by normal mucosa. Balloon dilatation was applied several times to prevent stenosis

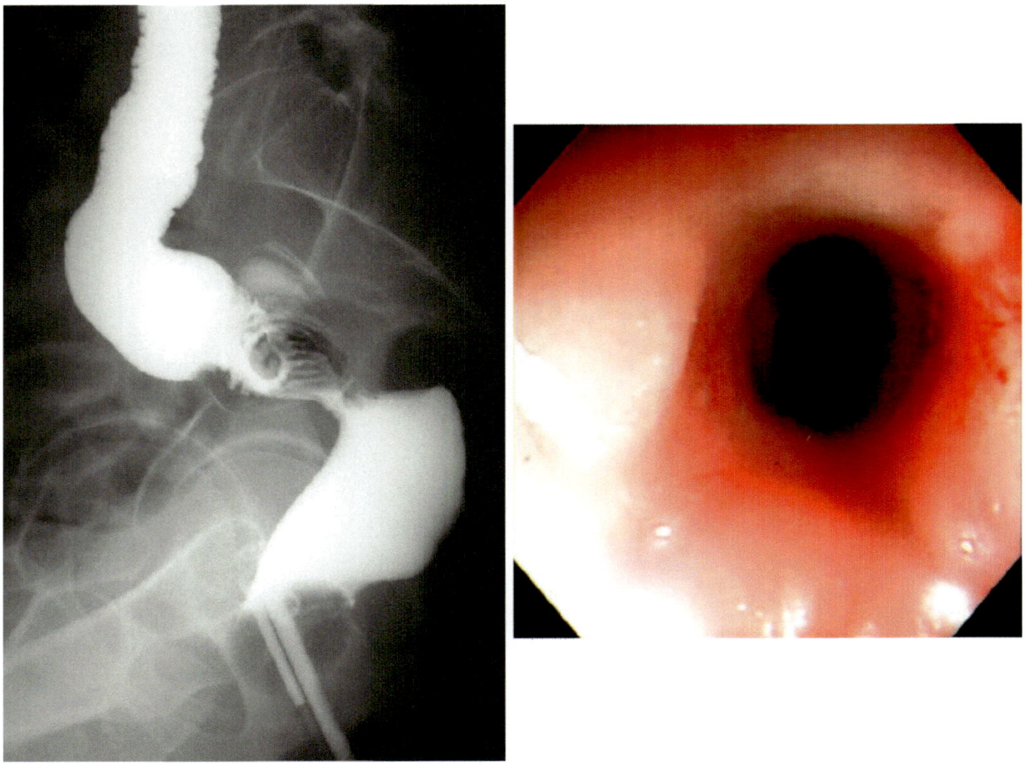

Fig. 16.29 A barium enema study and endoscopic view show good patency of the tract, which is now fully covered by normal mucosa. The patient was able to resume a normal life

cern about possible ineffective suturing and recurrence of leak as a result of multiple diverticula in the descending colon (Fig. 16.30). Therefore, the plan was to perform an MCA via the transverse colostomy; however, surgical staples created by automatic suture apparatus were identified in the stricture (Fig. 16.31). At that time, it was unknown if surgical staples would be severed by MCA. Nevertheless, MCA was performed, and the mated magnets were excreted 2 weeks later without any problems related to the surgical staples (Fig. 16.32). Radiographs

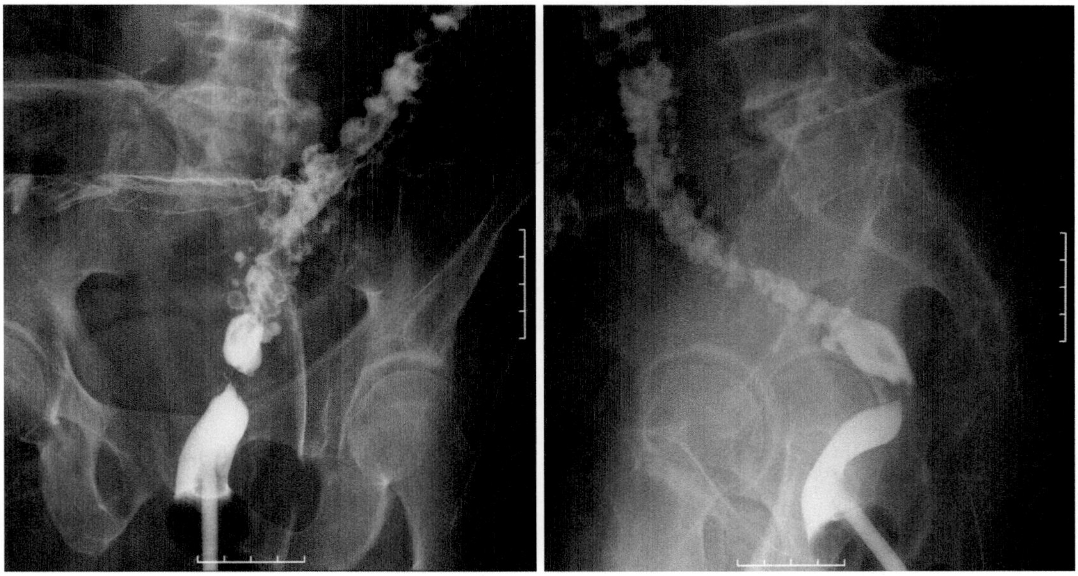

Fig. 16.30 An MCA between the descending colon and rectum. This patient developed an obstruction as a result of an anastomotic leak after low anterior resection for rectal cancer

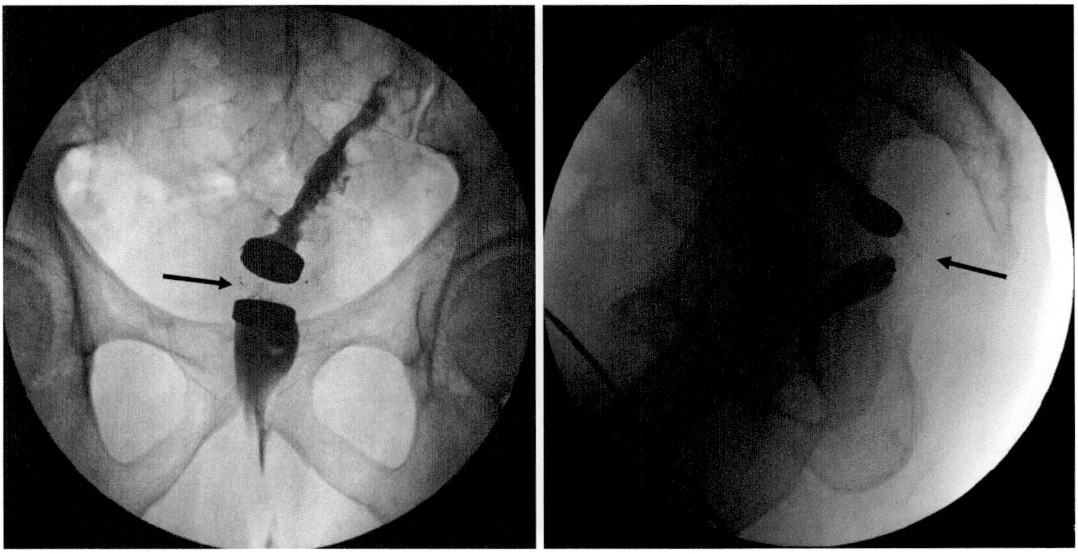

Fig. 16.31 Staples left by automatic suture apparatus can be seen at the obstruction site (*arrow*). The daughter magnet (20 mm in diameter, 5 mm in thickness) was transported over the guidewire through a transverse colostomy. The parent magnet (the same size as the daughter magnet) was carried into the rectum by digital manipulation. Finally, the two magnets were placed in position with no problems

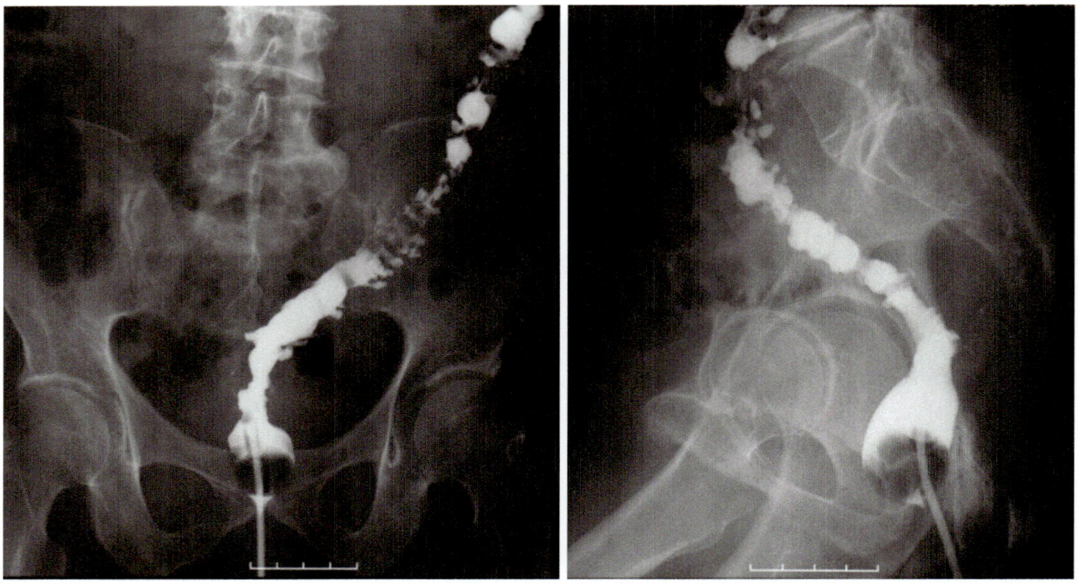

Fig. 16.32 The mated magnets were excreted 2 weeks later. A barium enema study confirming satisfactory passage of the contrast medium

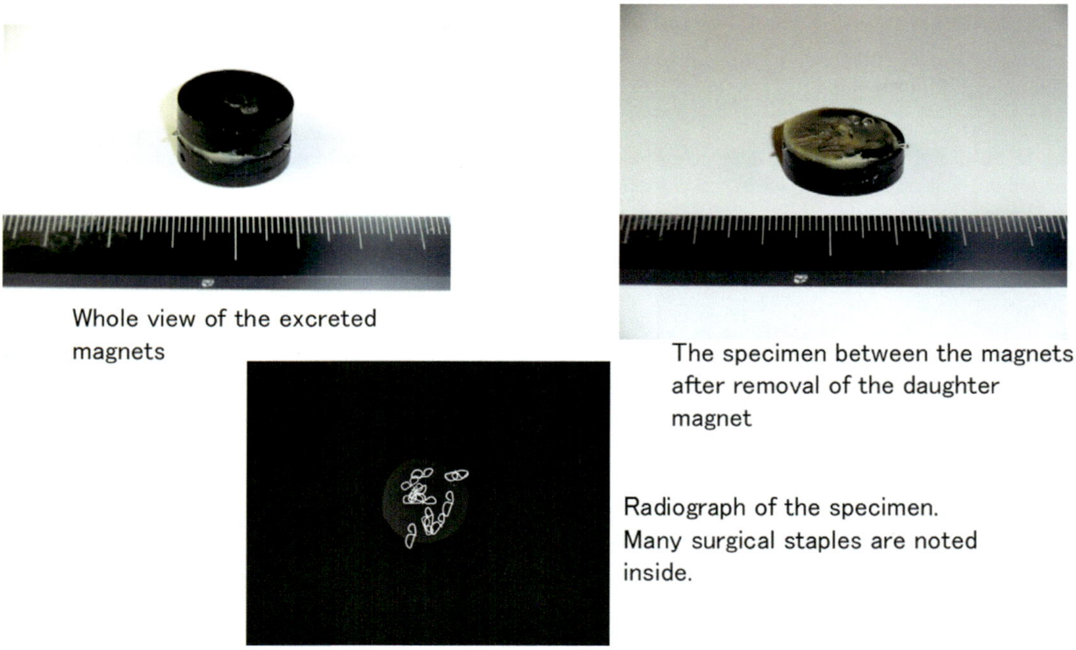

Fig. 16.33 Photograph showing a whole view of the excreted magnets and a radiograph of the specimen. There are many surgical staples in the specimen on the radiograph. Magnetic compression anastomosis is possible even if there are surgical staples between the magnets

revealed numerous surgical staples within the specimen (Fig. 16.33). Therefore, MCA is possible even if there are surgical staples between the magnets (Fig. 16.34). Balloon dilatation was applied on several occasions to prevent stenosis. Fecal passage was also thought to work as good

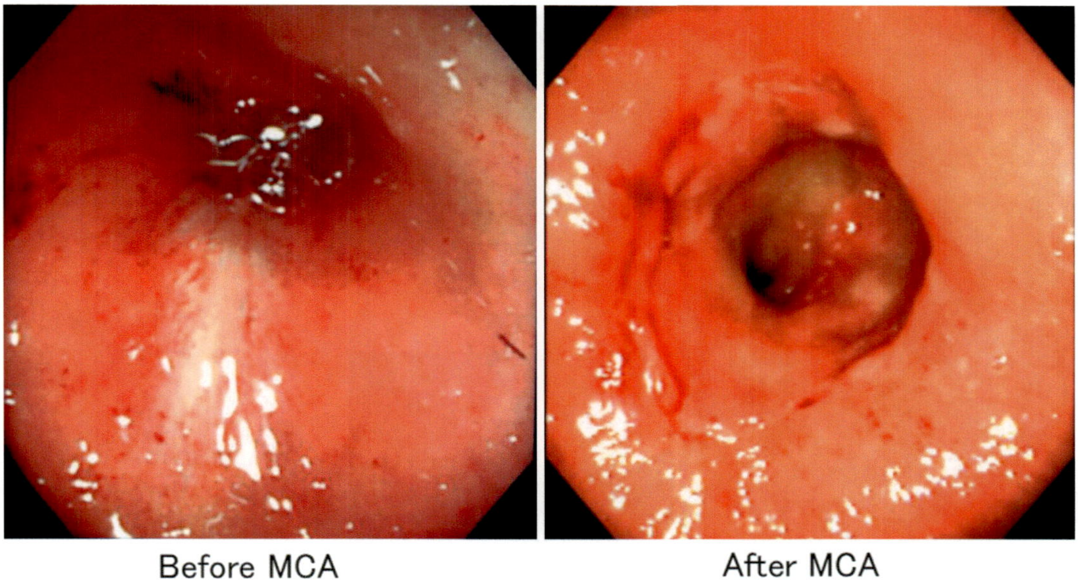

Fig. 16.34 An endoscopic view of the anastomosis site before and after MCA. Complete obstruction by several surgical staples can be seen before MCA. A newly created anastomosis without surgical staples is present after MCA

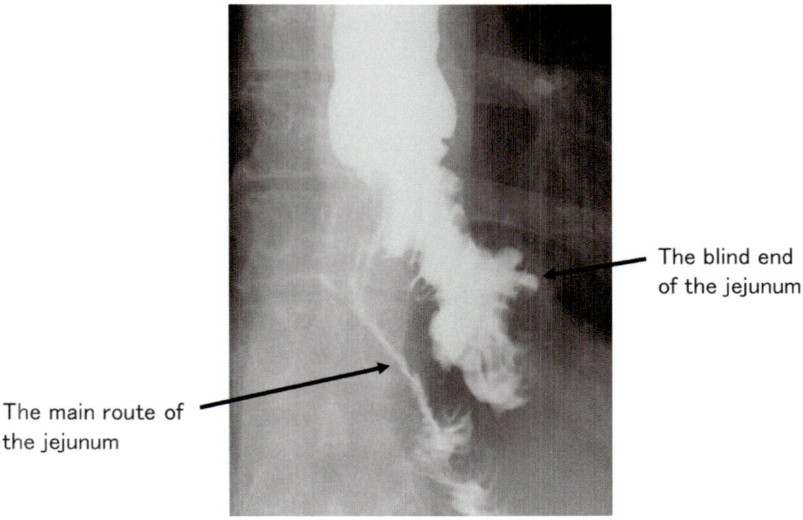

Fig. 16.35 Preoperative upper gastrointestinal study shows that the blind end of the jejunum has become a blind loop with multiple diverticula, which are dilating and pressing the true lumen of the jejunum. This was causing the patient to have difficulty with oral intake, and he developed aspiration pneumonia

dilatation force in this case. The patient returned to normal life after 3 weeks.

A Case of ρ-Anastomosis Between the Jejunum and Blind End of the Jejunum After Total Gastrectomy

The patient was a man in his 50s who had been experiencing difficulties with oral intake and developed aspiration pneumonia. He had undergone total gastrectomy with Roux-en-Y reconstruction for gastric cancer 10 years earlier. Postoperatively, a stricture gradually developed in the jejunum, causing elongation and formation of multiple diverticula in the blind end of the jejunum. The stricture also caused reflux of food materials and digestive juices, which led to the aspiration pneumonia (Fig. 16.35). We planned to create a ρ-anastomosis by MCA between the jejunum and blind end of the jejunum after total

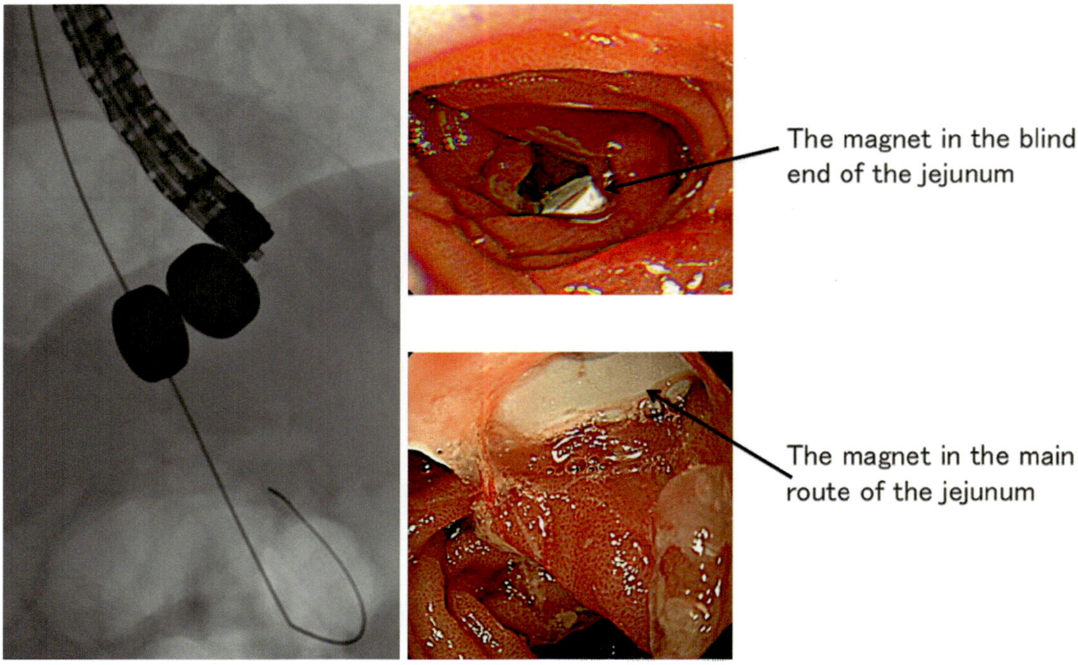

Fig. 16.36 Two disk magnets of the same size (15 mm in diameter, 5 mm in thickness) were placed to make a ρ-anastomosis between the blind end of the jejunum and the main route of the jejunum. An endoscopic view shows that each magnet was placed in a suitable position

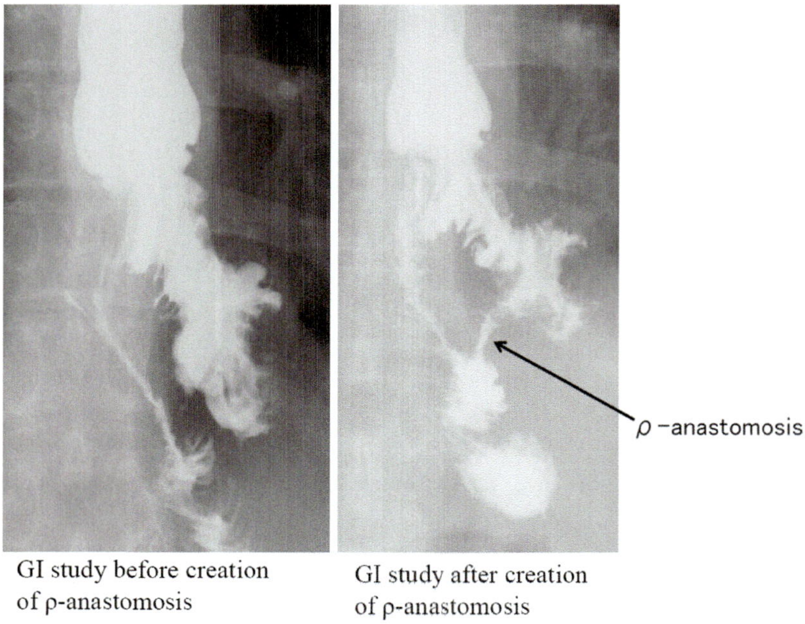

Fig. 16.37 After successful creation of a ρ-anastomosis between the blind end of the jejunum and the main route of the jejunum, the patient was able to resume oral intake and the aspiration pneumonia improved

gastrectomy (Fig. 16.36). After successful creation of the ρ-anastomosis between the blind end of the jejunum and the main route of the jejunum, a gastrointestinal study confirmed that the dilation of the blind portion had resolved, with flow of contrast medium into the main route of the jejunum via the ρ-anastomosis. The patient was able to resume oral intake and the aspiration pneumonia improved. He has returned to normal life and is doing very well (Fig. 16.37).

A Case of Ileocolostomy

The patient was a man in his 40s who was urgently admitted to hospital with a small bowel perforation. It was difficult to anastomose the small bowel loops in one sitting because of severe adhesions resulting from tuberculous peritonitis. Therefore, an ileostomy and an ascending colostomy were placed (Fig. 16.38). The patient was found to be HIV positive postoperatively. The surgeons hesitated to reoperate to perform an anastomosis because of the severe adhesions. Therefore, enteroenteric MCA was attempted between the ileostomy and colostomy because the ostomies were close in position (Fig. 16.39). The distance from each ostomy was so short that the two magnets could be carried by forceps. The two magnets mated closely in parallel such that there were no inclusions between the magnets (Fig. 16.40). The magnets were excreted 8 days later. Dilatation by digital manipulation was performed several times because the anastomotic site was very close to each ostomy. After successful creation of an ileocolostomy, each ostomy was closed surgically (Fig. 16.41).

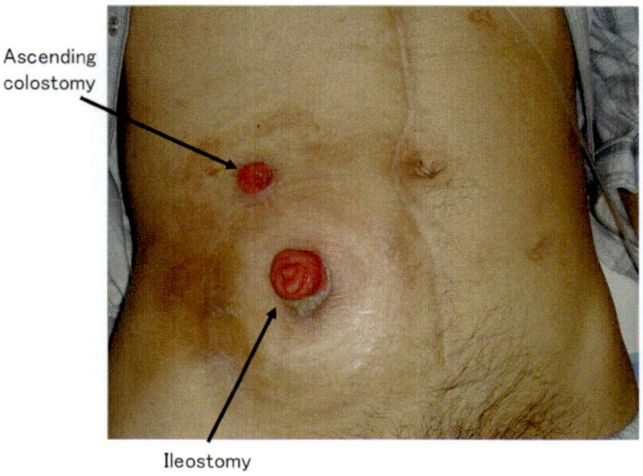

Fig. 16.38 Postoperative photograph of the abdomen of a patient in whom we needed to create an anastomosis between an ileostomy and an ascending colostomy

A Case of MCA Between An Esophagostomy and Gastric Tube

The patient was a man in his 60s who had undergone esophagectomy with gastric tube reconstruction. An anastomotic leak had developed, which was treated by esophagostomy. The plan

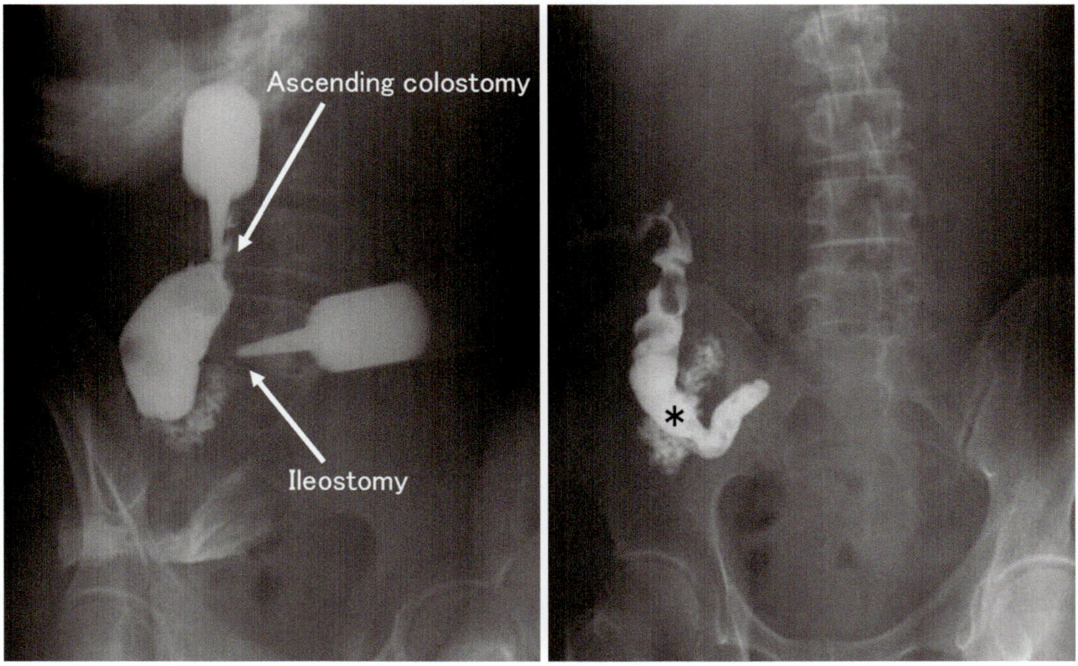

Fig. 16.39 Simultaneous colonography and ileography show those two loops are located close at the *asterisk* point

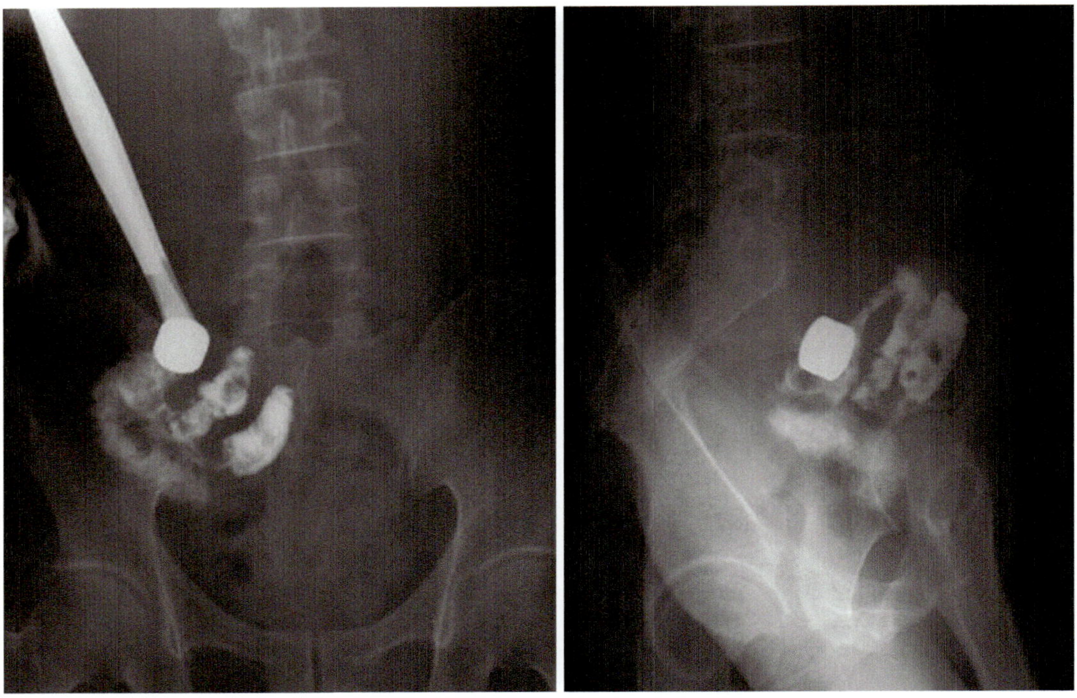

Fig. 16.40 The distance from each ostomy was so short that two magnets were able to be carried by forceps. The two magnets mated very close in parallel, so there were no inclusions between the magnets

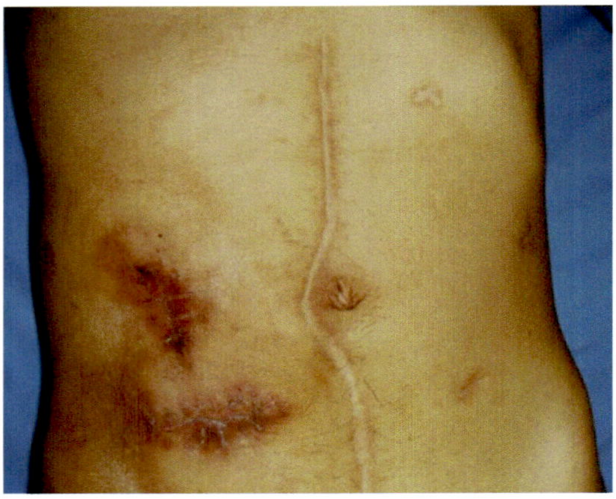

Fig. 16.41 The magnets were excreted 8 days later. After creating successful ileocolostomy, each ostomy was surgically closed

was to perform an MCA of the esophagostomy and gastric tube after all inflammation and leaking had settled. The parent magnet (12.5 mm in diameter, 5 mm in thickness) was transported from the jejunostomy over the guidewire, and the daughter magnet (the same size as the parent magnet) was placed via the esophagostomy by digital manipulation. However, the gap between the two magnets was wide (7 cm) and the magnets were unable to mate. Twelve disk magnets were then used as the daughter magnet, which resulted in successful mating (Fig. 16.42). The esophagostomy was closed after removal of the mated magnets. Balloon dilatation was performed once or twice a month for about a year, and local triamcinolone acetonide injections were administered via an endoscope on several occasions. An endoscopic study showed smooth elongation of the esophagus (confirmed in a biopsy specimen) connecting to the gastric tube (Fig. 16.43). Eventually, no further dilatation was needed, and the patient was able to resume eating normally.

A Case of Choledochoduodenostomy

The patient was a man in his 40s with a diagnosis of chronic alcohol-related pancreatitis who

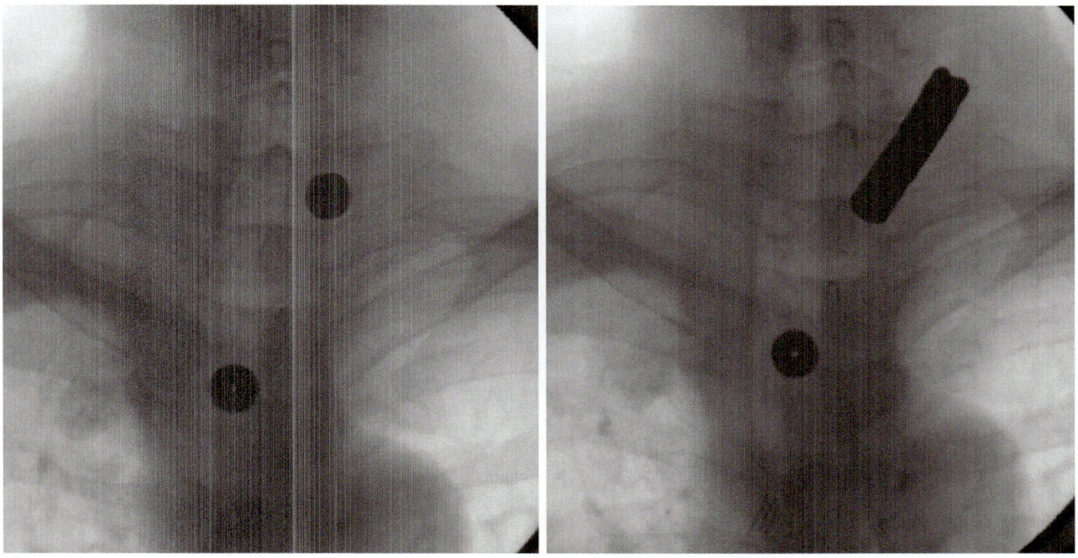

Fig. 16.42 The gap between the esophagostomy and the gastric tube is wide (about 7 cm), preventing mating of the two magnets. Twelve daughter magnets were applied in this case to increase magnetic power, which led to successful mating

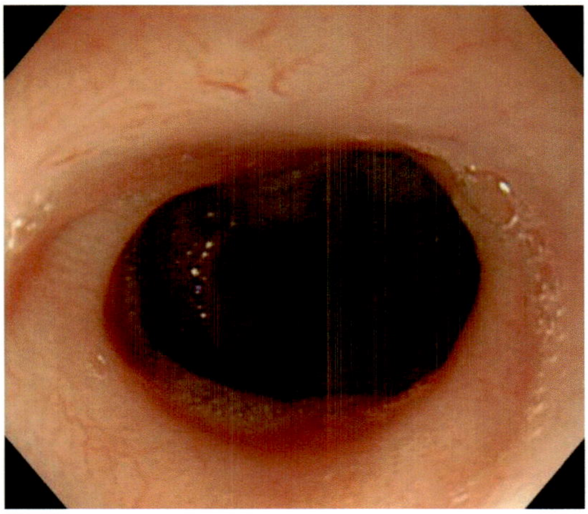

Fig. 16.43 After removal of the mated magnets, the esophagostomy was closed. Balloon dilatation was performed once or twice monthly for about a year, and a local injection of triamcinolone acetonide were administered via an endoscope on several occasions. Endoscopy showed a smooth anastomosis site with elongation of the esophagus. Finally, no further dilatation was needed, and the patient was able to resume eating normally at mealtimes

had had multiple hospital admissions for acute pancreatitis. Interventional relief consisting of an anastomosis between the dilated main pancreatic duct and stomach was planned (Figs. 16.44 and 16.45). The patient's episodes of acute pancreatitis had ceased completely after successful creation of the pancreaticogastrostomy. However, a few years later he developed obstructive jaundice due to fibrosis resulting from advanced chronic pancreatitis. Percutaneous transhepatic biliary drainage (PTBD) was performed (Fig. 16.46). An MCA between the CBD and duodenum was planned because the CBD was located beneath the second portion of the duodenum. The daughter magnet was carried via the PTBD route and the parent magnet was transported endoscopically. The magnets mated easily and passed into the duodenum after 2 weeks (Fig. 16.47). The internalized PTBD tube functioned as a tract between the CBD and duodenum and was exchanged every 2–4 weeks for approximately 6 months. Good flow of contrast medium from the CBD to the duodenum was noted when the PTBD tube was removed 6 months later (Fig. 16.48). Follow-up biliary scintigraphy 4 years later showed good flow into the bowel loops through the anastomotic site between the CBD and duodenum (Fig. 16.49).

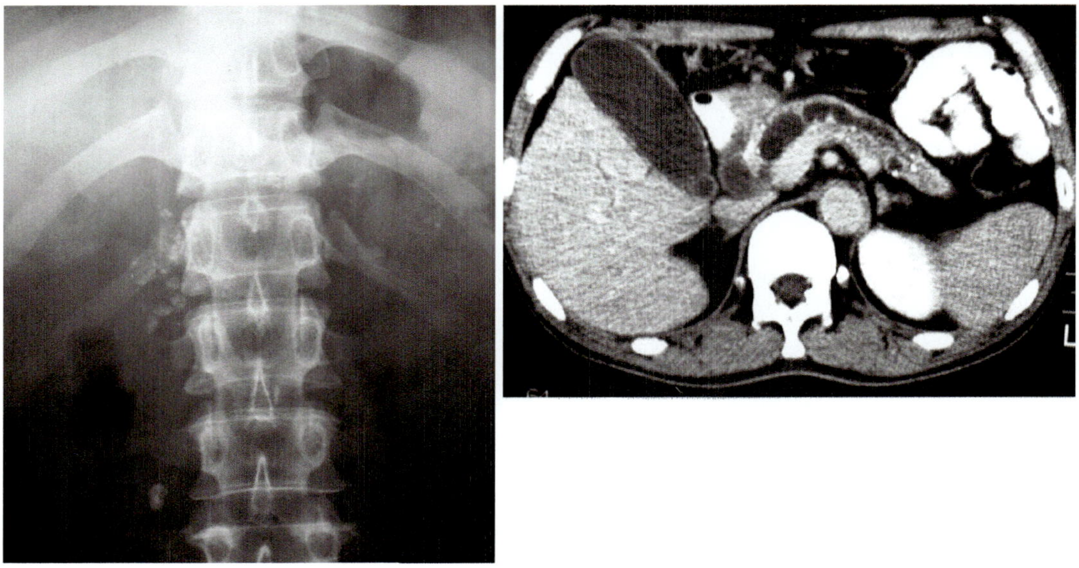

Fig. 16.44 A plain abdominal radiograph and a computed tomography scan showing typical images of chronic pancreatitis with pancreatic calcification and a dilated main pancreatic duct

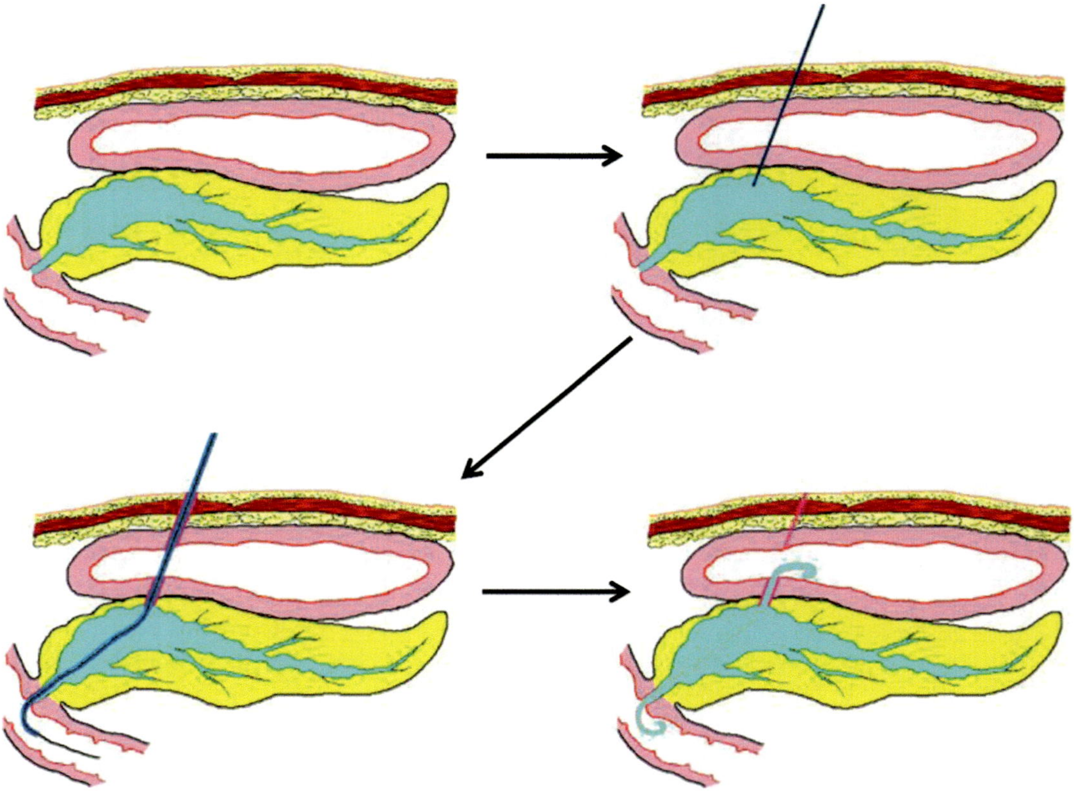

Fig. 16.45 Diagram showing how to create an interventional pancreaticogastrostomy

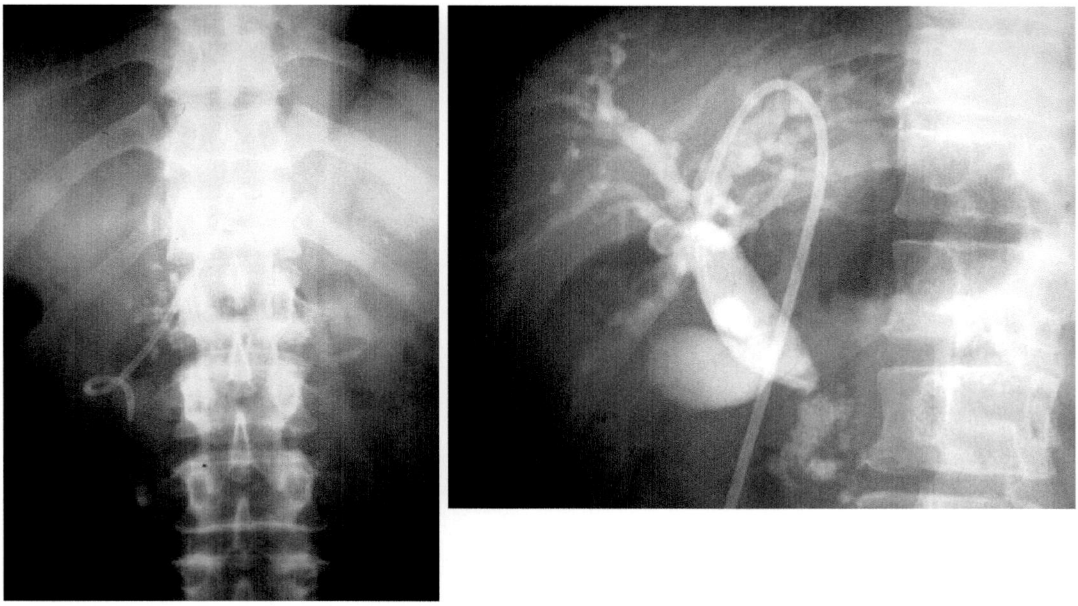

Fig. 16.46 Attacks of acute pancreatitis had ceased to occur in this patient after successful creation of a pancreaticogastrostomy. However, a few years later, fibrosis caused by the patient's chronic pancreatitis advanced and he developed obstructive jaundice. Therefore, percutaneous transhepatic biliary drainage was performed

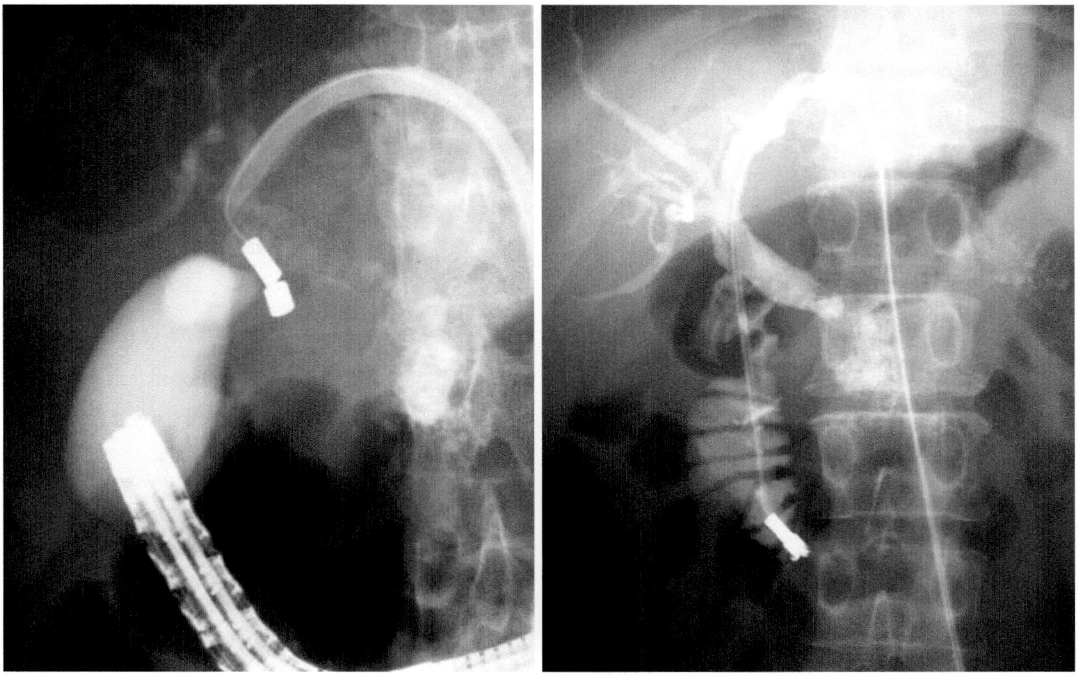

Fig. 16.47 The daughter magnet was carried via the percutaneous transhepatic biliary drainage route, and the parent magnet was transported endoscopically (*left*). The two magnets mated easily and passed into the duodenum after 2 weeks (*right*)

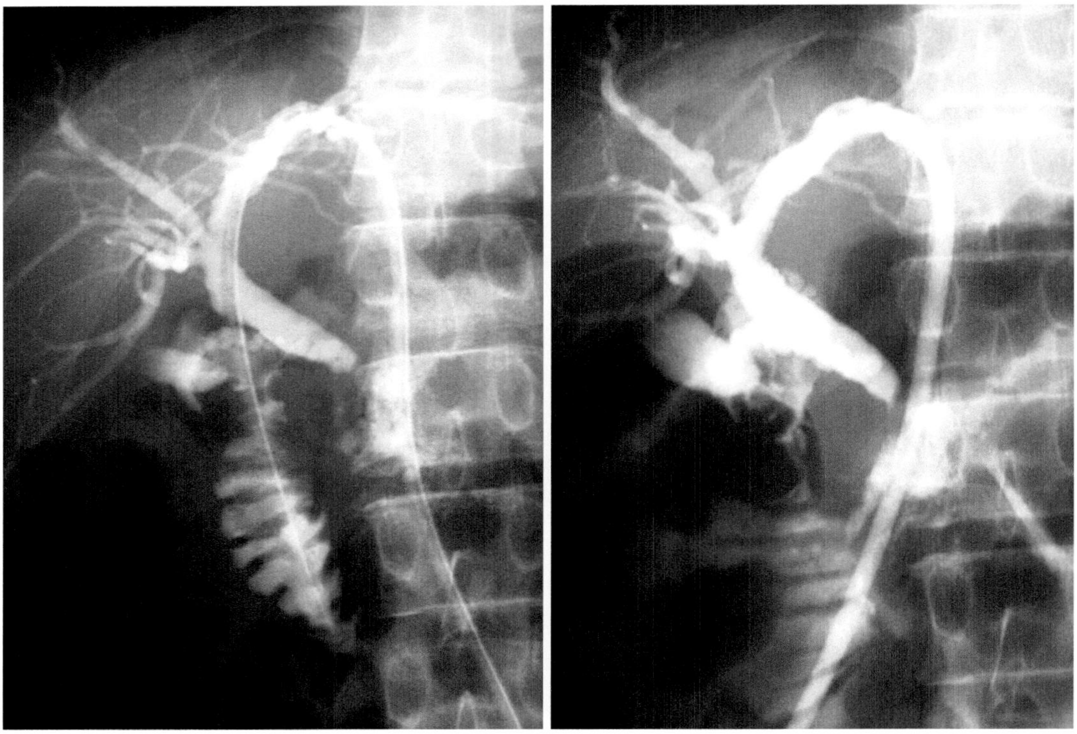

Fig. 16.48 After successful creation of an anastomosis between the common bile duct and duodenum, the tract was kept patent by the internalized percutaneous transhepatic biliary drainage tube, which was exchanged every 2–4 weeks for about 6 months (*left*). Good flow of contrast medium from the common bile duct to the duodenum was noted when the percutaneous transhepatic biliary drainage tube was removed after approximately 6 months

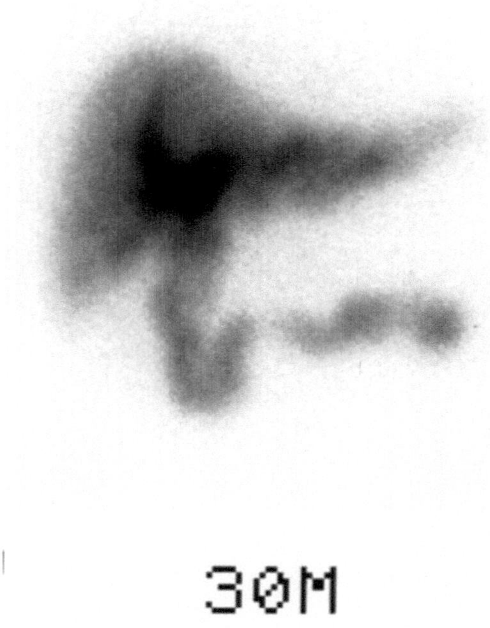

Fig. 16.49 Follow-up biliary scintigraphy showed good flow into the bowel loops through the anastomosis site between the common bile duct and duodenum 4 years later

A Case of MCA Between the Intrahepatic Bile Duct and a Roux-en-Y Jejunal Limb

The patient was a man in his 60s who developed obstructive jaundice as a postoperative complication of laparoscopic cholecystectomy. Therefore, a Roux-en-Y choledochojejunostomy was performed. However, his obstructive jaundice recurred 3 years later. A PTBD tube was inserted at that time. Cholangiography through the PTBD route showed complete obstruction at the anastomotic site (Fig. 16.50). The surgeons were reluctant to perform repeat surgery because of severe adhesions and instead planned an MCA between the intrahepatic bile duct and the Roux-en-Y jejunal limb. The parent magnet was transported under extracorporeal magnetic guidance along the ileus tube because no endoscope that could enter the small intestine was available at that time (Fig. 16.51). Successful creation of the MCA was confirmed by cholangiography through the

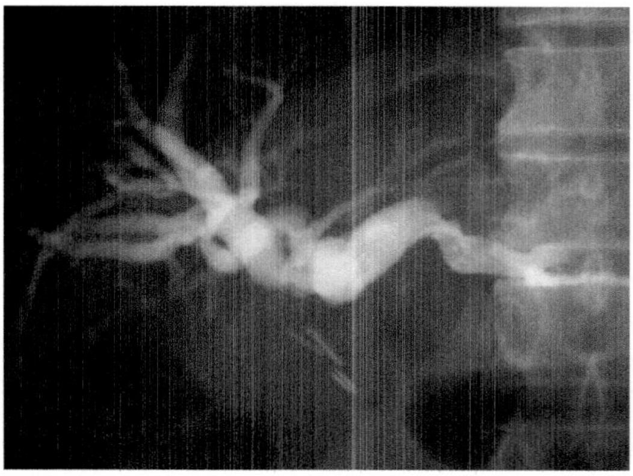

Fig. 16.50 Obstructive jaundice as a complication 3 years after laparoscopic cholecystectomy. Percutaneous transhepatic biliary drainage was performed. Cholangiography through the percutaneous transhepatic biliary drainage route showed complete obstruction at the anastomotic site. Repeat surgery was not desirable because severe adhesions were expected. A magnetic compression anastomosis (between the intrahepatic bile duct and a Roux-en-Y jejunal limb) was planned

PTBD route after 12 days. The mated magnets were released from the guidewire, which was attached to the daughter magnet, by pushing firmly over the guidewire. The mated magnets were excreted within a few days (Fig. 16.52). The tract was kept patent by an internalized tube stent for about a year. The tube was exchanged every 2–4 weeks on an outpatient basis.

A Case of Choledochocholedochostomy

The patient was a man in his 90s who had undergone an open cholecystectomy for gallstones. After surgery, complete obstruction of the CBD occurred as a result of cholangitis due to leakage, so PTBD was performed (Fig. 16.53). A biliobiliary MCA of CBD was planned. The daughter magnet was brought to the blind end of the CBD

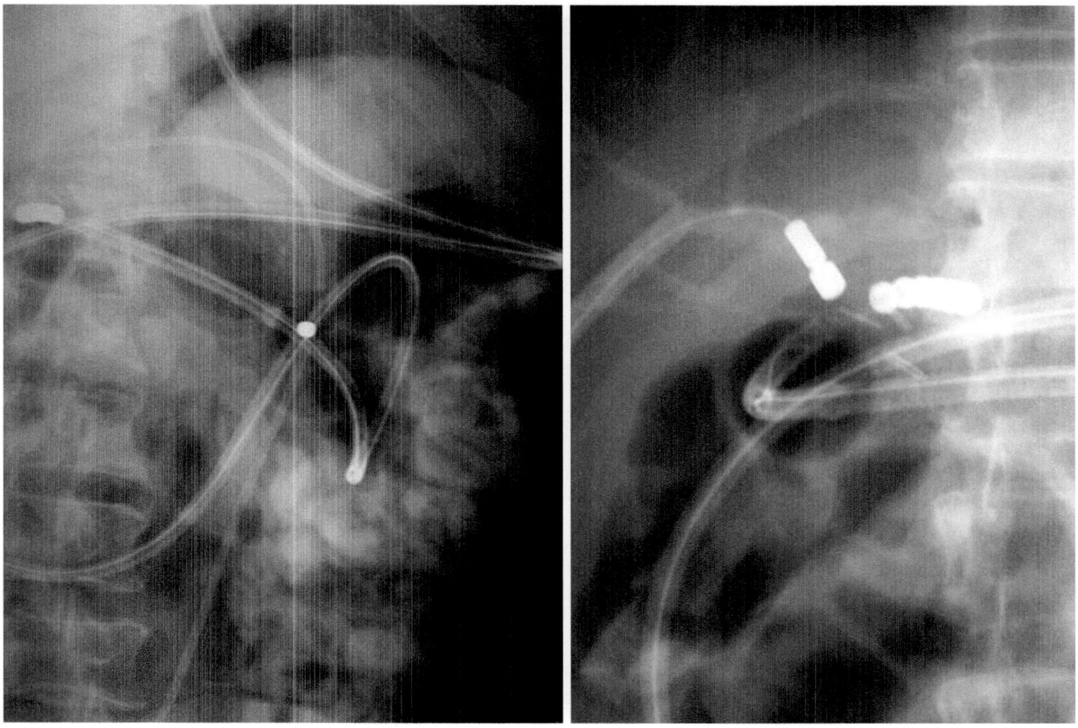

Fig. 16.51 The parent magnet was transported by extracorporeal magnetic guidance along the ileus tube, which was placed in the Roux-en-Y jejunal limb because a small intestine endoscope was not available at that time. Both magnets mated smoothly

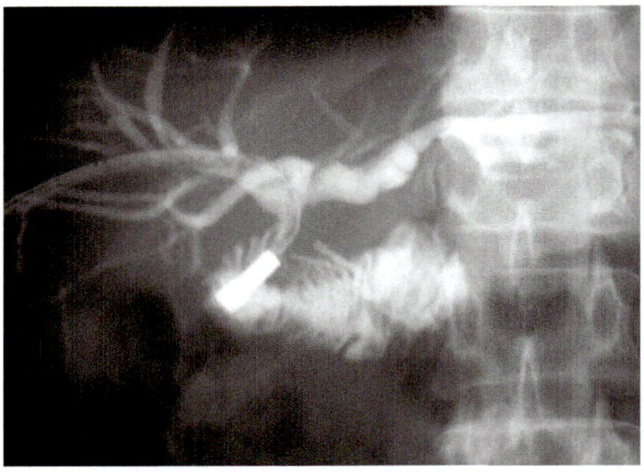

Fig. 16.52 Successful creation of a magnetic compression anastomosis was confirmed by cholangiography through the percutaneous transhepatic biliary drainage route. The mated magnets were released from the guidewire attached to the daughter magnet by pushing firmly on the pusher over the guidewire. The tract was kept patent by an internalized tube stent that was exchanged every 2–4 weeks and left in place for about 1 year

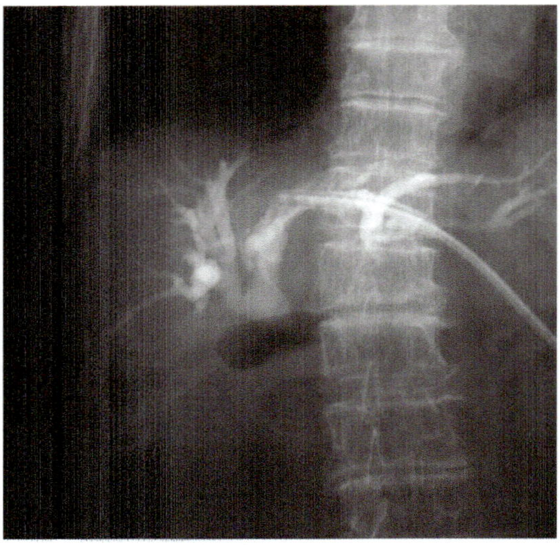

Fig. 16.53 Cholangiography through the percutaneous transhepatic biliary drainage route shows complete obstruction of the common bile duct

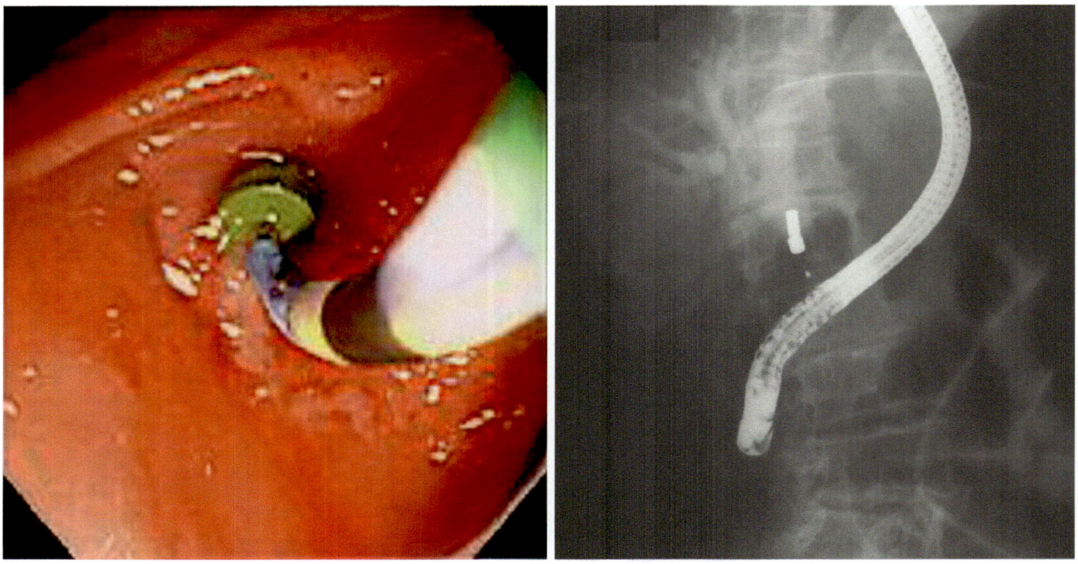

Fig. 16.54 The daughter magnet is brought to the blind end of the common bile duct through the percutaneous transhepatic biliary drainage route. The parent magnet is then transported endoscopically in the common bile duct through the ampulla of Vater (*left*). Two magnets were instantly mated (*right*)

via the PTBD route. The parent magnet was then transported endoscopically into the CBD through the ampulla of Vater. The two magnets mated immediately (Fig. 16.54). Successful anastomosis of the CBD was achieved after removal of the internalized tube stent from the PTBD, which was exchanged every 2–4 weeks for 6 months (Fig. 16.55). The patient was able to return to normal life without the need for repeat surgery.

A Case of MCA Between the Intrahepatic Bile Ducts

The patient was a woman in her 50s who had received a living donor left-lobe liver graft and hepaticocholedochostomy and developed a biliary occlusion 1 month following her transplant. A cholangiographic study via the PTBD and CBD routes revealed that the CBD was con-

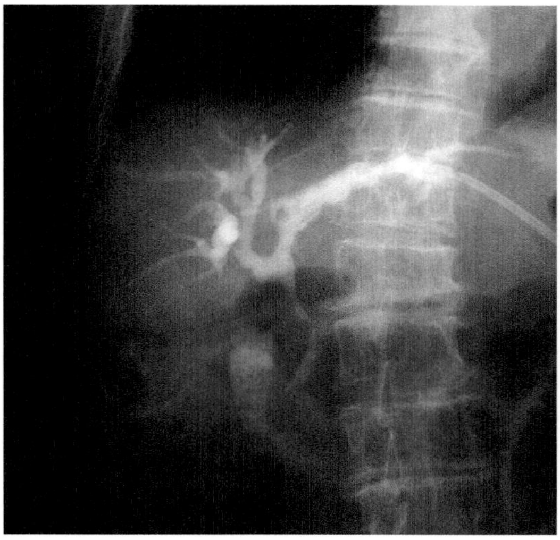

Fig. 16.55 After removal of the tube stent used for percutaneous transhepatic biliary drainage, which was exchanged every 4–6 weeks for about 6 months, successful anastomosis of the common bile duct was achieved

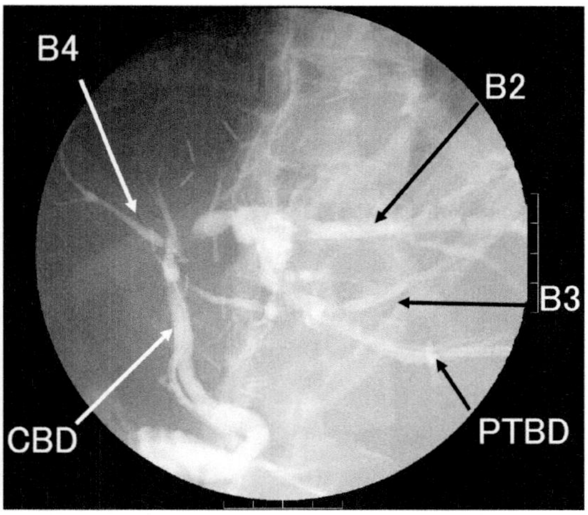

Fig. 16.56 Cholangiography via the percutaneous transhepatic biliary drainage and common bile duct routes. B4 connects to the common bile duct, but there is no connection between the common bile duct and B2 or B3. Therefore, a magnetic compression anastomosis between the intrahepatic bile ducts was planned

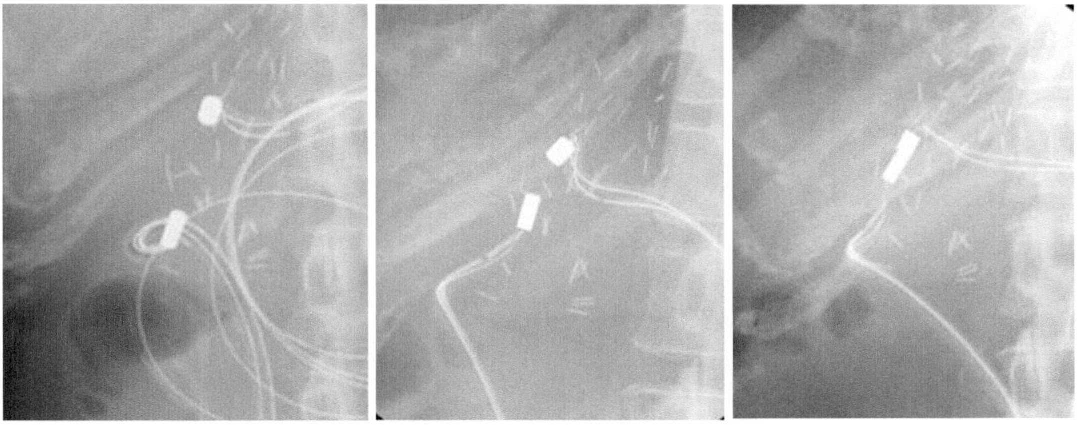

POD 0 POD 4 POD 28

Fig. 16.57 The magnets were inserted via the percutaneous transhepatic biliary drainage and common bile duct routes. There was still a wide gap of about 30 mm between the magnets on postoperative day 0. However, both magnets were perfectly mated on postoperative day 28

nected to B4 but not to B2 and B3 (Fig. 16.56). An MCA between the intrahepatic bile ducts was planned. The magnets were inserted via the PTBD and CBD routes. There was still a wide gap of about 30 mm between the magnets on postoperative day (POD) 1. However, both magnets were mated on POD 28 (Fig. 16.57). A fistulous tract was successfully created between the intrahepatic bile ducts, and an internalized tube stent was placed to maintain the patency of the tract (Fig. 16.58). The tube stent was exchanged every 2–4 weeks in the outpatient clinic and was removed uneventfully 1 year later.

A Case of Creation of a New Cystic Duct Between the Gallbladder and CBD by MCA

The patient was a woman in her 70s who had developed obstructive jaundice as a result of lower bile duct cancer. PTBD and percutaneous transhepatic gallbladder drainage (PTGBD) had been instituted to control cholecystitis and obstructive jaundice. She was not a candidate for surgery, and how to manage the PTBD and PTGBD to increase her quality of life posed a major problem (Fig. 16.59). Therefore, we devised a plan whereby a new cystic duct was created to bring together the gallbladder and CBD, after which an endoscopic retrograde biliary drainage stent was placed within the newly fashioned duct. The PTBD and PTGBD routes were able to be removed (Fig. 16.60).

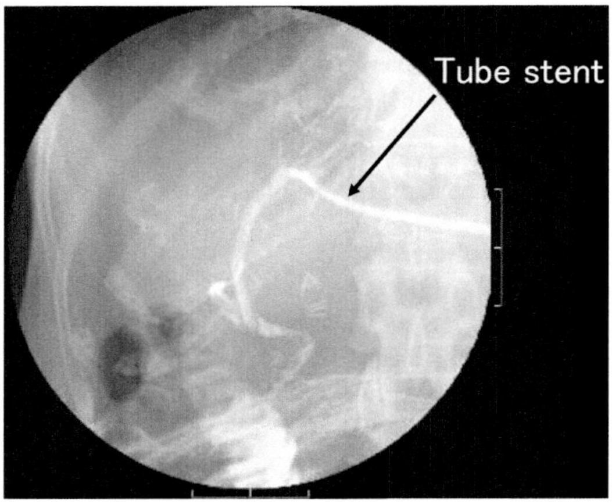

Fig. 16.58 Successful creation of the fistulous tract was accomplished, and a tube stent was placed to keep the tract patent

Magnetic Compression Revision for Stenosis

Next, we started to apply MCA as a treatment for stenosis in the gastrointestinal tract as well as creating a bypass route. Two disk magnets of the same size are usually used for this purpose. The parent magnet is transported across the stenosed site after balloon dilation of the stenosis. After mating, the stenotic site is pinched out by the two magnets. This strategy is very effective for an esophageal stricture, for which it is impossible to make a bypass route by MCA (Fig. 16.61) [17].

Representative Clinical Cases

A Case of Magnetic Compression Revision for Stenosis After Distal Gastrectomy

The patient was a woman in her 70s who had undergone distal gastrectomy with Roux-en-Y reconstruction. Postoperative oral intake was almost impossible because of complete obstruction at the anastomotic site between the stomach and jejunum. Endoscopic observation showed excess mucosa at the orifice, but no resistance to insertion of the endoscope. Balloon dilatation was performed unsuccessfully on many occasions (Fig. 16.62). We then planned MCRS to

Fig. 16.59 The percutaneous transhepatic gallbladder drainage route separate from the percutaneous transhepatic biliary drainage route. The patient had a lower bile duct cancer that was not indicated for surgery. To increase the patient's quality of life, the plan was to unify both routes and internalize via a new cystic duct, which was created by a magnetic compression anastomosis between the gallbladder and the common bile duct

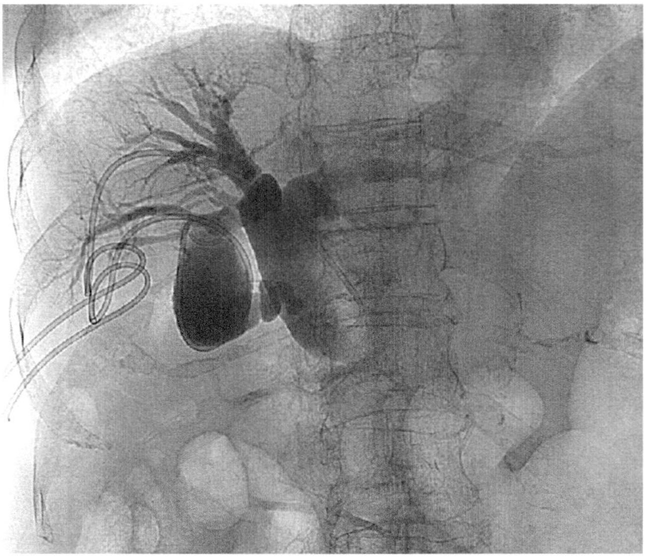

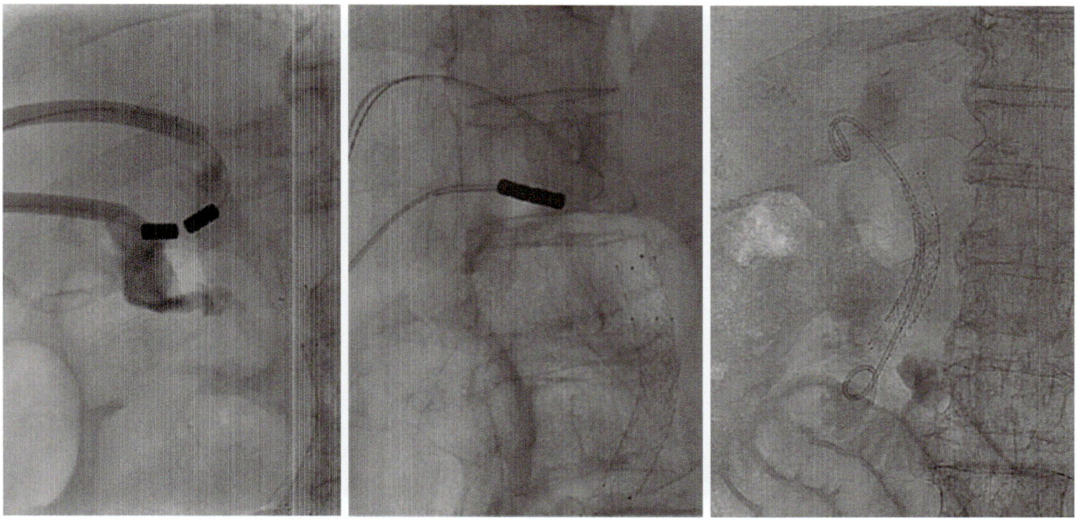

Fig. 16.60 The magnets were inserted separately via the percutaneous transhepatic gallbladder and biliary drainage routes. Both magnets mated and a new cystic duct was created between the gallbladder and common bile duct. An endoscopic retrograde biliary drainage stent was then placed through the new cystic duct. The percutaneous transhepatic gallbladder and biliary drainage tubes were then removed

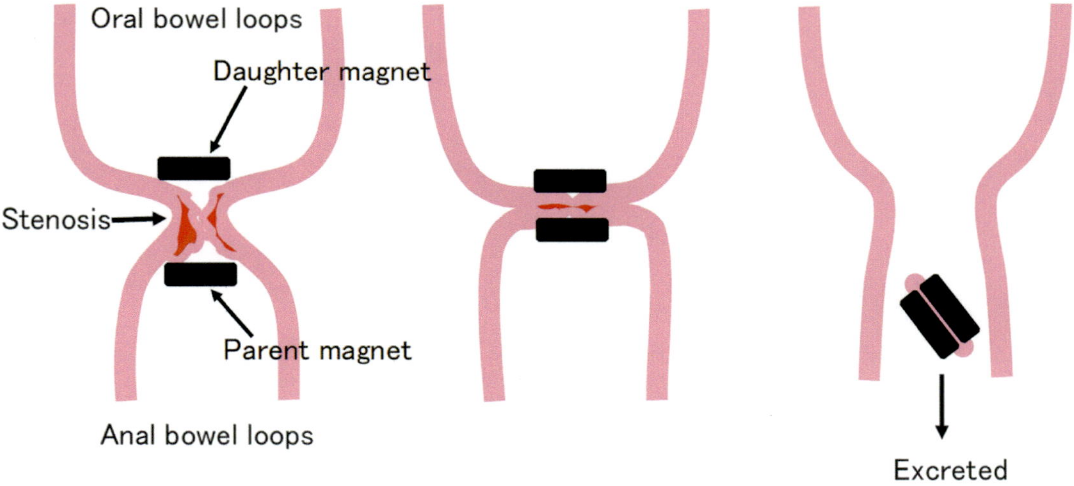

Fig. 16.61 Diagram showing the process of magnetic compression revision for stenosis. First, the parent magnet is transported across the stenosis, which is temporarily dilated by a balloon catheter. The daughter magnet is then positioned and the magnets are mated. The structure at the site of the stenosis is compressed by the magnets, which are finally removed from the gastrointestinal tract

address the excess mucosa. A cone coaxial transporter was devised to carry the pair of magnets (Fig. 16.63). This transporter allows the magnets to be retained in the center of the bowel lumen without bias such that the newly created tract runs in the center of the bowel lumen (Fig. 16.64). Good flow of contrast medium through the anastomotic site confirmed that the MCRS was successful. Endoscopy after MCRS confirmed disappearance of the excess mucosa and reappearance of the orifice that had previously been hidden. The patient was able to resume normal oral intake without the need for further surgery (Fig. 16.65).

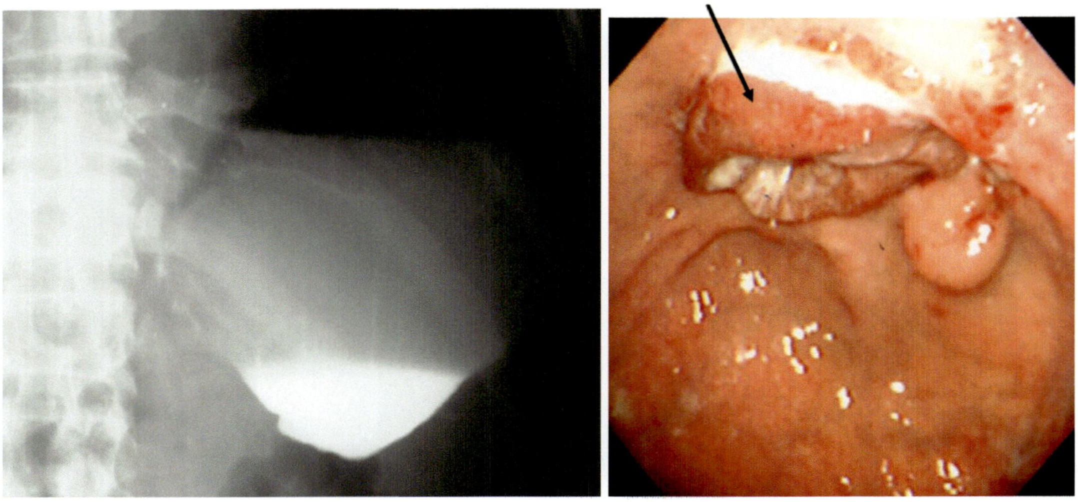

Fig. 16.62 Complete obstruction can be seen at the anastomosis on a gastrointestinal study after distal gastrectomy with reconstruction of a Roux-en-Y jejunal limb. Endoscopy shows that the lumen is filled with excess mucosa (*arrow*). However, the endoscope was inserted easily without resistance. Balloon dilatation was performed many times but unsuccessfully

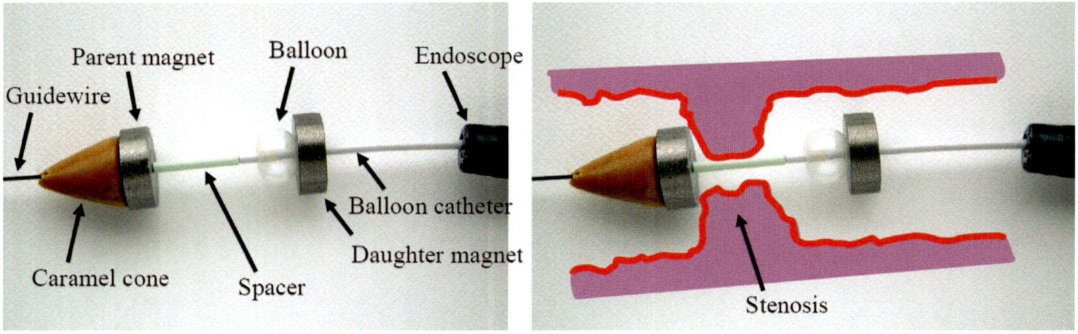

Fig. 16.63 Apparatus for cone coaxial transport of a parent and daughter magnet. The parent magnet is attached to the caramel-colored cone to make insertion easy. The magnets are positioned at either side of the stenosis. The advantage of this method is that the magnets are kept in the center of the bowel lumen without bias, so the newly created tract runs along the center of the bowel lumen

A Case of MCRS After Esophagectomy

The case was a man in his 50s who had undergone esophagectomy with reconstruction by colon interposition after a previous total gastrectomy. A year later, he developed a stricture at the anastomotic site after a leak-related infection (Fig. 16.66) and required bougie dilatation once or twice a week. At this time, he was eating very small amounts of food at 1.5-hour intervals because he could not eat a normal amount of food at his usual mealtimes. MCRS was planned to remove the stricture. The parent magnet was carried by a sideways transport and pulling up method because this type of stricture can be strong (Fig. 16.67). Using this method, the parent magnet works like an arrowhead that can be easily pushed through the gap in the stricture. The parent magnet works as an anchor for the strings used for pulling up after it is carried across the stricture (Figs. 16.68 and 16.69). The new tract was found to have a wide bore after successful MCRS. An endoscopic study showed improvement of the stricture (Fig. 16.70). The patient did not need further bougie dilatation and was able to resume eating normally.

Results

Technical Success

Mating of the magnets is almost always achieved when sufficient time is available. Three patients who received enteroenteric anastomoses succumbed to their underlying disease before movement of the magnets was seen. Successful creation of an anastomosis was confirmed in all, but 3 of 203 the remaining patients. The overall success rate was 98.5% for enteroenteric MCA (200/203 cases), 97.9% for bilioenteric or biliobiliary MCA (185/189 cases), and 87.5% for MCRS (28/32 cases).

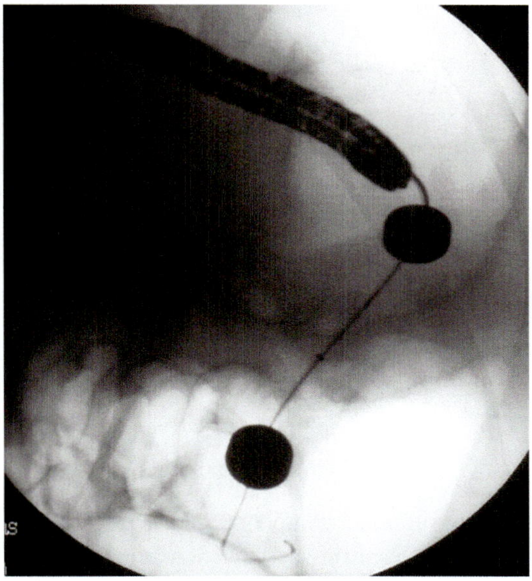

Fig. 16.64 A cone coaxial transporter was applied in this case. A parent magnet and daughter magnet were settled in good positions without any problem

Complications

Emergency laparotomy was required in a patient who received a colocolonic anastomosis after a loop of small bowel became trapped between magnets placed in two large bowel loops. Two further patients required corrective surgery after creation of the anastomosis because the transverse colon became trapped between the magnets in the stomach and duodenum. One patient who received an MCA between the ileum and colon for ileus required surgical removal of the mated magnets because they had passed into the blind iliac loop. Some patients complained of mild abdominal pain until the day after placement of the magnets, which was relieved by analgesics. Leakage was identified in one patient who received an MCA colocolostomy. Leakage was predicted in this case because the oral side of the colon showed

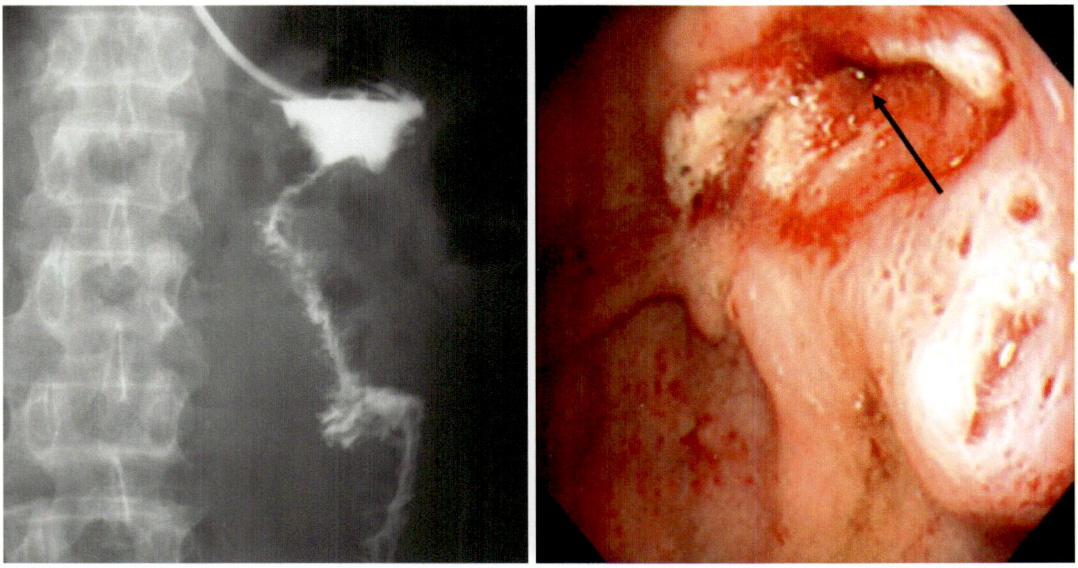

Fig. 16.65 Good flow of contrast medium through the anastomotic site was observed after successful magnetic compression revision for stenosis. Endoscopy after the procedure shows that the excess mucosa has disappeared, and the orifice, which was previously hidden in the excess mucosa, is now visible (*arrow*)

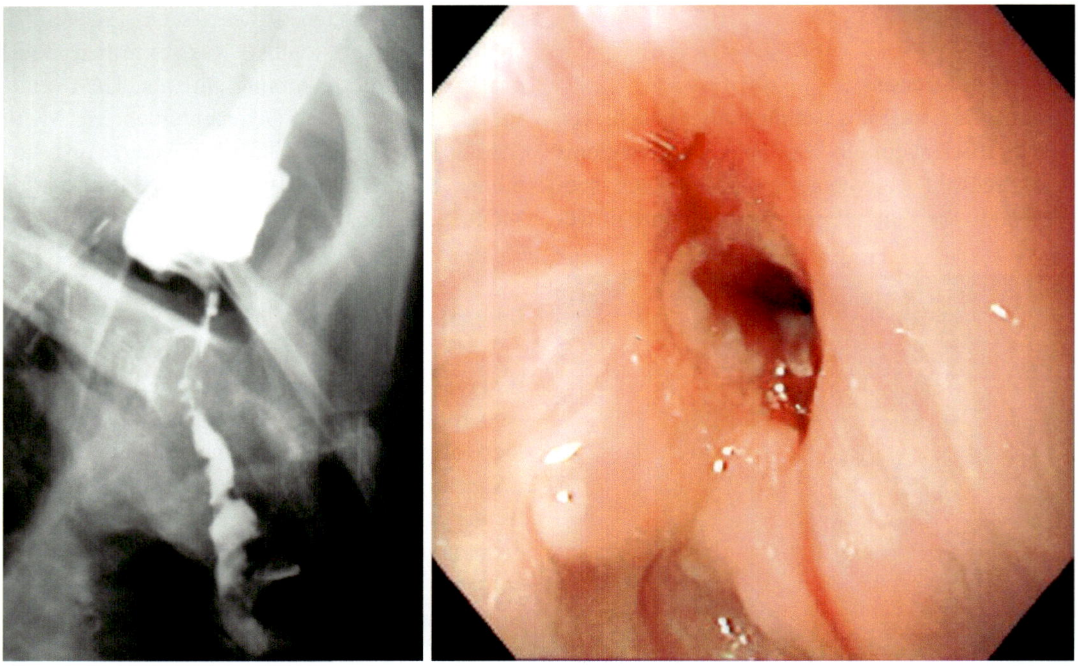

Fig. 16.66 Preoperative upper gastrointestinal and endoscopic studies show a marked stricture at the anastomotic site

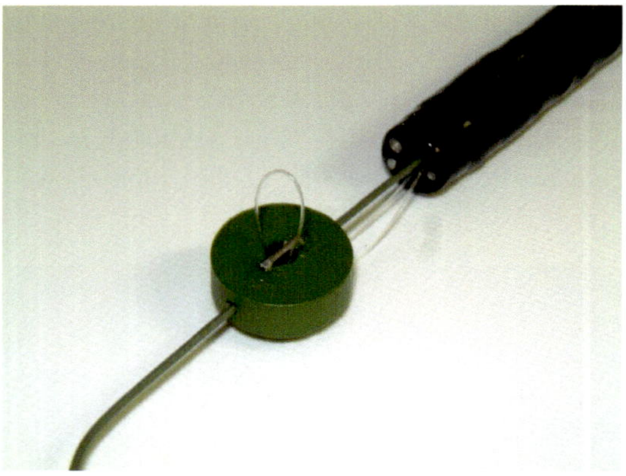

Fig. 16.67 Photograph showing the parent magnet attached over the guidewire from an endoscope for use of the sideways transport and pulling up method

marked dilatation without decompression. This was treated by percutaneous drainage. No other complication has been encountered so far.

Discussion

Although the original concept of mechanical compression anastomosis was first proposed as far back as 1821 [1] and refined in 1892, the magnets available at that time were not strong enough to apply sufficient compression to create an anastomosis. After strong permanent magnets became available, Saveliev and Cope proposed the use of MCA in 1993 and 1995, respectively [2–4]. However, there were still many problems to solve such as whether the magnets were safe, the incidence of leaks, an effective method for delivering the magnets to various sites in the bowel, and prevention of acute occlusion. Accordingly, this method did not enter clinical use until our early efforts in 1997 [5, 6].

MCA can be performed only when the two target points for anastomosis are relatively close to each other. The magnets strongly attract each other when the distance between them is 3 cm or less. If the distance between the target points for anastomosis is about 3 or 4 cm on plain abdominal radiographs or abdominal CT scans, an endoscope can be used to push one of the magnets to within 3 cm of the other, so that mating is facilitated. Mating of the magnets was achieved at this distance in many cases, so it can be considered as a reasonable standard. Of course, there may be cases in the future where anastomosis cannot be achieved even at a shorter distance or in which anastomosis is possible over a longer distance. Enteroenteric MCA can be attempted over a

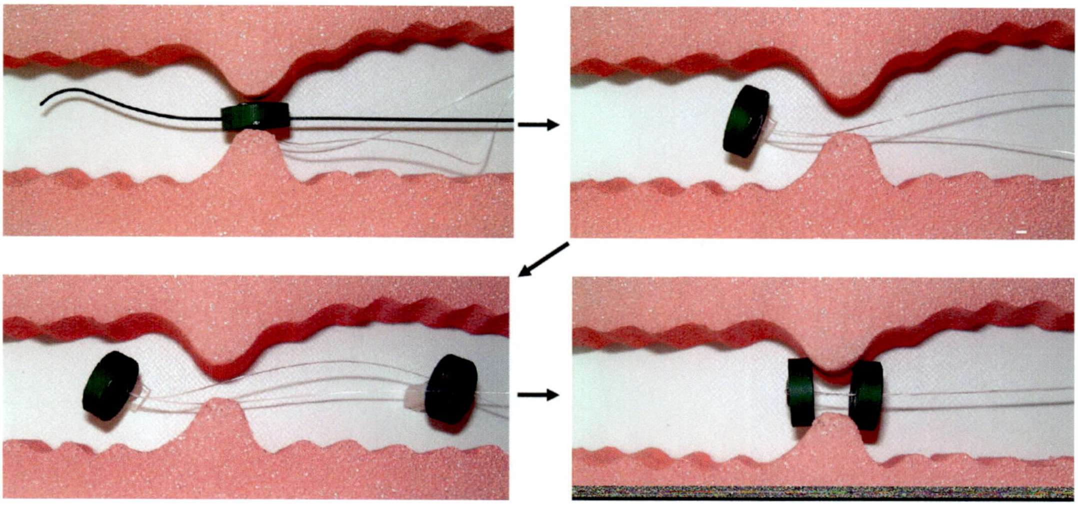

Fig. 16.68 Photographs showing the mechanism of the sideways transport and pulling up method. Sideways transport allows the parent magnet to enter a narrow tight stricture

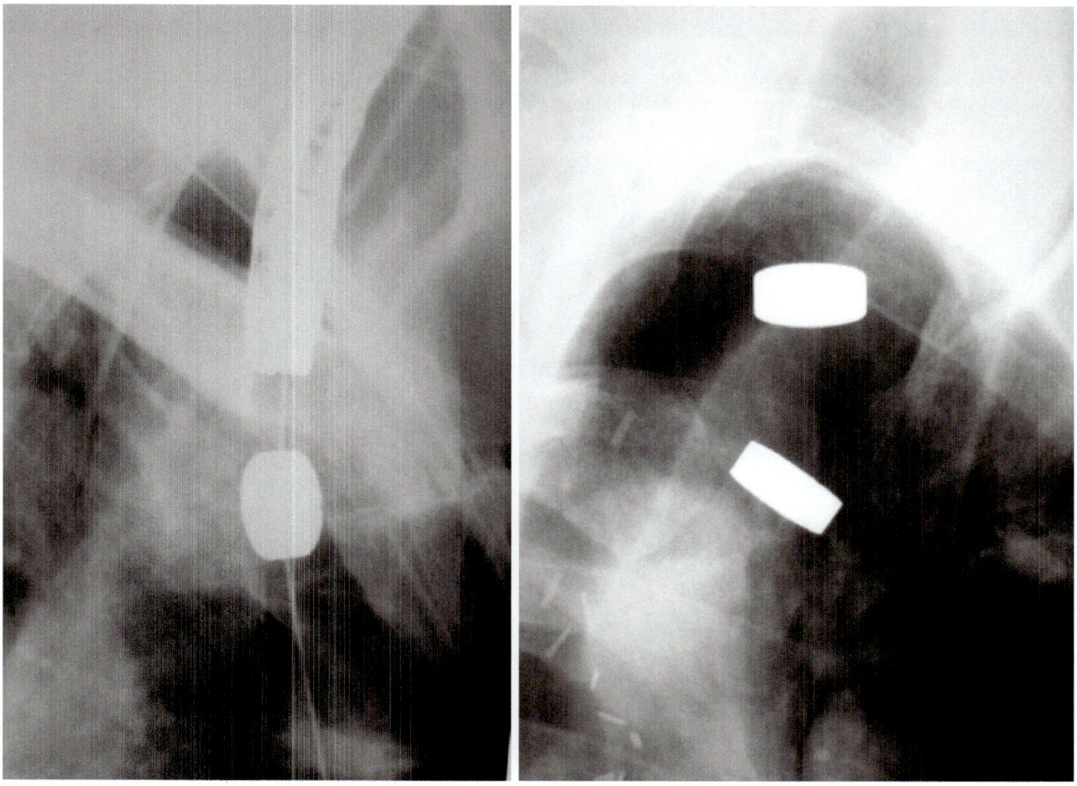

Fig. 16.69 The parent magnet is pushed by an endoscope to cross the stricture at the anastomotic site (*left*). After successful placement of the parent magnet, which is pulled up using the strings, the daughter magnet is sent over the strings (*right*)

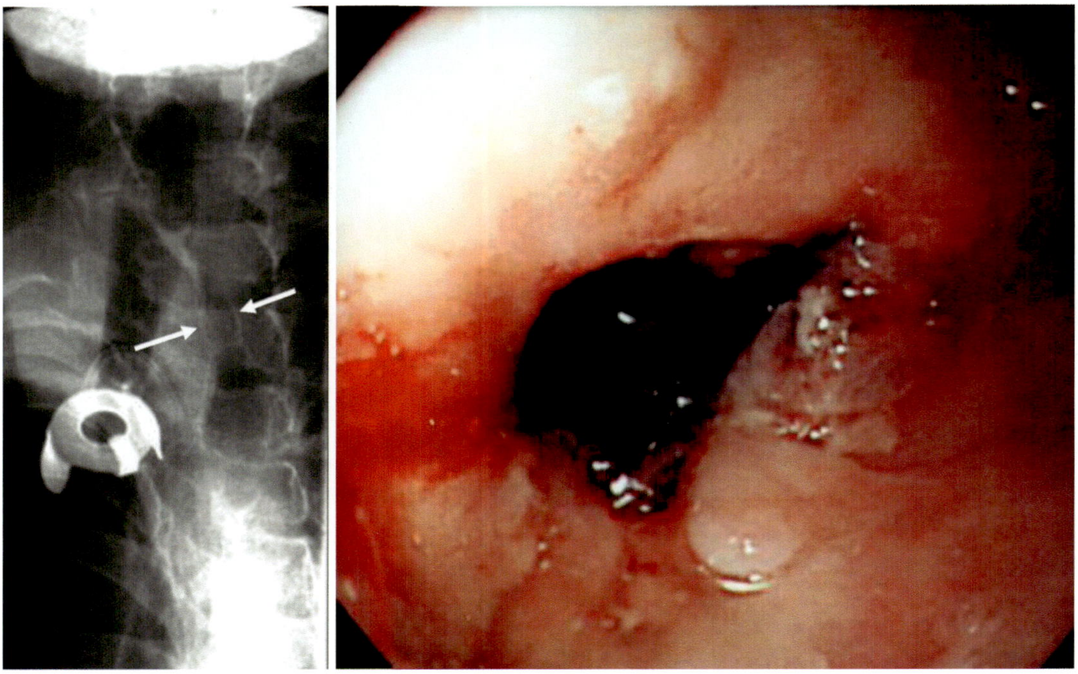

Fig. 16.70 The new tract had a wide bore after magnetic compression revision for stenosis (between the *white arrows*). Endoscopy after the procedure shows marked improvement of the stenosis

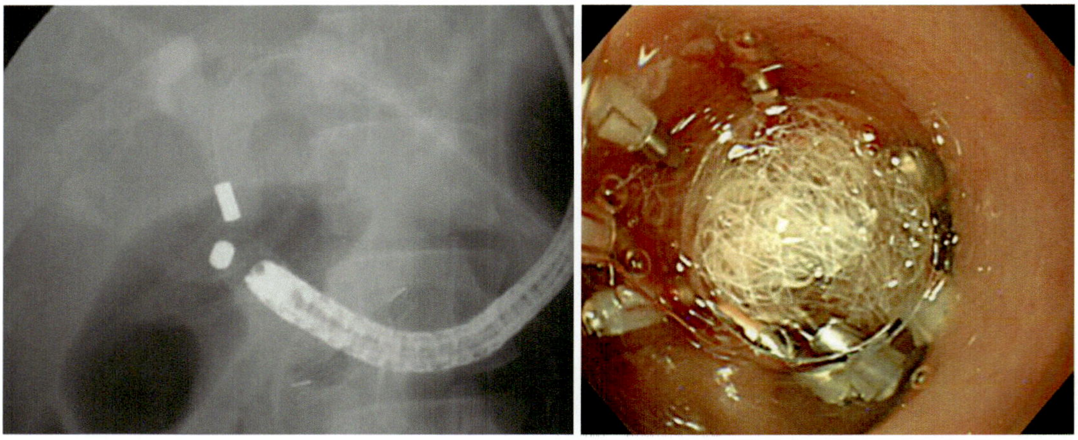

Fig. 16.71 A case of choledochoduodenostomy. It was impossible to mate the magnets because of a wide gap due to the presence of the falciform ligament. The parent magnet was finally fixed into the duodenum by gauze and clips using excellent endoscopic technique

longer distance because the intestine is more mobile, which makes it possible to create an anastomosis. Bilioenteric MCA is also possible at a distance of more than 3 cm if both magnets are held in place for several days. However, it is difficult to keep the parent magnet in place for this length of time because of peristalsis. In such cases, we fix the parent magnet to the bowel wall endoscopically using gauze and clips (Figs. 16.71 and 16.72).

There are two types of rare-earth magnets, namely, samarium-cobalt and neodymium-iron-

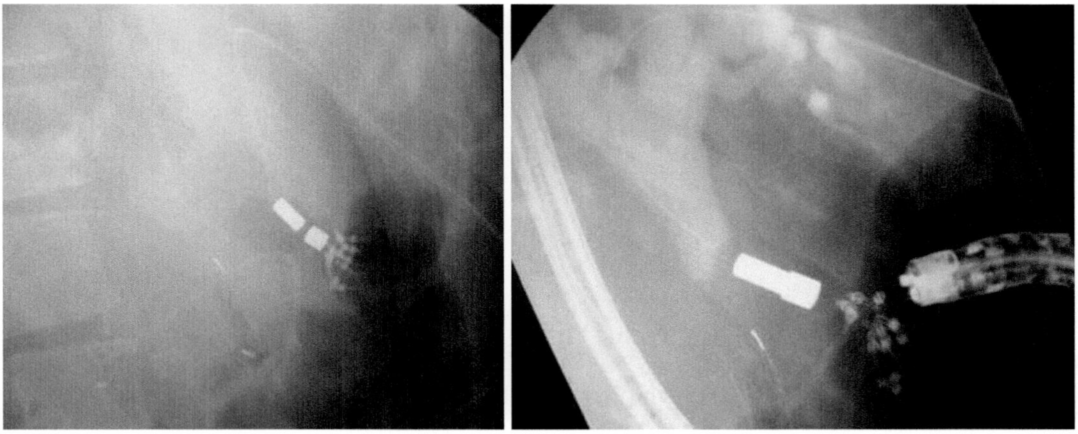

Fig. 16.72 The magnets were finally mated after 3 days. The fistulous tract was successfully created 10 days later. The tract was kept patent by a tube stent

boron. We use samarium-cobalt magnets because they have been confirmed in several experiments to be more stable, more heat resistant, and biologically safe. The neodymium-iron-boron magnet is usually plated with nickel to prevent oxidation, so is corrosive and biologically toxic. No allergic reactions to the samarium-cobalt magnet have been observed. All magnets were removed or excreted from the body within 2 weeks to a few months, so the potential long-term effects of the magnetic force need not be considered. Mild blunt pain was observed after insertion of the magnets in 12% of enteroenteric MCA cases. This pain was thought to be related to pinpoint ischemia caused by compression of the magnets in the bowel loop. The progress of the MCA is clearly indicated by the position of the magnets on follow-up plain radiography, a decrease in discharge of bile juice, and the color of secretions.

We did not coat the surface of the magnet with resin or paint in our first 2 or 3 years of performing MCA procedures. However, after encountering a case in which the magnet was eroded by gastric juices (Fig. 16.73), we started coating the magnets with nylon resin to protect them from these juices. No further cases of erosion have occurred since we started taking this precaution.

The magnet has a side hole and a top hole. The side hole is mainly used for transport of the magnet over the guidewire or when crossing a stricture, as with sideways transport and the pulling up method. The top hole is used for pulling up to pinch the stenosis in MCRS (see Fig. 16.15). These magnets are not commercially available currently, but will be available for clinical use in the future.

There is inevitably a risk of stenosis every time an MCA is created. Stenosis occurred after the first bilioenteric anastomosis was performed, so the MCA was repeated. The anastomotic site was dilated using a balloon immediately after the magnets moved, which may have damaged the mucosa of the duodenum and CBD when the anastomosis was created, thereby leading to the stenosis. We placed a tube stent to maintain the patency of the tract for 6 months after this case instead of using balloon dilatation as in bilioenteric or biliobiliary MCA cases. However, a stenosis occurred in another bilioenteric MCA case 6 months after removal of a tube stent; MCA was not repeated in this case because we were able to place a tube stent immediately via the PTBD route. The tube stent was kept in place for about 12 months thereafter. There have been no other cases of stenosis requiring balloon dilatation since we started placing a tube stent for 12 months. The tube stent needs to be exchanged every 2–4 weeks in the outpatient clinic to keep it clean. There have been no recurrences of stenosis from the second case of bilioenteric anastomosis

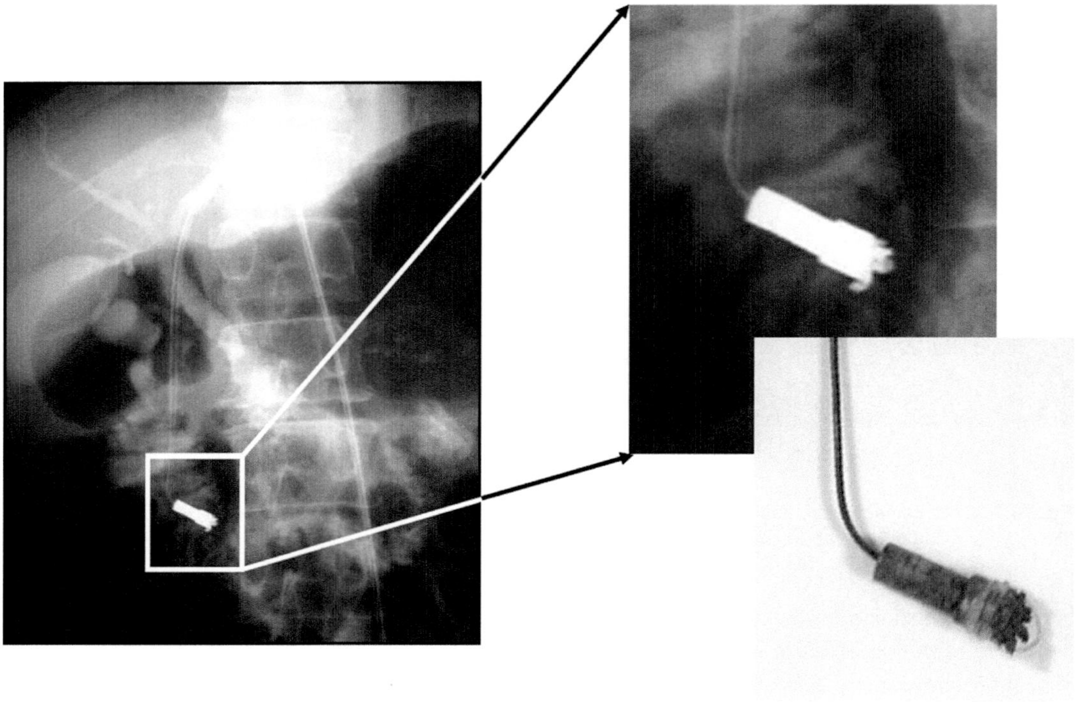

Fig. 16.73 The same case as shown in Figs. 16.44–16.49. The parent magnet appeared to be eroded on a plain radiograph. The mated magnets were removed after successful creation of the anastomosis and observed in detail. The magnets were found to be very sensitive to gastric acid even they are made of a sintered ceramic

onward and no complications, such as retrograde cholangitis, during follow-up. Therefore, it seems reasonable to continue using our present bilioenteric or biliobiliary MCA strategy.

Stenosis may also occur in cases with enteroenteric MCA. Stenosis develops in more than 80% of gastroduodenal or gastrojejunal MCA cases after removal of the mated magnets. Endoscopic investigations show that early detachment of the mated magnets seems to be the cause of the stenosis. Areas without mucosal union occur when the mated magnets are detached prematurely; these areas become ulcerated and then contract when scar tissue forms, leading to restenosis (Figs. 16.74 and 16.75).

Our accumulated experience suggests that stenosis occurs in about 10–20% of cases soon after creation of a total enteroenteric anastomosis. Our immediate objective is to solve this problem. Based on our endoscopic findings, it seems that a stenosis is most likely to occur when the magnet starts to move before the anastomotic site is sufficiently covered by mucosa. One solution may be to use weaker magnets so that the anastomosis

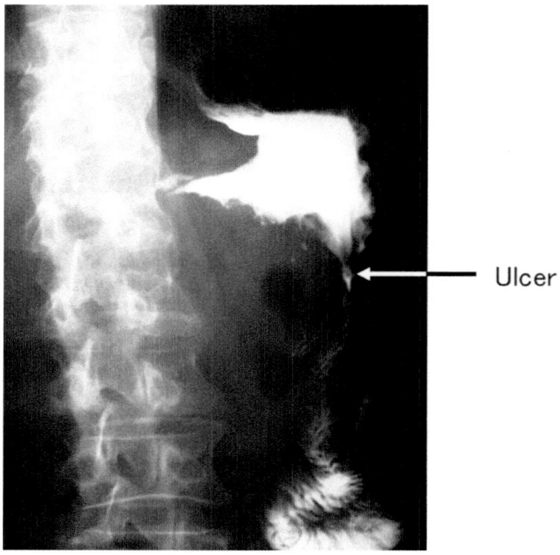

Fig. 16.74 An ulcer is seen at the anastomotic site on a gastrointestinal study after removal of the mated magnets (*arrow*)

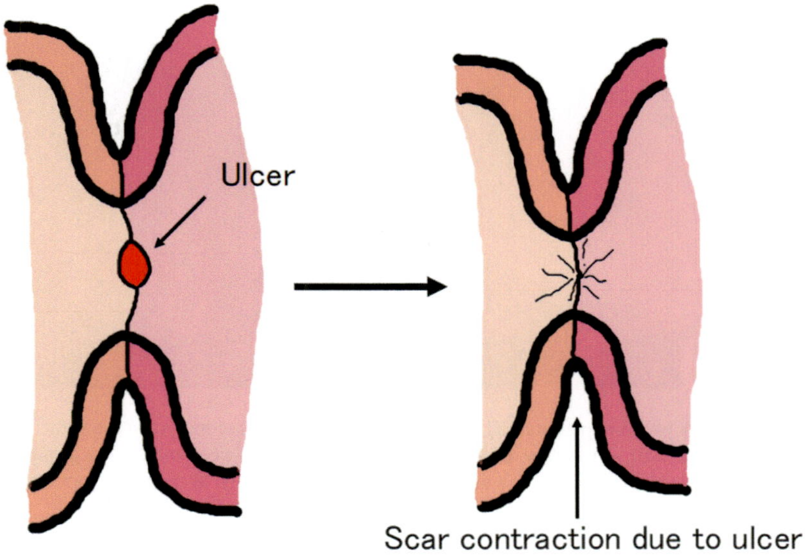

Fig. 16.75 Early detachment of the mated magnets produces an ulcer, which could cause scar contraction and stenosis

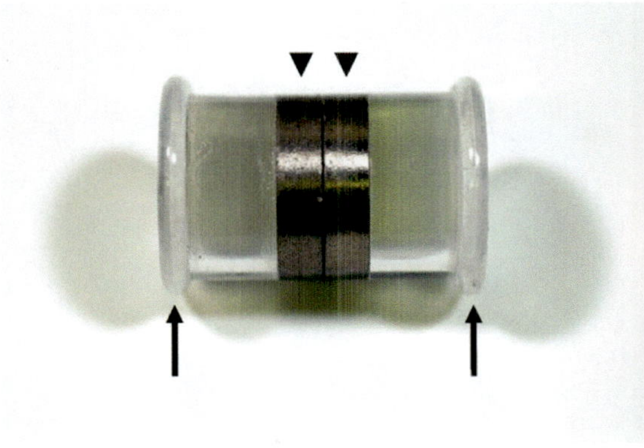

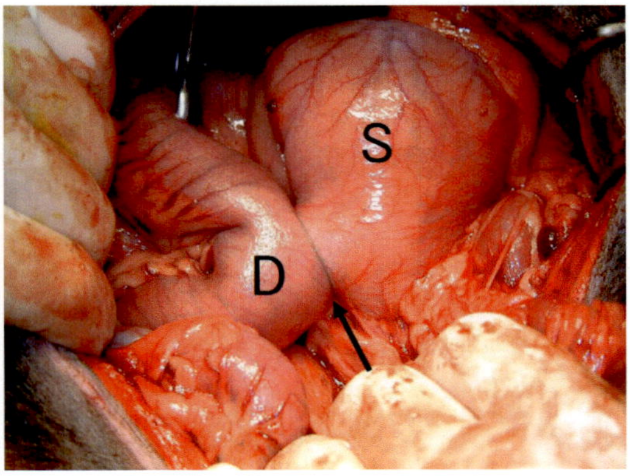

Fig. 16.76 Two flanged cylindrical stents are mated. The stents are always used as a pair. Each stent is a cylinder with a 3200-gauss samarium-cobalt permanent magnet at one end (*arrowheads*) and a flange at the other (*arrows*). The cylindrical stent and its flange are made of silicon rubber (*left*). The parent flange tube stent is in the duodenum (D) and the daughter stent is in the stomach (S). Note that the mated magnets are compressing the walls (*arrow*) of the stomach and duodenum (*right*)

takes longer to form, thereby allowing sufficient time for development of the mucosa. Another solution would be to attach a flanged cylindrical stent to the magnets (15 mm in diameter) so that they remain in place for longer after creation of the anastomosis (Fig. 16.76). We have performed mongrel canine experiments to determine whether there is a relationship between the risk of ulceration and the amount of time the flanged cylindrical stent is left in place after MCA gastroduodenostomy [13, 14]. Ulceration at the anastomotic site did not occur when the stent was indwelling for 4 weeks, but did occur when it was indwelling for 2 weeks (Figs. 16.77 and 16.78). We used a flanged cylindrical stent in one patient with a satisfactory result; however, delivery of the stent was problematic, and we do not plan to use this type of stent again until a more straightforward delivery method is found. If we use a larger disk magnet, the rate of stenosis may decrease. However, there is a limit to the size of the magnet that can be used, which is at most about 20 mm in diameter. The best way to prevent acute stenosis is frequent balloon dilatation

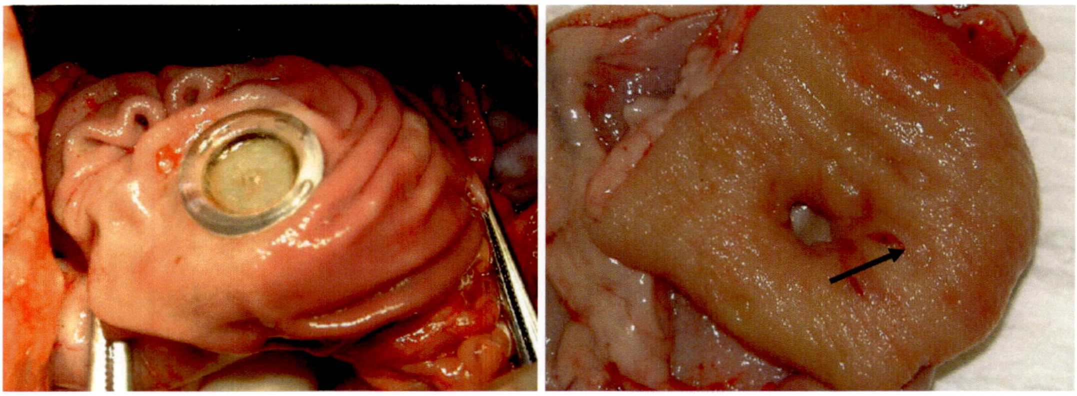

Fig. 16.77 A photograph obtained by opening a mongrel canine gastric wall at the time of sacrifice. The flanged cylindrical stents are still in place at the anastomotic site in a dog from the 2-week indwelling group (*left*). A macroscopic view from the duodenal side in a dog from the 2-week indwelling group. An ulcer (*arrow*) can be clearly seen at the anastomotic site (*right*)

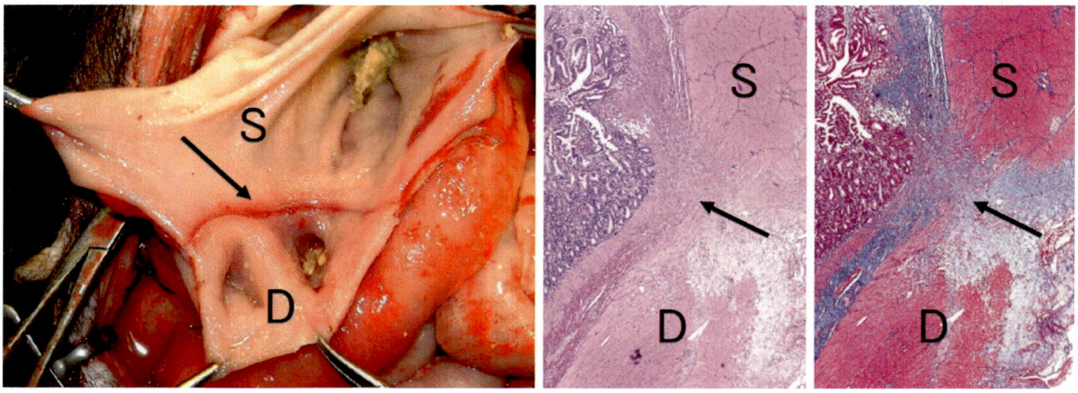

Fig. 16.78 Smooth mucosal union can be seen with no ulceration at the anastomotic site in the 4-week indwelling group. The fine red line (*arrow*) between the gastric (S) and duodenal (D) mucosa may represent fresh mucosa (*left*). Photomicrograph showing that the anastomotic site (*arrows*) is fully covered by fresh mucosa, although muscular union is still underway. The left specimen is hematoxylin-eosin stained and the right is Masson's trichrome-stained. The upper part is the stomach (S) and the lower part is the duodenum (D) on each photomicrograph (*right*)

(FBD; see Fig. 16.24), which is necessary once or twice weekly for several weeks. We have encountered very few stenoses since adopting this method, even in patients with gastroduodenal or gastrojejunal anastomoses. Although FBD can be performed easily in the upper gastrointestinal tract, it is more difficult to perform in deeper intestinal structures, such as the ileum or colon. In addition to FBD, it is also important to recover oral intake and close a colostomy as soon as possible because passage of food or feces works as a bougie at the anastomotic site. Two cases of leakage after FBD were noted when the anastomotic site was expanded excessively; percutaneous drainage was required in both cases. Therefore, it is important to gradually dilate the anastomotic site when performing FBD.

Only two of our cases have needed endoscopic local injection of triamcinolone acetonide to control contraction of scar tissue. However, it is unknown how effective these were, given that several attempts were required to hit the injection.

We have performed more than 20 MCA procedures involving the jejunum and blind end of the jejunum to treat stenosis that developed in the jejunum after total gastrectomy. Our experience has been that the probability of stenosis occurring somewhere in the jejunum after total gastrectomy is about 1 in 300–500 cases. We did have one interesting case of jejunal stenosis after total gastrectomy [23]. This patient developed complete obstruction of the jejunum 1 year after total gastrectomy with Roux-en-Y reconstruction. The obstructed site was only 4 cm below the surgical anastomosis line, not in the main route of the jejunum. MCRS was performed, after which the patient was able to resume eating (Fig. 16.79). We believe that stenosis may occur in the jejunum because the osmotic pressure is difficult to adjust at this site after total gastrectomy. In such cases, repeat surgery is difficult because the operative site is very deep and good results cannot be expected in the presence of severe peritoneal adhesions. MCRS should be considered rather than repeat surgery in such circumstances.

Anastomotic leak is one of the complications of a surgical anastomosis procedure. However, we have encountered almost no leaks after MCA or MCRS. There was only one case of leakage after MCA in a patient in whom colocolostomy was performed to straddle a colon cancer at the splenic flexure because the oral side of the markedly dilated colon was not decompressed, and the leak was predicted.

Damaged to vessels trapped between the magnets is frequently raised as a potential problem with this MCA method. A number of animal experiments have shown that even relatively large vessels that supply the stomach and intestinal tract undergo gradual involution when compressed by the magnets, and new vessels are created that bypass the site of compression to maintain blood flow. However, in our experiments in rats, compression of major vessels, such as the superior mesenteric artery, by the magnets resulted in a mortality rate of up to 60%, suggesting that an anastomosis with the potential to affect large vessels should be performed with the utmost care. In practice, gastroduodenal anastomosis raises such a possibility. Fortunately, we have not experienced this complication. When an enteroenteric MCA is performed, the patient should be observed carefully for severe abdominal pain immediately after the procedure to predict such an event. Bilioenteric or biliobiliary anastomosis rarely involves blood vessels because the magnets are small. Therefore, investigating blood flow in the hepatic artery and portal vein by abdominal ultrasonography does not make much sense.

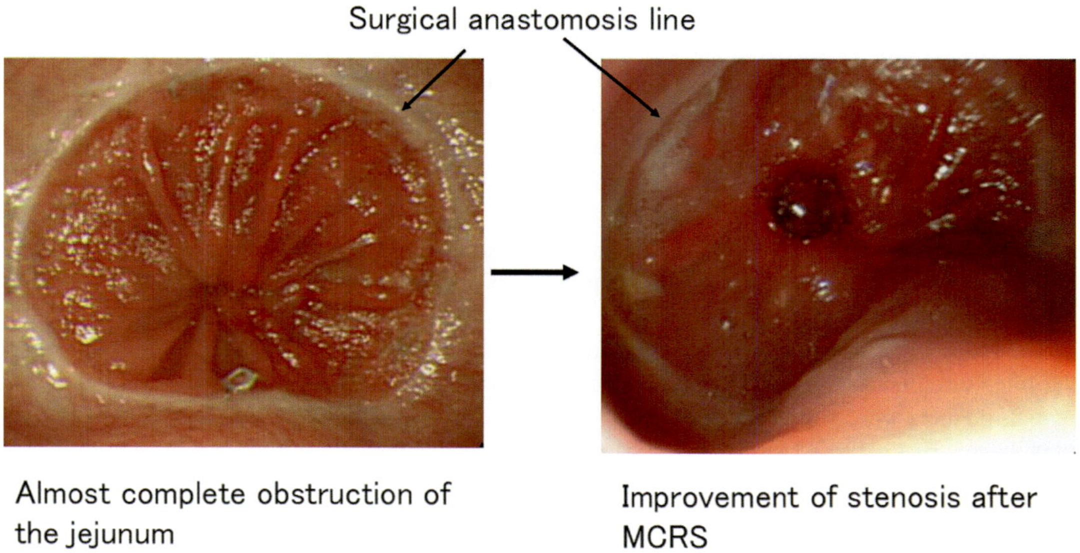

Fig. 16.79 Endoscopic studies show almost complete obstruction of the jejunum 4 cm below the surgical anastomosis line. Good patency is observed after MCRS

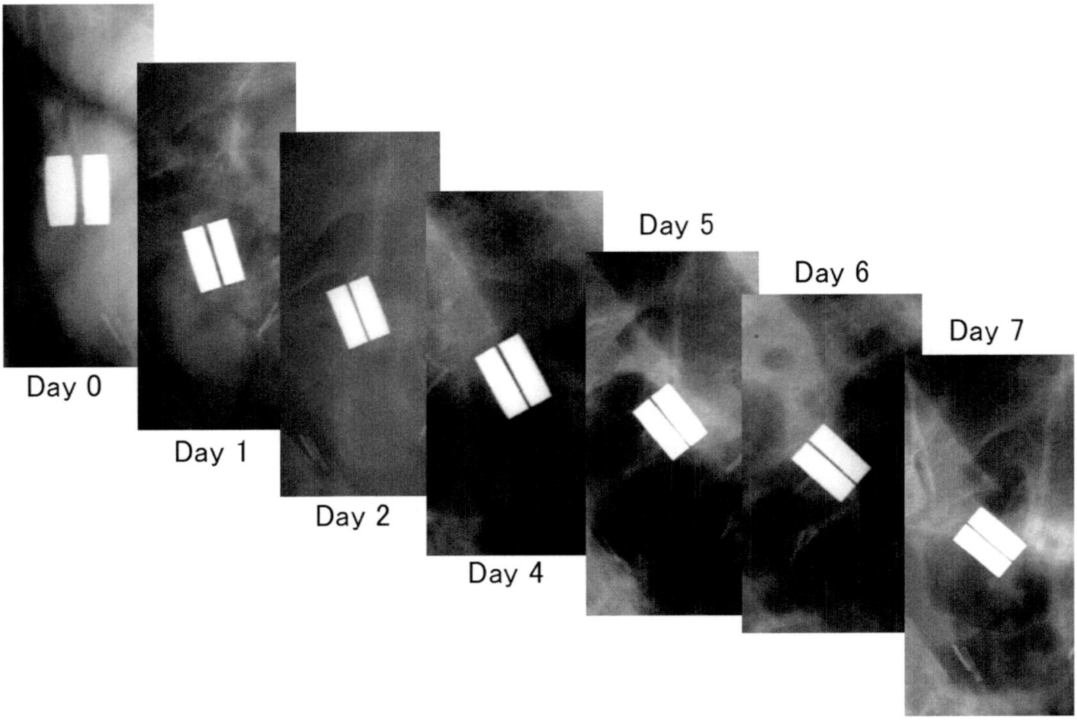

Fig. 16.80 Changes in the angle between the axis of the magnets and the vertical axis confirm successful magnetic compression anastomosis

In the case of bilioenteric MCA, the Roux-en-Y jejunal limb could not be reached with an endoscope at the time we started performing these procedures, so a different method was used to place the parent magnet in the jejunal limb. Our method of extracorporeal magnetic guidance via which the parent magnet is transported alongside the ileus tube was primitive but was very easy to perform and efficient because the correct direction was indicated by the tube and the intestinal tract was straightened, making it simple to move the magnet. Extracorporeal magnetic guidance was performed by alternating of the poles to move the intracorporeal parent magnet forward or across the plica circulares. The poles of the extracorporeal magnets were simply alternated by flipping the magnets back and forth (see Fig. 16.20). Today, a parent magnet can be easily transported into the Roux-en-Y jejunal limb because an endoscope that can enter the small intestine has become available in the past 10 years. This method is expected to be useful when MCA is performed in deep bowel loops, where a small intestine endoscope does not reach in all clinical situations.

In many cases of enteroenteric MCA, an interesting finding is that there is a change in angle between the axis of the mated magnets and the vertical axis (Fig. 16.80). Endoscopic observation revealed that this phenomenon is attributable to the many holes opening around the rim of the magnet, which finally connect and become like the lid of a can (Fig. 16.81). This finding is a good indicator of how well enteroenteric MCA is proceeding.

In bilioenteric or biliobiliary MCA cases, the guidewire attached to the daughter magnet shows a similar change in that the bending of the guidewire is gradually extended. This is because the mated magnets are pushed out to the other side by the guidewire. This finding is also a good indicator of how bilioenteric or biliobiliary MCA is proceeding (Fig. 16.82).

Some patients underwent an MCA or MCRS procedure after implantation of a pacemaker

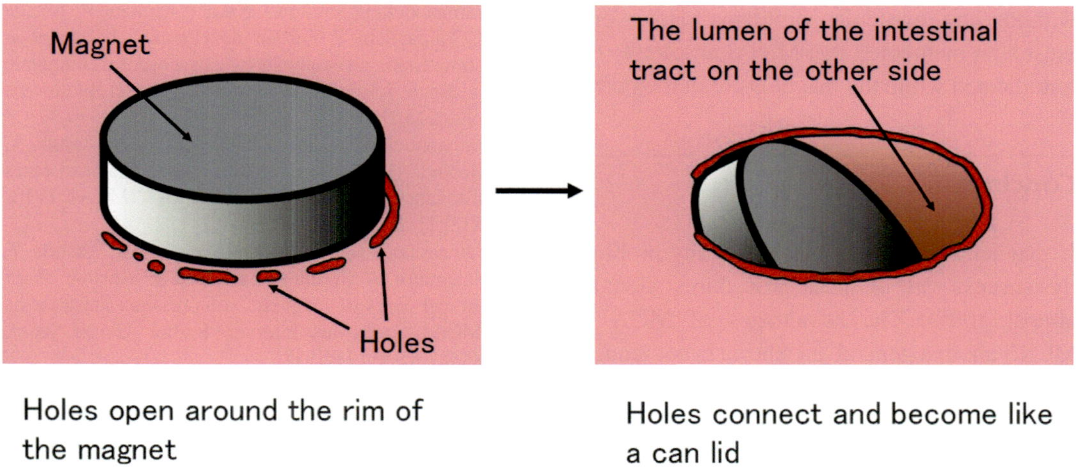

Fig. 16.81 Diagrams showing why changes in the angle between the axis of the magnets and the vertical axis appears in the process of magnetic compression anastomosis

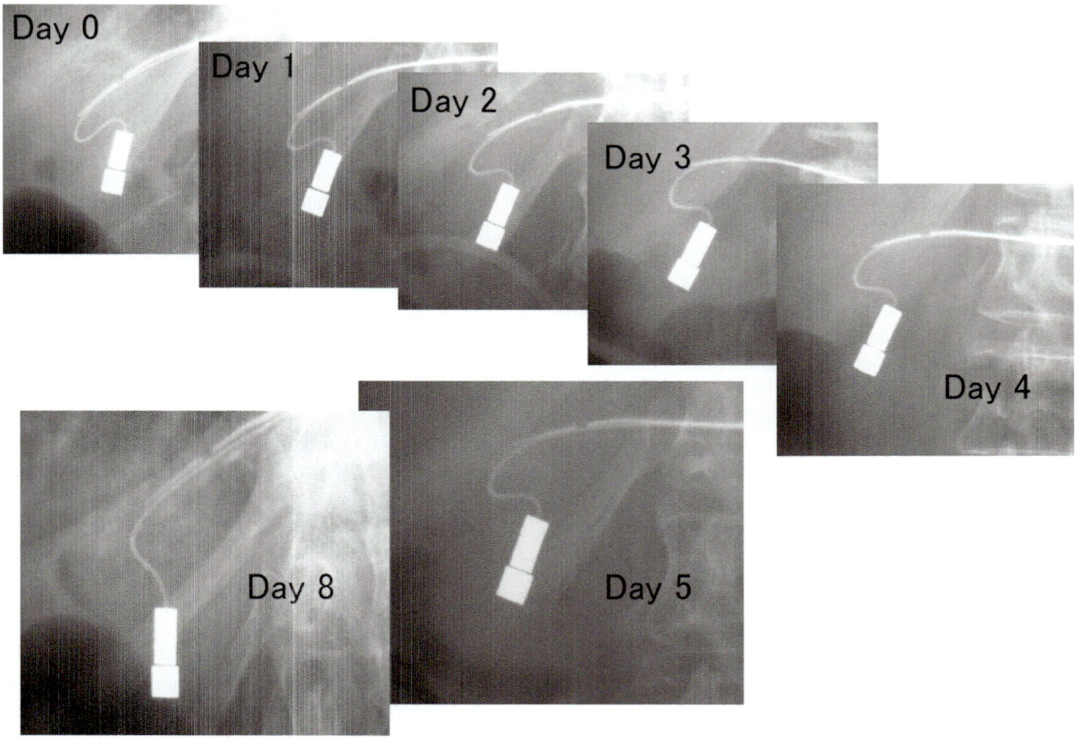

Fig. 16.82 Changes in the bending of the guidewire are a good indicator of how bilioenteric or biliobiliary magnetic compression anastomosis is proceeding

without any particular problems. However, it must be remembered that MRI is absolutely contraindicated while the magnets are in the body.

Conclusion

If magnets can be mated without any problems, the success rate of these procedures should be almost 100%. The advantages of MCA and MCRS are that general anesthesia is not required, the anastomosis can be performed without laparotomy, and no leak occurs. However, there are still many unknown with this new method. No absolute contraindications to MCA or MCRS have been found in our experience so far. However, its limits have yet to be determined, and further research is needed before this method can be used in other clinical settings.

References

1. Murphy JB. Cholecysto-intestinal, gastro-intestinal, entero-intestinal and approximation without suture. Med Record (NY). 1982;42:665–76.
2. Saveliev VS, Avaliani MV, Bashirov AD. Endoscopic magnetic cholecystodigestive anastomosis. Personal technique for palliative treatment of distal bile duct obstruction. J Laparoendosc Surg. 1993;3:99–113.
3. Cope C. Creation of compression gastroenterostomy by means of the oral, percutaneous, or surgical introduction of magnets: feasibility study in swine. JVIR. 1995;6:539–45.
4. Cope C. Evaluation of compression cholecystogastric and cholecystojejunal anastomoses in swine after peroral and surgical introduction of magnets. JVIR. 1995;6:546–52.
5. Yamanouchi E, Kawaguchi H, Endo I, Arakawa H, Yamaguchi T, Sakuyama K. A new interventional method: magnetic compression anastomosis with rare-earth magnets. Cardiovasc Intervent Radiol (United States). 1998;21(Suppl(1)):S155.
6. Yamanouchi E, Kawaguchi H, Endo I, Arakawa H, Yamaguchi T, Sakuyama K. A new interventional method of anastomosis with magnets: magnetic compression anastomosis in five clinical cases. Radiology. 1998;209(P):567.
7. Yamanouchi E, Sugiura T, Nakamura R, Kushiya H, Sakai F, Okawa T, et al. Further development of magnetic compression anastomosis by extracorporeal magnetic guidance: three clinical cases in bowel loops. Cardiovasc Intervent Radiol (United States). 1999;22(Suppl(2)):S174.
8. Yamanouchi E, Sugiura T, Sakai F, Kumano R, Takada K, Yamaguchi T. Further development of magnetic compression anastomosis by extracorporeal magnetic guidance: four clinical bowel loop cases. Radiology. 1999;213(P):302.
9. Yamanouchi E, Sugiura T, Nakamura R, Yasuda Y, Machida H, Fujimura M. Review of 22 clinical cases of magnetic compression anastomosis (MCA). JVIR. 2000;11(2):265.
10. Yamanouchi E, Machida H, Sugiura T, Yasuda Y, Nakamura R, Fujimura M, Sakai F. Review of 25 clinical cases of magnetic compression anastomosis (MCA). Cardiovasc Intervent Radiol (United State). 2000;23(Supp 1):S157.
11. Yamanouchi E, Sugiura T, Yasuda Y, Machida H, Nakamura R, Sakai F, et al. Review of 30 cases of magnetic compression anastomosis (MCA). Radiology. 2000;217(P):584.
12. Yamanouchi E, Ikeda T, Nakamura R, Kumano R, Izumo T, Daimon T, Ueno M, Kobayashi K. Review of 40 clinical cases of magnetic compression anastomosis (MCA). Cardiovasc Intervent Radiol (United State). 2000;24(Supp 1):S190.
13. Machida H, Yamanouchi E, Sugiura T, Yasuda Y, Nakamura R, Fujimura M, Sakai F. A proposal for a new stent (Eigorotta Yamachicchi Stent) with magnetic compression anastomosis. Cardiovasc Intervent Radiol (United State). 2000;23(Supp 1):S157.
14. Yamanouchi E, Kumano R, Sugiura T, Matsumoto J, Hayakawa M, Imanishi Y, Ikeda T, Nakamura R, Kobayashi KC, Omae K, Iinuma Y, Oonishi T. A proposal of a new stent (Eigorotta Yamachicchi Stent) for magnetic compression anastomosis (MCA). Radiology. 2001;221(P):106.
15. Takao S, Matsuo Y, Shinchi H, Nakajima S, Aikou T, Iseji T, Yamanouchi E. Magnetic compression anastomosis for benign obstruction of the common bile duct. Endoscopy. 2001;33(11):988–90.
16. Yamanouchi E, Kumano R, Sugiura T, Matsumoto J, Hayakawa M, Imanishi Y, Ikeda T, Nakamura R, Kobayashi KC, Omae K, Iinuma Y, Oonishi T. Review of 43 clinical cases of magnetic compression anastomosis (MCA). Radiology. 2001;221(P):107.
17. Yamanouchi E, Kumano R, Nakayama M, Omae K, Iinuma Y, Matsumoto J, Oonishi T, Hayakawa M, Imanishi Y. Magnetic compression revision anastomosis for stenosis. Cardiovasc Intervent Radiol (United States). 2002;25(Suppl(2)):S209.
18. Yamanouchi E, Kumano R, Kobayashi K, Hattori T, Matsumoto J, Oonishi T, Hayakawa M, Tani I. Treatment for bowel or biliary obstruction by magnetic compression anastomosis. J Nippon Med Sch. 2002;69(5):471–5.
19. Yamanouchi E, Kumano R, Kobayashi K, Hattori T, Matsumoto J, Oonishi T, Hayakawa M, Tani I. Review of 59 clinical cases of magnetic compression anastomosis (MCA). Radiology. 2002;225(P):220–1.
20. Okajima H, Kotera A, Takeichi T, Ueno M, Ishiko T, Hirota M, Asonuma K, Yamanouchi E, Inomata Y. Magnet compression anastomosis for bile duct

stenosis after duct-to-duct biliary reconstruction in living donor transplantation. Liver Transpl. 2005;11(4):473–5.
21. Itoi T, Yamanouchi E, Ikeda, Sofuni A, Tsuchiya T, Tsuchida A, Kasuya K, Moriyasu F. Magnetic compression anastomosis: a novel technique for canalization of severe hilar bile duct strictures. Endoscopy. 2005;37:1248–51.
22. Nakaseko Y, Shiba H, Yamanouchi E, Takano Y, Sakamoto T, Imazu H, Ashida H, Yanaga K. Successful treatment of stricture of duct-to-duct biliary anastomosis after living-donor liver transplantation of the left lobe: a case report. Transplant Proc. 2017;49:1644–8.
23. Kamada T, Ohdaira H, Takeuchi H, Takahashi J, Marukuchi R, Suzuki N, Narihiro S, Hoshimoto S, Yoshida M, Yamanouchi E, Suzuki Y. Magnetic compression anastomosis for nonanastomotic stenosis of the proximaljejunum after total gastrectomy with Rouxen-Y reconstruction: a case report. Surgical Case Reports 2020;6:167.
24. Kamada T, Ohdaira H, Takeuchi H, Takahashi J, Ito E, Suzuki N, Narihiro S, Yoshida M, Yamanouchi E, Suzuki Y. New Technique for Magnetic Compression Anastomosis Without Incision for Gastrointestinal Obstruction. Journal of the American College of Surgeons. 2020;232:170–77.

Use of Magnetically Controlled Growing Rod Implants for the Spine

17

Michel Gagner

Scoliosis needs surgical correction when the spinal curve surpasses 45 or 50 degrees, especially after skeletal maturity, particularly if it causes loss of lung function. Typically, a posterior fusion has been a standard treatment for scoliosis, and orthopaedic surgeons will use segmental pedicle screw constructs with hooks and wires.

Anterior approaches had been performed for thoracolumbar and lumbar scoliosis with thoracoscopic and/or laparoscopic-assisted techniques using anterior instrumentation for the thoracic curve employing video-assisted thoracoscopic surgery techniques but faded out for more fashionable posterior approaches. Selected severe idiopathic scoliosis cases may need manifold vertebral wedge osteotomies without fusion. This chapter will review the literature published on magnetically controlled growing rod (MCGR) to decrease the complications related to frequent surgical rod lengthenings and diminish numerous surgeries that follow.

Animal models were used to develop technical aspects of magnetic rods. Akbarnia et al. have employed a porcine model, randomly assigned to a MCGR device group and a sham group. A total of eight animals were operated on, and the MCGR group experienced weekly adjustments with a total of 49 mm of distraction across the ununited vertebral levels, prearranged for a 7-week period with an average adjustment of 7 mm per week. Radiographic images of the MCGR apparatus exposed an average distraction of 39 mm (range 32–46 mm), resulting in attainment of 80% of projected spinal height [1].

A couple of years later, Cheung et al. reported in the Lancet on the use of magnetically controlled growing rods for non-invasive outpatient distractions in five patients, two of whom have reached 24 months follow-up. Their mean degree of scoliosis, measured by Cobb angle, was 67° before implantation and 29° at 24 months. Length of the instrumented segment of the spine increased by a mean of 1.9 mm with each distraction. Throughout follow-up, patients had no discomfort, had excellent functional outcomes, and no device-related complications were noted at the time of publication [2].

Then Hickey reported on six patients with the magnetically controlled growing rod system MAGEC, Ellipse (Figs. 17.1 and 17.2). NuVasive, Inc. paid $410 million to acquire Ellipse Technologies in January 2016. It has become the leader in spine technology innovation, which includes access, implants and fixation systems, biologics, software for surgical planning, navigation and imaging solutions, magnetically adjustable implant systems for spine and orthopaedics (Figs. 17.3 and 17.4), and intraoperative monitoring services. With more than $1 billion in net sales, NuVasive has 2800 employees and distributes in more than 50 countries.

M. Gagner (✉)
Hôpital du Sacré-Cœur de Montréal, Montréal, QC, Canada

Chief of Surgery, Westmount Square Surgical Center, Westmount, QC, Canada

M. Gagner (ed.), *Magnetic Surgery*, https://doi.org/10.1007/978-3-030-73947-8_17

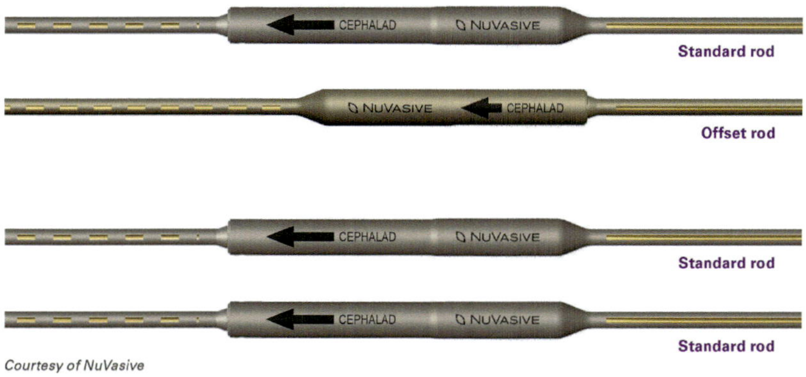

Fig. 17.1 MAGEC® Rods. (©2016. NuVasive Specialized Orthopedics, Inc. All rights reserved. NuVasive and Speed of Innovation are registered trademarks of NuVasive, Inc. MAGEC is a registered trademark of NuVasive Specialized Orthopedics, Inc. NuVasive Specialized Orthopedics, Inc. is a trademark of NuVasive, Inc.)

In patients who had MAGEC as a primary procedure, mean preoperative Cobb angle was 74°, with post-operative Cobb angle of 42° $p \leq 0.001$, a 43% correction 2 years later (Fig. 17.5). Spinal development rate was 6 mm per year, and in terms of complications, only one screw pull-out, and a single rod fracture were documented [3].

Ellipse Technologies was founded in 2005 and had developed two major products, the MAGEC–EOS spinal bracing and distraction system for treatment of early-onset scoliosis (EOS), and the PRECICE® limb-lengthening system for treatment of limb length discrepancy. These devices have been utilized to treat more than 5000 patients worldwide.

When NuVasive Inc. acquired the company, they assessed the market to be approximately $1.2 billion, with the MAGEC system potentially affecting 690,000 annual procedures. But Ellipse itself had only revenues of approximately $40 million in 2015.

Jenks et al. proceeded to publish a NICE medical technologies guidance report. The Medical Technologies Advisory Committee at the National Institute for Health and Care Excellence (NICE) selected the MAGEC system for evaluation. The meta-analysis distinguished cost savings of £12,077 per patient with MAGEC rods compared with conventional rods, over 6 years. NICE issued a positive recommendation as supported by the evidence [4]. Cost comparisons have also been evaluated by Rolton et al. over a projected 5-year period. The initial expenditure for insertion for MCGR was £12,913 more than the conventional rods. There was substantial cost savings for each lengthening which, projected over the 5-year lifetime, amounted to a cost savings of over £8000 per patient [5].

Stokes et al. did an elegant study to look at replacing pre- and post-distraction spine radiographs to verify lengthening using ultrasonography. All patients were imaged via ultrasound, ease of rod identification was established, and the reliability and reproducibility of optimal reference point selection were assessed blindly by three operators. Measurement of the rod's neck distance on ultrasound demonstrated a high degree of reliability ($a = 0.99$; $p < 0.001$). Consequently, the algorithm using ultrasonography instead of X-rays had been successfully executed [6].

More clinical data with early experience followed. The University of Hong Kong reported their experience with MCGR on 32 participants from 16 regions. They found that adolescent idiopathic scoliosis and congenital scoliosis patients had less favourable outcomes. They suggested some modifications on the rod configuration, timing, frequency, technique, and amount of distraction. Risk factors for distraction failure include larger patients, internal magnets too close

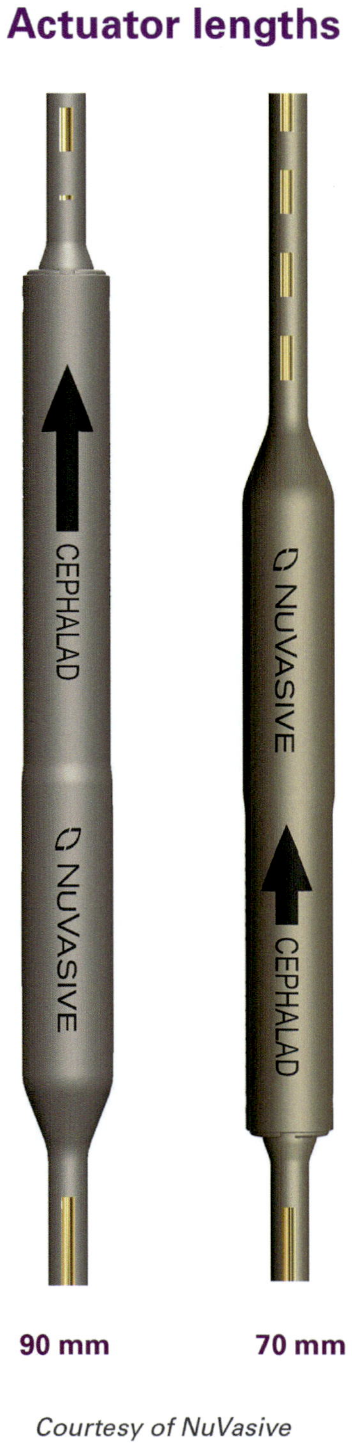

Fig. 17.2 MAGEC® Actuators. (©2016. NuVasive Specialized Orthopedics, Inc. All rights reserved. NuVasive and Speed of Innovation are registered trademarks of NuVasive, Inc. MAGEC is a registered trademark of NuVasive Specialized Orthopedics, Inc. NuVasive Specialized Orthopedics, Inc. is a trademark of NuVasive, Inc.)

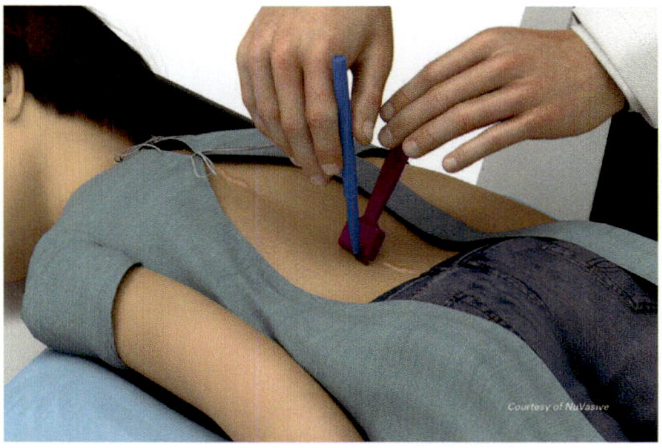

Fig. 17.3 Use of rod magnet location. (©2016. NuVasive Specialized Orthopedics, Inc. All rights reserved. NuVasive and Speed of Innovation are registered trademarks of NuVasive, Inc. MAGEC is a registered trademark of NuVasive Specialized Orthopedics, Inc. NuVasive Specialized Orthopedics, Inc. is a trademark of NuVasive, Inc.)

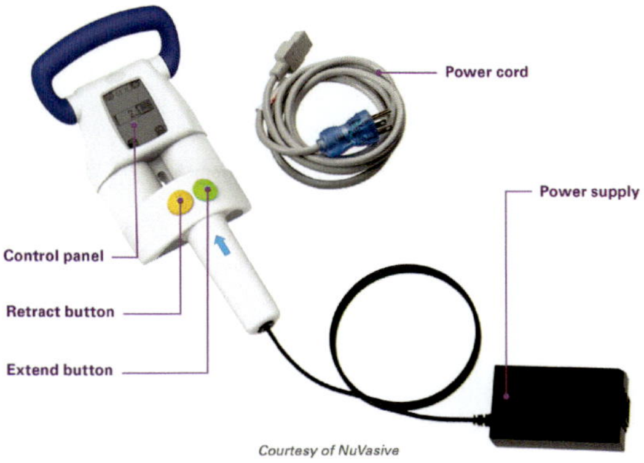

Fig. 17.4 External remote controller. (©2016. NuVasive Specialized Orthopedics, Inc. All rights reserved. NuVasive and Speed of Innovation are registered trademarks of NuVasive, Inc. MAGEC is a registered trademark of NuVasive Specialized Orthopedics, Inc. NuVasive Specialized Orthopedics, Inc. is a trademark of NuVasive, Inc.)

to each other, and magnets too close to the apex of the major curve [7]. Cheung et al. also identified factors for rod slippage, in a study of 22 patients with MCGR and six distraction episodes. Increased height, weight, body mass index, older age, increased T1–12 and T1-S1 lengths, and less distance between magnets were significantly associated with early rod slippage [8].

Special groups were studied, and the technology applied to children with spinal muscular atrophy (SMA), which were then assessed for control of spinal deformity in a group of patients

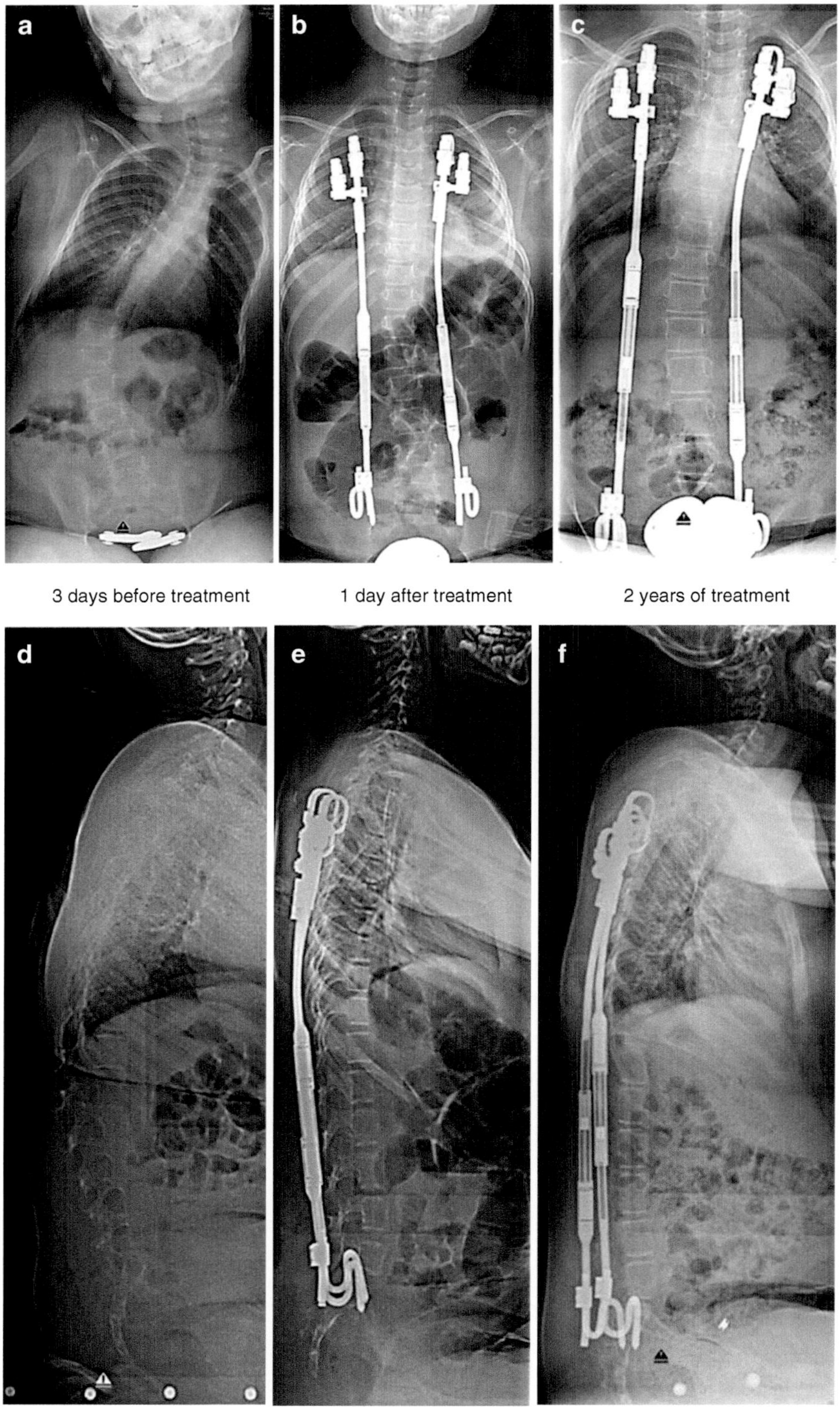

Fig. 17.5 (**a**–**c**) Postero-anterior views and (**d**–**f**) lateral views, with the magnetically controlled devices. (From Lorenz HM, et al. [9]. JB JS Open Access under the terms of the Creative Commons Attribution-Non-Commercial-No Derivatives License 4.0 (CCBY-NC-ND))

managed with magnetically controlled implants for 2 years. The mean main curve of patients decreased from 70° before implantation of the magnetically controlled device to 30° after implantation of the device. Correction was continued during the follow-up period, with a mean curve of 31° at the time of the latest follow-up at 2.2 years. Pelvic obliquity was improved by 76% (from 17° to 4°) and remained constant during follow-up. Thoracic kyphosis could not be corrected within the studied period. Spinal length of the children increased by >50 mm immediately after device implantation and gradually increased at a rate of 13.5 mm/year. over the sequence of treatment. Implantation of this externally controlled bilateral magnetic rod with rib-to-pelvis fixation signifies a harmless and extremely efficient approach to influence spinal deformity in children with SMA, attaining appropriate and stable curve correction as well as intensified spinal length [9].

Joyce et al. looked at the explanted rods to learn about the mechanical defects and improve designs of those in the near future. Explanted MAGEC rods from seven spinal centres were obtained for independent examination. Thirty-four MAGEC rods, from 18 children, explanted for failure of rod lengthening and distraction, were assessed. All MAGEC rods showed localized marks, which were labelled "growth marks" as they signified growth of the rod in vivo on the extending component. After carving open, titanium wear debris was uncovered inside all 34 (100%) MAGEC rods. Ninety-one percent of MAGEC rods showed measurable wear of the extending bar, towards the magnet end. Considerable damage to the radial bearing was ascertained inside 74% of MAGEC rods, O-ring seal failure was seen in 53% of cases, and in 44% of MAGEC rods, the drive pin was fractured. The metallosis reported clinically around some MAGEC rods may come from high volumes of titanium wear debris, along with O-ring seal damage [10]. Rushton also looked at 45 explanted MAGEC rods from 25 cases. The mean age at insertion was 8.6 years and rods were in patients for a mean of 2.7 years. As control, two unused MAGEC rods produced a mean force of 45.3 and 50.2 Ibf, above the manufacturer's reported standard. Of the 45 explanted rods, 10 (22%) yielded a force greater or equal to manufacturer's standard, mean 46.7 Ibf. Six rods (13%) produced some force but less than the maker's standard, with a mean of 34.8 Ibf, and surprisingly, 29 rods (64%) produced no force. The rod duration was significantly negatively correlated with the force produced on testing ($r = -0.63$, $P < 0.005$), as 12 rods implanted longer than 38 months did not deliver any force. Hence, the majority of explanted rods produced no force, whilst others produced reduced force. These outcomes raised questions concerning the longevity of the implant [20].

Gilday studied if desired lengthening can reliably be achieved, or if prior spine instrumentation and large tissue depths affect lengthening. They examined 31 patients with a mean age of 8.1 years with major curves measuring 60 degrees at the time of MCGR insertion. Total length increment relative to the scheduled distraction was 86%. Length increases for patients with and without prior surgery were similar at 87% and 86%. Total lengthening was inversely proportional to tissue depth ($r = 0.38$, $P < 0.01$); indeed, the lower lengthening achieved was 2.1%/mm of tissue depth. Expansions in rod length were 14% lower than the planned distraction. Larger distance between the rod and the skin negatively altered the magnitude of distraction [11].

Thakar et al. concentrated on the analysis of complications after magnetically controlled growing rods in early-onset scoliosis. This was a systematic review using PUBMED, Medline, Embase, Google Scholar, and the Cochrane Library. Fifteen studies (336 patients) were included (42.5% male, average age 7.9 years, mean follow-up 29.7 months). Improvement was achieved in all studies, from a preoperative 64.8° to 34.9°, as was growth advancement ($p = 0.001$). With an overall complication rate of 44.5% and a revision rate of 33%, the most common complications revealed anchor pull-out (11.8%), implant failure (11.7%), and rod breakage (10.6%). There were no significant differences between primary (39.8%) and conversion (33.3%) procedures, and a non-statistically significant increased complication rate with single rods (40 vs. 27%) [12].

Poon et al. were concerned about the negative consequences of growing rod treatments and evaluated the maximal force generated at different lengths with 12 MCGRs (90-mm actuator length). The maximal lengthening force measured in pounds-of-force generated by each rod was recorded at expansion lengths of 0, 25, and 40 mm. At 0 mm, the mean maximum force was 46.8 lb., at 25 mm of expansion, the mean maximum force was 44.9 lb., and at 40 mm of lengthening, the mean maximum force was 43.2 lb. Mathematically, there was a statistically significant reduction in the maximal force engendered with progressive MCGR lengthening, at an average decrease of 0.089 lb. of force ($p = 0.003$) per mm of lengthening. Poon concluded that the decrease in the force produced might result in diminished spine length gained with each subsequent MCGR lengthening [13].

Then longer term studies began to be published. A Subramanian cohort had a longer follow-up (47 months), over 6 years in 31 children, and remarked that the mean Cobb angle was 54° preoperatively and 37° at the latest follow-up ($p < 0.001$). The mean T1-S1 height increased from 287 mm to 338 mm ($p < 0.001$) and the mean sagittal balance abridged from 68 mm preoperatively to 18 mm at the latest follow-up. The mean Activity Scale for Kids (ASKp) scores rose in all areas, with standing skills and personal care being significant at the latest follow-up ($p < 0.05$). The advances in Cobb angle, TK and T1-S1 heights were not correlated to gender, the aetiology of the EOS, or conversion from a conventional growing rod system. A total of 21 children developed 23 complications at a rate of 0.23 per patient per year. Complications obtained at a mean of 38 months after the initial surgery obliged 22 further procedures. Finally, children who acquired a complication were more likely to be younger, have complicated EOS, and have a single rod [14].

The Hung study looked at primary versus conversions in 383 MCGR patients, 272 (71%) were primary and 111 (29%) were conversion. There was no statistically significant difference in Cobb rectification at 1 year or between follow-up at one and 2 years. Significantly greater height gains were seen in primary than in converted patients in the one-year follow-up cohort. There was a higher rate of complications in the conversion group than in the other group; however, the difference was not statistically significant. Overall, most complications were implant-related, and no loss of curve correction happened in whichever group [15].

Direct medical costs have also been reviewed recently [16]. A recent study by Oetgen demonstrated that the average overall charge for MCGR implantation was 1.5 times greater than traditional rods TGR implementation ($p = 0.04$). Average charges were statistically comparable across all groups, except implant costs, which were significantly higher for MCGR (MCGR: $31,621 vs. TGR: $8966, $p < 0.0001$). The average percentage reimbursement of total charges was similar between surgeries, MCGR 43% vs. TGR 46%, ns. MCGR implantation has a significantly higher charge than TGR, due to the prohibitive expense of MCGR implants. Despite this, institutional reimbursement is analogous between surgical operations. Whilst MCGRs appeared to be "cost-effective" after 3 years, their results imply that health care institutions assume the cost of this new technology whilst payers gain the long-term financial profit [18]. Hasharvadna found similar costs in their analysis [19].

Pepke et al. looked at the sagittal profile of patients with an implanted MCGR, in a retrospective study of patients with scoliosis from 2012 to 2018. In 21 patients, they found a significant coronal correction of the structural and compensatory curves ($p < 0.01$), and sagittal profile revealed a significant decrease of TK ($p < 0.001$) and T9SPi ($p = 0.002$) with a concurrent increase of T1T3 angle ($p = 0.015$) and T1T4 angle ($p = 0.015$). No significant changes of the sagittal parameters of cervical, lumbar, and spinopelvic parameters were noted [17].

Is there an association between the diameter of MCGR constructs and the rate of rod fracture? A study by Roye BD took 527 patients with 1054 rods, of which 552 (52.4%) rods had a diameter of less than or equal to 5 mm and 461 (43.7%) rods had a diameter of greater than 5 mm. Twenty (1.9%) total rod fractures occurred: 9 (1.6%) rods with diameters of ≤5 mm, 10 (2.2%) rods with diameters of >5 mm, and 1 uncategorized rod ($p = 0.529$). No difference in the rate of rod fracture or survival distribution was found between rod diameters of >5 mm and ≤ 5 mm even after stratification by ambulatory status, major coronal curve, weight, or location of anchors. Hence, rod fracture appears to be a rare event in dual MCGR constructs and rod diameter does not seem to be associated with the incidence or rate of rod fracture [21].

Doany published an analysis of the quality of life in patients harbouring magnetic rods. Inclusion criteria were: ≤10 years of age at index procedure, major curve ≥30°, no previous spine surgery, minimum 1-year post-operative follow-up. The 24-item early-onset scoliosis questionnaire (EOSQ-24) was employed to assess quality of life in 44 children with scoliosis, of whom 25 had traditional rods TGR and 19 MCGR. The groups were comparable in sex, but patients were older (14.0 vs. 8.8 years) and had lengthier follow-up (101.3 vs. 34.3 months) in TGR ($P < 0.01$). The study found that scores of economic burden and overall satisfaction in MCGR were significantly higher to those in TGR [22].

Analyses of rod failures by Panagiotopoulou et al. showed that one-third of retrieved magnetic rods had a fractured pin, surface degradation on the extendable telescopic rod, and considerable corrosion along the internal mechanism. They recommended that orthopaedic surgeons consider that any inability of magnetically controlled growth rods to distract may be due to corrosive debris building up inside the mechanism, thereby preventing normal function [23].

Cheung recently published a 6 years follow-up cohort of only 10 scoliosis patients, with mean 6.1 yr. of follow-up. Steady improvements in T1–12, T1-S1, and instrumented segment were observed. Rate of lengthening reduced after the first year of use but improved back to initial rates after rod exchange. Seven of the ten patients experienced complications, with reoperation rate of 40% for rod distraction failure and proximal foundation problems [24].

Lebon looked specifically at post-operative long-term complications in 30 patients with a median age at surgery was 9.1 years. Of the 24 complications experienced by patients: 7 were proximal pull-outs of the hooks, 3 rod breakages, 6 failures of the lengthening (of which 4 were complete blockages and 2 were complete blockages followed by backtracking), 1 proximal junctional kyphosis, 1 wound dehiscence, 1 superficial infection, 1 deep infection requiring implant removal, 1 pulmonary embolism, 1 pulmonary insufficiency, 1 secondary lumbar scoliosis, and 1 painful outpatient distraction. Eight patients had a gradual shortfall of effectiveness of distractions, and with a substantial complication rate, 13 revisional surgeries in 9 patients were observed [25].

Yoon also investigated whether ultrasound (U/S) is an alternative to radiography when measuring magnetically controlled growth rod length. The average rod lengths were 1.322 cm with U/S and 1.329 cm with radiography. The mean total effective radiation dose of the pre-lengthening and post-lengthening PA spinal radiographs was 0.26 mSv. U/S allows patient monitoring and accurate MCGR measurement whilst decreasing patients' radiation exposure [26].

According to Choi, traditional growing rods have a reported wound and implant complication rate as high as 58% and should be compared with MCGR patients. Of the 30 primary and 24 conversion procedures with a mean duration of follow-up 19.4 months, 21 (38.8%) of 54 patients had a complication. Fifteen (27.8%) patients had at least one revisional surgery, in which 6 (11.1%) had damaged rods; 6 (11.1%) patients experienced one episode of absence or loss of lengthening. Seven patients (13.0%) had either proximal or distal fixation-related complication at a mean of 8 months. Two patients (3.7%) had infections requiring drainage. It showed that compared with traditional growing rods, MCGR had a lower infection rate (3.7% vs. 11.1%). MCGR did not appear to prevent common implant-related complications such as rod or foundation failure [27].

Cheung looked at the three-dimensional (3D) changes in deformity correction with MCGR distractions. A total of 10 EOS patients were studied during a mean post-operative follow-up of 34 months. Six patients had rod exchange at mean 29.5 months after initial implantation. Despite constant expansions in body height and arm span, the main variations in coronal and rotational profiles only happened at the initial rod implantation surgery with only minor changes taking place with successive follow-ups. No changes in pelvic parameters were examined, hence, 3D changes with MCGR are chiefly observed with initial rod implantation and no significant changes are witnessed with distractions. It was concluded that MCGR may thwart deformity progression in the axial plane [28].

Guan recently evaluated the efficacy and safety of MCGR in treating early-onset scoliosis. In total, 13 studies (n = 249) were included, with a mean of 22-month follow-up. Scoliosis correction was well preserved, perfecting from 36.4 degrees at post-initial to 37.1 degrees at last follow-up. Kyphosis evolved from 28.8 degrees at post-initial to 34.4 degrees at last follow-up ($P = 0.024$). Annual T1-S1 and T1-T12 longitudinal extensions were 8.7 and 4.7 mm/year, respectively. With more follow-up, no weakening was observed in annual extension of T1-S1 ($P = 0.4680$) or T1-T12 ($P = 0.8053$). The occurrences of alignment-related, implant-related, and wound-related complication were 3.5%, 30.1%, and 6.9%, correspondingly. No correlation was observed between complication and term of follow-up, and rate of unplanned surgery was 24%. MCGR was found to be efficient in the maintenance of coronal correction and preservation of spine growth [29].

On February 13, 2020, NuVasive Inc. issued a voluntary recall of the MAGEC X magnetically controlled growing rod device. The actuator end cap was noted to detach from the lengthening apparatus in 0.5% of devices. When the end cap dislodged from the lengthening mechanism, the internal threads become exposed to body fluids and may lead to extravasation of metallic wear debris. The MAGEC X devices were pulled off the market by NuVasive to further investigate and tackle the root cause of the matter. This is a class II FDA recall that withdraws the device from the international market and does not pertain to the prior MAGEC rod model branded MAGEC 1.5. Stay tuned for more progress on magnetic rods.

References

1. Akbarnia BA, Mundis GM Jr, Salari P, Yaszay B, Pawelek JB. Innovation in growing rod technique: a study of safety and efficacy of a magnetically controlled growing rod in a porcine model. Spine (Phila Pa 1976). 2012;37(13):1109–14.
2. Cheung KM, Cheung JP, Samartzis D, et al. Magnetically controlled growing rods for severe spinal curvature in young children: a prospective case series. Lancet. 2012;379(9830):1967–74.
3. Hickey BA, Towriss C, Baxter G, et al. Early experience of MAGEC magnetic growing rods in the treatment of early onset scoliosis. Eur Spine J. 2014;23(Suppl 1):S61–5.
4. Jenks M, Craig J, Higgins J, et al. The MAGEC system for spinal lengthening in children with scoliosis: a NICE medical technology guidance. Appl Health Econ Health Policy. 2014;12(6):587–99.
5. Rolton D, Richards J, Nnadi C. Magnetic controlled growth rods versus conventional growing rod systems in the treatment of early onset scoliosis: a cost comparison. Eur Spine J. 2015;24(7):1457–61.
6. Stokes OM, O'Donovan EJ, Samartzis D, Bow CH, Luk KD, Cheung KM. Reducing radiation exposure in early-onset scoliosis surgery patients: novel use of ultrasonography to measure lengthening in magnetically-controlled growing rods. Spine J. 2014;14(10):2397–404.
7. Cheung JP, Cahill P, Yaszay B, Akbarnia BA, Cheung KM. Special article: update on the magnetically controlled growing rod: tips and pitfalls. J Orthop Surg (Hong Kong). 2015;23(3):383–90.
8. Cheung JPY, Yiu KKL, Samartzis D, Kwan K, Tan BB, Cheung KMC. Rod lengthening with the magnetically controlled growing rod: factors influencing rod slippage and reduced gains during distractions. Spine (Phila Pa 1976). 2018;43(7):E399–405.
9. Lorenz HM, Badwan B, Hecker MM, et al. Magnetically controlled devices parallel to the spine in children with spinal muscular atrophy. JB JS Open Access. 2017;2(4):e0036. Published 2017 Nov 28.
10. Joyce TJ, Smith SL, Rushton PRP, Bowey AJ, Gibson MJ. Analysis of explanted magnetically controlled growing rods from seven UK spinal centers. Spine (Phila Pa 1976). 2018;43(1):E16–22.
11. Gilday SE, Schwartz MS, Bylski-Austrow DI, et al. Observed length increases of magnetically controlled growing rods are lower than programmed. J Pediatr Orthop. 2018;38(3):e133–7.
12. Thakar C, Kieser DC, Mardare M, Haleem S, Fairbank J, Nnadi C. Systematic review of the complications associated with magnetically controlled growing rods for the treatment of early onset scoliosis. Eur Spine J. 2018;27(9):2062–71.
13. Poon S, Spencer HT, Fayssoux RS, Sever R, Cho RH. Maximal force generated by magnetically controlled growing rods decreases with rod lengthening. Spine Deform. 2018;6(6):787–90.

14. Subramanian T, Ahmad A, Mardare DM, Kieser DC, Mayers D, Nnadi C. A six-year observational study of 31 children with early-onset scoliosis treated using magnetically controlled growing rods with a minimum follow-up of two years. Bone Joint J. 2018;100-B(9):1187–200.
15. Hung CW, Vitale MG, Samdani A, et al. Outcomes of primary and conversion magnetically controlled growth rods are different at two-year follow-up: results of North American release. Spine Deform. 2019;7(5):829–35.
16. Luhmann SJ, McAughey EM, Ackerman SJ, Bumpass DB, McCarthy RE. Cost analysis of a growth guidance system compared with traditional and magnetically controlled growing rods for early-onset scoliosis: A US-based integrated health care delivery system perspective. Clinicoecon Outcomes Res. 2018;10:179–87. Published 2018 Mar 16.
17. Pepke W, Almansour H, Diebo BG, Akbar M. Correction of the spine with magnetically controlled growing rods in early onset scoliosis: A pre-to-post analysis of 21 patients with 1-year follow-up [published online ahead of print, 2019 Sep 10]. Korrektur der Wirbelsäule mit magnetisch kontrollierten mitwachsenden Stäben bei Patienten mit Early-onset-Skoliose : Prä-Post-Analyse von 21 Patienten mit 1-Jahres-Follow-up [published online ahead of print, 2019 Sep 10]. Orthopade. 2019; https://doi.org/10.1007/s00132-019-03801-x.
18. Oetgen ME, McNulty EM, Matthews AL. Cost-effectiveness of magnetically controlled growing rods: who really benefits? Spine Deform. 2019;7(3):501–4.
19. Harshavardhana NS, Noordeen MHH, Dormans JP. Cost analysis of magnet-driven growing rods for early-onset scoliosis at 5 years. Spine (Phila Pa 1976). 2019;44(1):60–7.
20. Rushton PRP, Smith SL, Forbes L, Bowey AJ, Gibson MJ, Joyce TJ. Force testing of explanted magnetically controlled growing rods. Spine (Phila Pa 1976). 2019;44(4):233–9.
21. Roye BD, Marciano G, Matsumoto H, et al. Is rod diameter associated with the rate of rod fracture in patients treated with magnetically controlled growing rods? [published online ahead of print, 2020 Jun 19]. Spine Deform. 2020; https://doi.org/10.1007/s43390-020-00161-x.
22. Doany ME, Olgun ZD, Kinikli GI, et al. Health-related quality of life in early-onset scoliosis patients treated surgically: EOSQ scores in traditional growing rod versus magnetically controlled growing rods. Spine (Phila Pa 1976). 2018;43(2):148–53.
23. Panagiotopoulou VC, Tucker SK, Whittaker RK, et al. Analysing a mechanism of failure in retrieved magnetically controlled spinal rods. Eur Spine J. 2017;26(6):1699–710.
24. Cheung JPY, Yiu K, Kwan K, Cheung KMC. Mean 6-year follow-up of magnetically controlled growing rod patients with early onset scoliosis: a glimpse of what happens to graduates. Neurosurgery. 2019;84(5):1112–23.
25. Lebon J, Batailler C, Wargny M, et al. Magnetically controlled growing rod in early onset scoliosis: a 30-case multicenter study. Eur Spine J. 2017;26(6):1567–76.
26. Yoon WW, Chang AC, Tyler P, Butt S, Raniga S, Noordeen H. The use of ultrasound in comparison to radiography in magnetically controlled growth rod lengthening measurement: a prospective study. Eur Spine J. 2015;24(7):1422–6.
27. Choi E, Yaszay B, Mundis G, et al. Implant complications after magnetically controlled growing rods for early onset scoliosis: a multicenter retrospective review. J Pediatr Orthop. 2017;37(8):e588–92.
28. Cheung JPY, Cheung PWH, Cheung KMC. The effect of magnetically controlled growing rods on three-dimensional changes in deformity correction. Spine Deform. 2020;8(3):537–46. https://doi.org/10.1007/s43390-020-00055-y.
29. Guan D, Zhang Y, Xu J. Clinical outcome of magnetically controlled growing rod in early-onset scoliosis: a systematic review. Clin Spine Surg. 2020;33(4):150–5.

Magnetic Anal Sphincter for Fecal Incontinence

18

Michel Gagner

Introduction

The problem of fecal incontinence is growing due to multiple factors, it can be caused by trauma (childbirth), surgery, neurological, or other. Proper diagnosis is important with confirmatory anal manometry. Over the years, multiple surgical therapies have been suggested and tried including injection of biomaterials into the anal canal, radiofrequency treatment of the anal canal, repair of anal muscle injuries, sacral nerve stimulation, artificial bowel sphincter, muscle transposition to reinforce the anal sphincter, and creation of a stoma. Magnets have been introduced in the last two decades to palliate this problem; however, some have abandoned due to problems or erosions and migrations [1, 2]. Recently, we have seen a resurgence in using a new type of magnets assembly; the literature is reviewed here, including some recent comparisons to other treatments for fecal incontinence.

Literature Review

Mauro Bortolotti and colleagues have been doing pioneering work in this area, and their 2008 paper concerning an original magnetic device to reinforce the hypotonic anal sphincter and thwart fecal incontinence is an important contribution. The device itself consists of two small magnetic plaques surgically inserted in the wall of the anal canal between the external and internal anal sphincters with the opposite polarities face to face, so that when they are attracting themselves they close the anal lumen (Fig. 18.1). Bortolotti evaluated different materials with different magnetic forces (neodymium > ferrite > plastoferrite), in three swine, in which the endoanal pressure was measured with a manometric catheter before and after magnet implantation. The endoanal pressure after the insertion of neodymium magnets was 79.7 ± 13.1 (mean ± SD), after ferrite magnets, it was 42.1 ± 5.6 mmHg, and after plastoferrite magnets, it was 21.6 ± 4.6 mmHg, all significantly higher than the pressure documented in basal conditions (1.72 ± 0.71 mmHg). Bortolotti et al. were able to demonstrate that the implantation of magnets in the wall of the anal canal can create a high pressure zone to provide fecal continence and that the strength can be modulated by using magnets of various attraction force to allow a measured correction [3].

Lehur and colleagues also pushed the envelope with a design of their own [4], more recently studied in long-term effectiveness and safety of this innovative treatment in a prospective multicenter pilot study, performed at four clinical sites in Europe and the United States [5]. The cohort encompassed patients with severe fecal incontinence for ≥6 months who had previously failed

M. Gagner (✉)
Hôpital du Sacré-Cœur de Montréal, Montréal, QC, Canada

Chief of Surgery, Westmount Square Surgical Center, Westmount, QC, Canada

M. Gagner (ed.), *Magnetic Surgery*, https://doi.org/10.1007/978-3-030-73947-8_18

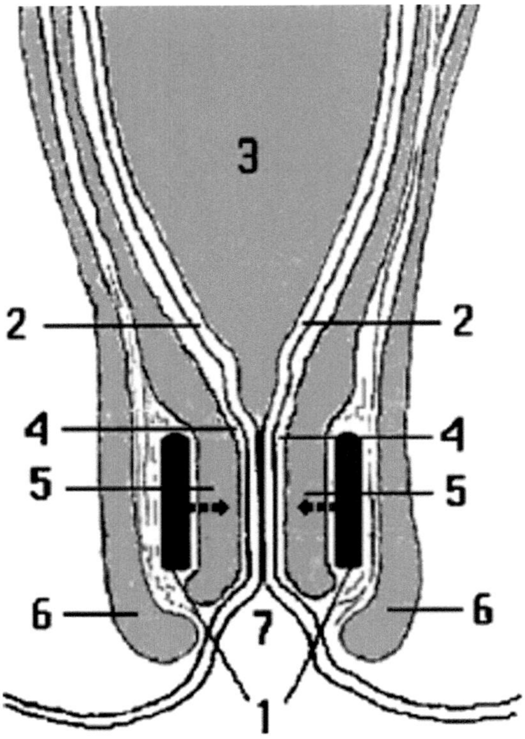

Fig. 18.1 Bortolotti magnets parts, side diagram of the anal positions. (From Bortolotti et al. [3]. Reprinted with permission from Springer Nature)

conservative therapy and were implanted with a magnetic anal sphincter device between 2008 and 2011. A total of 35 patients (34 women) underwent magnetic anal sphincter augmentation. The median length of follow-up was 5.0 years (range, 0–5.6 years), with 23 patients completing assessment at 5 years. Eight patients underwent a subsequent surgery (7 device explantations) because of device failures or complications, 7 of which occurred in the first year. Therapeutic success rates with patients who underwent device explantation or stoma creation counted as treatment failures were 63% at year 1, 66% at year 3, and 53% at year 5. In patients who retained their device, the number of incontinent episodes per week and Cleveland Clinic incontinence scores significantly decreased from baseline, and there were significant improvements in all 4 scales of the Fecal Incontinence Quality of Life instrument. There were 30 adverse events reported in 20 patients, most commonly defecatory dysfunction (20%), pain (14%), erosion (11%), and infection (11%). It was concluded that magnetic anal sphincter augmentation provided excellent outcomes in patients who retained a functioning device at long-term follow-up, but in my opinion, it was not a great result. Protocols to reduce early complications will be important to improve overall outcomes [5].

The size and dimension of the anal canal appears to play a significant role and surgeons and devices may need to adapt to the variability [6]. Measuring the anal circumference exactly with a sizing tool represents a crucial step of the procedure because it determines the correct size and success of the definite implant. There has been an improvement in the latest device for standardization of the procedure to facilitates the learning curve and avoid the need for radiological on-table control [6].

Once the device is implanted, satisfaction may decrease over time. In the short term, implantation of a magnetic anal sphincter (MAS) is a safe and effective treatment for fecal incontinence (FI), and patient satisfaction remains high in the medium term. Data on 23 women, median age 64 (35–78) years, implanted with a MAS device between December 2008 and September 2012, were reviewed from a prospective database. Assessment was based on significant improvement of incontinence scores – the Cleveland Clinic Florida Incontinence Severity (CCF-IS) score, fecal incontinence quality of life (FIQoL) score – and patient satisfaction at 6, 12, 24, and 36 months after surgery. The device was removed in two patients owing to complications, and the median follow-up was 17.6 months. The median preoperative CCF-IS score was 15.2 and fell to 6.9, 7.7, 7.8, and 5.3 at 6, 12, 24, and 36 months, respectively. The median FIQoL score significantly ($P < 0.001$) improved from 1.97 preoperatively to 3.19, 3.11, 2.92, and 2.93, respectively, at the same time periods. Sixteen of the 23 patients were pleased; lack of improvement was the key reason for dissatisfaction. Respectable initial results tend to remain stable over time, and about two-thirds of patients are content following implantation [7].

The competing technology is the soft silicone type of implant, and a published study on the long-term results of a successive series of patients implanted with the Acticon Neosphincter (AMS Minnetonka, Minnesota) (Fig. 18.2), which is non-magnetic, from May 1996 to Jan 2010 was described on 52 patients with severe fecal incontinence for a mean of 10.6 years. Indications for implantation were sphincter destruction (45), pudendal neuropathy (12), congenital malformation (7), and perineal colostomy (4). The mean follow-up period was 64 months; nevertheless, 26 patients (50%) required revisions after a mean of 58 months, with 73% due to a leaking cuff from a presumed microperforation. Fourteen patients (27%) required definitive explantation after a mean of 15 months, with the majority (43%) due to infection. And 9 patients were lost to follow-up. In 35 patients (67%) with an activated device, there were significant improvements in both median Wexner ($P < 0.0001$) and quality-of-life scores ($P = 0.0286$). There was a significant change between preoperative resting anal pressures and closed pressures at activation ($P < 0.0001$), and latest follow-up ($P < 0.0001$). It was concluded that with vigilant patient selection, painstaking surgical technique, and committed surveillance, favorable long-term results can be achieved with satisfactory rates of revision and explantation [8].

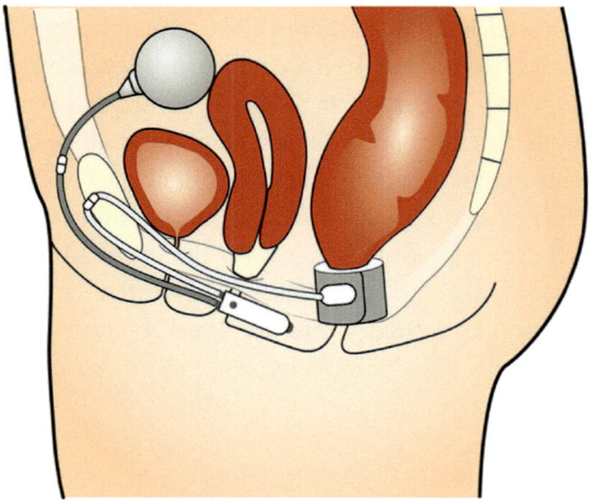

Fig. 18.2 American Medical Systems (AMS) artificial anal sphincter, positioned in the female pelvis. (From Thomas and Vaizey [21]. Reprinted with permission from Springer Nature)

The magnetic anal sphincter and the artificial bowel sphincter were finally compared, but without a RCT. From December 2008 to June 2010, 10 female patients, median age 65 years, with severe fecal incontinence for a median of 7.5 years, were implanted with the magnetic anal sphincter. They were compared with 10 female patients implanted with the artificial bowel sphincter and were matched for age, etiology, duration of incontinence, and preoperative functional scores. Patients with the magnetic anal sphincter had a briefer median operative time (62 vs. 97.5 min, $P = 0.0273$), hospitalization stay (4.5 vs. 10 days, $P < 0.001$), and follow-up period (8 vs. 22.5 months, $P = 0.0068$), without a statistically significant change in 30-day complications (4 vs. 2, $P = 0.628$) and revision/explantation (1 vs. 4, $P = 0.830$). Both groups achieved substantial advances in continence ($P < 0.0002$) and quality-of-life scores ($P < 0.009$). In a comparison of baseline resting anal pressures, patients with the artificial bowel sphincter had significantly greater pressures with inflation ($P = 0.0082$), and those with MAS had a significant upsurge as well ($P = 0.0469$). At the last follow-up, both cohorts had similar quality-of-life scores ($P = 0.374$); patients with the artificial bowel sphincter had higher (median) closed-cuff anal pressures compared with the anal resting pressure of those with a magnetic anal sphincter (89 vs. 58.5 cmH_2O, $P = 0.0147$) together with more constipation (4 vs. 1, $P = 0.830$) and a trend toward better incontinence scores ($P = 0.0625$). This was a nonrandomized study with small patient numbers. In the short term, the magnetic anal sphincter and the artificial bowel sphincter were equally effective in re-establishing continence and quality of life [9].

Comparison with sacral stimulation and magnetic anal sphincter (MAS) has been looked at also. From December 2008 to December 2010, 12 women, median age 65 years, having fecal incontinence for a median of 6.5 years, were implanted with a MAS. A control group was used, consisting of 16 women, of comparable age, preoperative function scores, indications, and duration of incontinence, and implanted with a sacral pulse generator. The duration of follow-up was similar MAS = 18 months vs. SNS = 22 months; with a $p = 0.318$. Four patients with MAS suffered a 30-day complication, and the device was removed from one patient in each group. A significant enhancement in incontinence ($P < 0.001$) and quality-of-life scores ($P < 0.04$) ensued in both groups. The mean anal resting pressure improved significantly in patients implanted with a MAS ($P = 0.027$). Hence, one can conclude that in this nonrandomized study of devices in fecal incontinence patients, MAS was as effective as sacral stimulation in improving continence and quality of life, with similar complications [10].

Another paper looked at the safety profile of the magnetic new device implanted in patients with fecal incontinence [11]. After surgical implantation in patients with fecal incontinence of more than two episodes per week at three trial centers in Europe and the United States, patients were evaluated and followed. The device itself was placed around the anal canal through an anterior incision. In total, 14 patients were implanted with the device, all being women with a mean age of 63 years and with a median follow-up of 6 months [12]. There have been no intraoperative unfavorable events and the mean hospital stay was 3 days. Three patients had the device explanted, two were removed and one passed spontaneously. Five patients with 6-month follow-up demonstrated a mean reduction in the number of average weekly incontinence occurrences from 7.2 to 0.7 (91%) and a mean decrease in Wexner Continence Score from 17.2 to 7.8 (55%). Compared to baseline, quality of life greatly expanded in all domains of the fecal incontinence quality of life (FIQoL) scoring system. Two patients at 1-year follow-up both reported perfect continence, but erosion has been the most important problem [1].

Are the erosion rates higher in the esophagus than the anal canal? In fact, the erosion rates into the esophagus is an important complication and is reported to occur at lower incidences (0.1–0.15%) than for the anal canal [13]. A recent review obtained from the device manufacturer, Torax Medical, Inc., as well as the manufacturer and user facility device experience (MAUDE) database was studied in detail. The study period was a decade, from February 2007 through July 2017, and included all devices placed internationally. In total, 9453 devices were positioned, with 29 reported cases of erosions after a median time to presentation of 26 months after implantation, most occurring between 1 and 4 years after placement [14]. Therefore, the calculated risk of erosion was 0.3% at 4 years. Most patients faced dysphagia-prompting review, and the treatment was device explantation which all had successfully extirpated, mostly using an endoscopic removal of the visible intraluminal part and laparoscopic removal of the remaining parts. At a median follow-up of 58 days postremoval, there was no morbidity and 24 patients have reverted to baseline. Four patients recounted ongoing mild dysphagia. Erosion of the LINX device is a significant but sporadic complication that has been safely handled via minimally invasive approaches without long-term concerns [14].

On January 5, 2016, Torax Medical received FDA approval for its FENIX® continence restoration system to treat fecal incontinence, under a humanitarian device exemption (HDE) [19]. Torax was aiming predominately at women with an injury associated with childbirth. The FENIX device is a Magnetic Sphincter Augmentation (MSA) technology that has been proven to be effective in treating gastroesophageal reflux disease (GERD) with their LINX reflux management system. The FENIX device was successively launched in Europe in 2011, it comprised of a small, flexible band of interlinked titanium beads with magnetic cores (Figs. 18.3 and 18.4) [15]. The magnetic beads expand from each other with defecation pressure to allow for the intended passage of stool [18] (Fig. 18.5). The system begins functioning instantly after implantation and does not require activation by the patient or postoperative adjustments.

The FENIX® continence restoration system for the treatment of fecal incontinence was implanted on April 2016 in the first US patients by Dr. Paul Pettit, Associate Professor at the Mayo Clinic in Jacksonville, FL, and subsequently assisted robotics were used to perform intrapel-

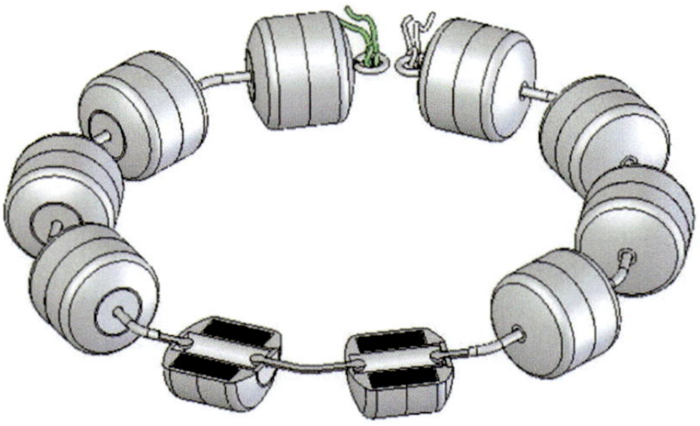

Fig. 18.3 Fenix implant. (From US Food and Drug Administration [19])

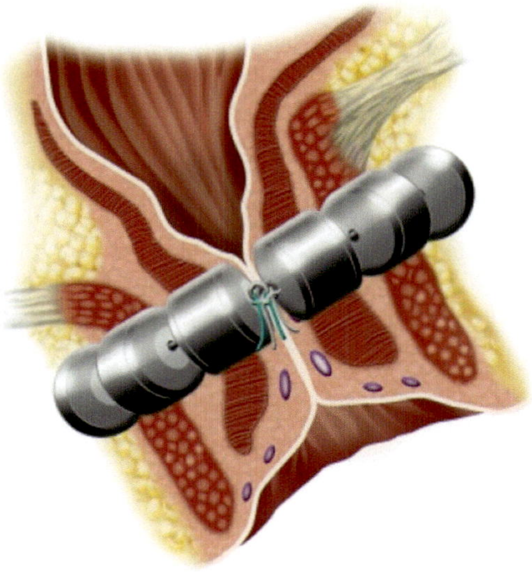

Fig. 18.4 Fenix position in the anal canal. (From US Food and Drug Administration [19])

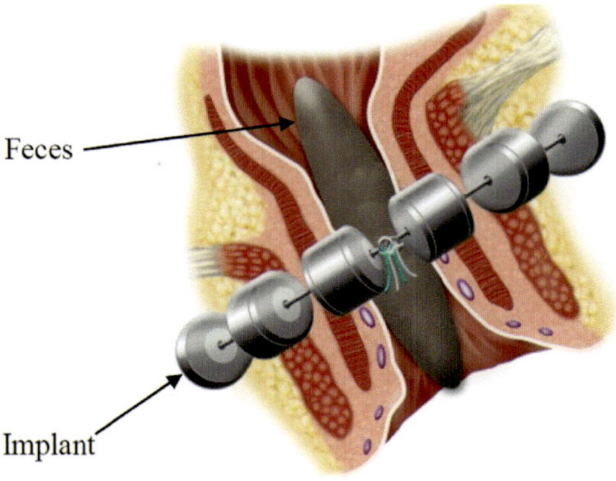

Fig. 18.5 During defecation, the magnets are extended. (From US Food and Drug Administration [19])

vic indications [16, 17]. But on February 17, 2017, Ethicon Johnson & Johnson acquired Torax for an undisclosed amount after having invested $25 million in series E. In a coup de théâtre, on April 27, 2017, Torax Medical announced the discontinuation of sales and clinical studies of the FENIX® continence restoration system. This decision was apparently solely a business decision based on fit with Torax and Ethicon's strategic business plans and was not due to any safety concerns with the FENIX system. It is unclear if this decision will be reversed in the near future, or if it did counteract with other Ethicon businesses or plans for fecal incontinence. This is reminiscent of the compression anastomotic device demise, from Niti Technologies Ltd., by Covidien a few years ago.

Professor Lehur from Nantes France went into a recent requisitory editorial about how the industry is killing the artificial sphincter, and colorectal surgeons, engineers, and device companies need to get together again and retool the artificial sphincter for 30 million patients that are incontinent worldwide. He went on to write and say that the two original companies of the Acticon Neosphincter and Fenix were purchased recently by others who chose to preserve vending the AMS-800 and LINX devices for reasons other than fecal incontinence, while withdrawing from the market of the fecal incontinence devices [20].

References

1. Bortolotti M. The magnetic anal sphincter: a seductive promise still not kept. Color Dis. 2015;17(1):89–90.
2. Lehur PA, Barussaud ML. The magnetic anal sphincter: a seductive promise still not kept. Color Dis. 2015;17(5):452.
3. Bortolotti M, Ugolini G, Grandis A, et al. A novel magnetic device to prevent fecal incontinence (preliminary study). Int J Color Dis. 2008;23:499–501.
4. Mantoo S, Meurette G, Podevin J, Lehur PA. The magnetic anal sphincter: a new device in the management of severe fecal incontinence. Expert Rev Med Devices. 2012;9(5):483–90.
5. Sugrue J, Lehur PA, Madoff RD, et al. Long-term experience of magnetic anal sphincter augmentation in patients with fecal incontinence. Dis Colon Rectum. 2017;60(1):87–95.

6. Kim M, Lehur PA. How to size the anal canal circumference when implanting a magnetic anal sphincter for fecal incontinence. Evolution and update of a new surgical technique. Dis Colon Rectum. 2016;59(9):901–3.
7. Barussaud ML, Mantoo S, Wyart V, Meurette G, Lehur PA. The magnetic anal sphincter in faecal incontinence: is initial success sustained over time? Color Dis. 2013;15(12):1499–503.
8. Wong MT, Meurette G, Wyart V, Glemain P, Lehur PA. The artificial bowel sphincter: a single institution experience over a decade. Ann Surg. 2011;254(6):951–6.
9. Wong MT, Meurette G, Stangherlin P, Lehur PA. The magnetic anal sphincter versus the artificial bowel sphincter: a comparison of 2 treatments for fecal incontinence. Dis Colon Rectum. 2011;54(7):773–9.
10. Wong MT, Meurette G, Wyart V, Lehur PA. Does the magnetic anal sphincter device compare favourably with sacral nerve stimulation in the management of faecal incontinence? Color Dis. 2012;14(6):e323–9.
11. Lehur PA, McNevin S, Buntzen S, Mellgren AF, Laurberg S, Madoff RD. Magnetic anal sphincter augmentation for the treatment of fecal incontinence: a preliminary report from a feasibility study. Dis Colon Rectum. 2010;53(12):1604–10.
12. Lehur PA. The anal artificial sphincter in severe anal incontinence. Int J Surg Investig. 1999;1(3):268–9.
13. Faucheron JL, Sage PY, Trilling B. Erosion rate of the magnetic sphincter augmentation device is much higher for anal incontinence than for antireflux. J Gastrointest Surg. 2019;23(2):389–90.
14. Alicuben ET, Bell RCW, Jobe BA, et al. Worldwide experience with erosion of the magnetic sphincter augmentation device. J Gastrointest Surg. 2018;22(8):1442–7.
15. Williams AE, Croft J, Napp V, et al. SaFaRI: sacral nerve stimulation versus the FENIX magnetic sphincter augmentation for adult faecal incontinence: a randomised investigation. Int J Color Dis. 2016;31(2):465–72.
16. DeStephano CC, Chen AH, Pettit PD. The Fenix system for fecal incontinence: an overview and surgical demonstration. J Minim Invasive Gynecol. 2017;24(7):1078.
17. Espinal M, DeStephano CC, Guha P, Gajarawala SP, Chen AH, Pettit PD. Robotic placement of the FENIX continence restoration system in a patient with previous radiation to the pelvis: a case report. J Minim Invasive Gynecol. 2018;25(3):528–32.
18. Stokes WE, Jayne DG, Alazmani A, Culmer PR. A biomechanical model of the human defecatory system to investigate mechanisms of continence. Proc Inst Mech Eng H. 2019;233(1):114–26.
19. US Food and Drug Administration. Humanitarian device exemption (HDE). FENIX® Continence Restoration System. The summary of safety and effectiveness data. https://www.accessdata.fda.gov/cdrh_docs/pdf13/H130006b.pdf
20. Lehur PA, Christoforidis D, Meurette G. Artificial sphincters to treat severe fecal incontinence: currently in a deadlock. Dis Colon Rectum. 2020;63(8):1017–9.
21. Thomas G, Vaizey C. Surgery. In: Collins B, Bradshaw E, editors. Bowel dysfunction. Cham.: Springer; 2016. p. 225–39. https://doi.org/10.1007/978-3-319-43214-4_14.

19 Magnetic Satiety System: The Use of Magnets to Assist in Combating Obesity

Shahriar Sedghi, Katherine Kendrick, Sheng-Chiang Lee, Samuel Engle, Kenji Yoshida, and Betsy Smith

Obesity Epidemic

Obesity is routinely defined as an excess of body weight for height [1]. This is quantified as a body mass index (BMI), which is calculated by body weight in kilograms divided by height in meters squared. In adults, a BMI of greater than or equal to 25 is considered overweight, and a BMI of 30 is considered obese. Current estimates predict that that the rapid rise in obesity will continue to soar and that 3/4 of the American population will likely be overweight or obese by 2020 [2, 3]. A report by the Trust for America's Health and the Robert Wood Johnson Foundation found, using a model of population and trends, that half of US adults will be obese by 2030 [1]. In 2014, the National Health and Nutrition Examination Survey found that more than one-third (36.5%) of US adults aged 20 and older and 17% of children and adolescents aged 2–19 were obese. These figures are on the rise. The rapid rise in obesity over the twentieth century is concerning because obesity is associated with a decrease of lifespan by 4–7 years, increased risk of nearly every chronic disease, as well as increased morbidity and mortality [1].

Obesity has been found to contribute to more than 3 million deaths per year [4]. It is now the leading cause of morbidity and mortality in Western societies [5]. It has been found that, in men aged 25–34 years with a BMI >40 kg/m^2, there is a 10-fold excess mortality compared with their normal weight counterparts [6]. The current US generation is predicted to have a shorter life expectancy than their parents, due to the association of obesity and risk of nearly every chronic disease known [3]. Diseases associated with obesity include metabolic syndrome, diabetes mellitus, hypertension, coronary artery disease, sleep apnea, stroke, gastroesophageal reflux disease, certain malignancies, and fatty liver disease [5–7]. Obesity is additionally associated with increased aging [6]. The increase in obesity and obesity-related disease is taking a toll on healthcare costs. Obesity currently accounts for 17% of healthcare costs in the United States. Healthcare costs are significantly increased for both obese males and females [8]. The total US healthcare

S. Sedghi (✉)
Appetec INC, Gastroenterology Associates of Central Georgia, Macon, GA, USA

K. Kendrick
Department of Internal Medicine, Navicent Health/Mercer University School of Medicine, Macon, GA, USA

S.-C. Lee
Appetec INC, Macon, GA, USA

S. Engle
Business Development, Synectic Medical Product Development, Woodbridge, CT, USA

K. Yoshida
Clinical/Research, Gastroenterology Associates of Central Georgia, Macon, GA, USA

B. Smith
Department of Internal Medicine, Mercer University School of Medicine, Macon, GA, USA

M. Gagner (ed.), *Magnetic Surgery*, https://doi.org/10.1007/978-3-030-73947-8_19

spending is estimated at $2.7 trillion [1]. An additional cost is related to loss of productivity in the workplace. When examined in 2012, a company's annual healthcare cost and lost productivity in the highest vs lowest BMI groups was reported to be $6,313 with an average of 7.5 missed days versus $4,258 with an average of 4.5 days, respectively [8].

The question seldom asked is, why is there an obesity epidemic? After the 1980s, there was a significant rise in obesity [8, 9]. The increase has been attributed to "built environment," which includes the development of products that reduce physical activity that is, elevators, escalators, online entertainment, and television [8]. The built environment also includes the industrialization of food production, allowing access to inexpensive, highly processed, nutrient-poor food, as a major contribution. The consumption of sugar was rare prior to 1900, around 4–6 pound per year; currently, the average person consumes ~160 pounds per year [8]. It has been shown that added sugar is not only highly addictive but is also associated with obesity [8, 10]. Billions of dollars each year are allocated to advertising calorie-rich and nutrient-poor foods to children [8].

We now have such high numbers of obese and overweight people that the perception of "normal" is being altered. Social networks are contributing to the standardization of this new norm of being obese or overweight in our population [11]. Restaurants tend to be valued for large portion sizes, and large sugar-filled drinks are considered normal. Eating high-calorie food has been shown to lead to overeating, independent of macronutrient content or portion size [4, 12]. Also concerning is that the Western diet is metabolically toxic, as studies have shown that high-fat foods cause damage to regions of the brain that regulate food intake and can cause insulin resistance [4, 13–15]. Efforts to address the obesity epidemic as a public health issue in the United States have been labeled by many as paternalistic, undemocratic, excessive, and inappropriate. The societal expenses of obesity are considered as acceptable as the cost of personal freedom and choice [8]. It is imperative that any current or future treatment for obesity takes historical and etiological factors into consideration for their innovation to be successful.

Underlying Mechanisms of Obesity

The underlying cause of obesity is disruption of the homeostatic balance between energy intake and energy expenditure. When homeostatic mechanisms controlling food intake are poorly adapted to the unique modern environment of "plenty," both excess energy and reduced exercise result in obesity [16]. The intake of calories is controlled by complex interactions between the gut and central nervous system that are mediated by neural and hormonal signals [7, 16–20]. The brain interprets peripheral signals from the gut and adipose tissue regarding the need for energy intake and responds to such signals by increasing or decreasing food intake as needed. Intricate neuronal networks are housed within key brain areas such as the hypothalamus and brainstem; gut hormones (i.e., ghrelin, leptin, PYY, and GLP-1) act upon these neural networks which subsequently connect to other areas of the brain involved in feelings of reward and desire. Involvement of such centers within the brain is crucial to the body's response to hunger, satiation, and adjustment of energy intake [21, 22] (Fig. 19.1). Although such mechanisms are used to maintain the delicate balance between energy intake and expenditure, the reward system located in the ventral tegmental area (VTA) of the brain can override this homeostatic mechanism when presented with desirable food that is not necessary for energy balance, and the pleasure that is perceived by eating high-calorie foods reinforces the behavior [4]. Studies have shown the VTA is rich with dopaminergic neurons that are stimulated by food intake [4, 23, 24]. These are the same areas activated by psychoactive drugs, which tells us that food addiction is real[4]. The reward area of the brain also receives inputs from the brainstem and hypothalamus and is adjusted by vagal nerve stimulation [4, 23–25]. The drive for food intake is fundamental to survival [16]. However, the existence of this drive in the context of a surplus of energy within the modern environment has led to the obesity epidemic.

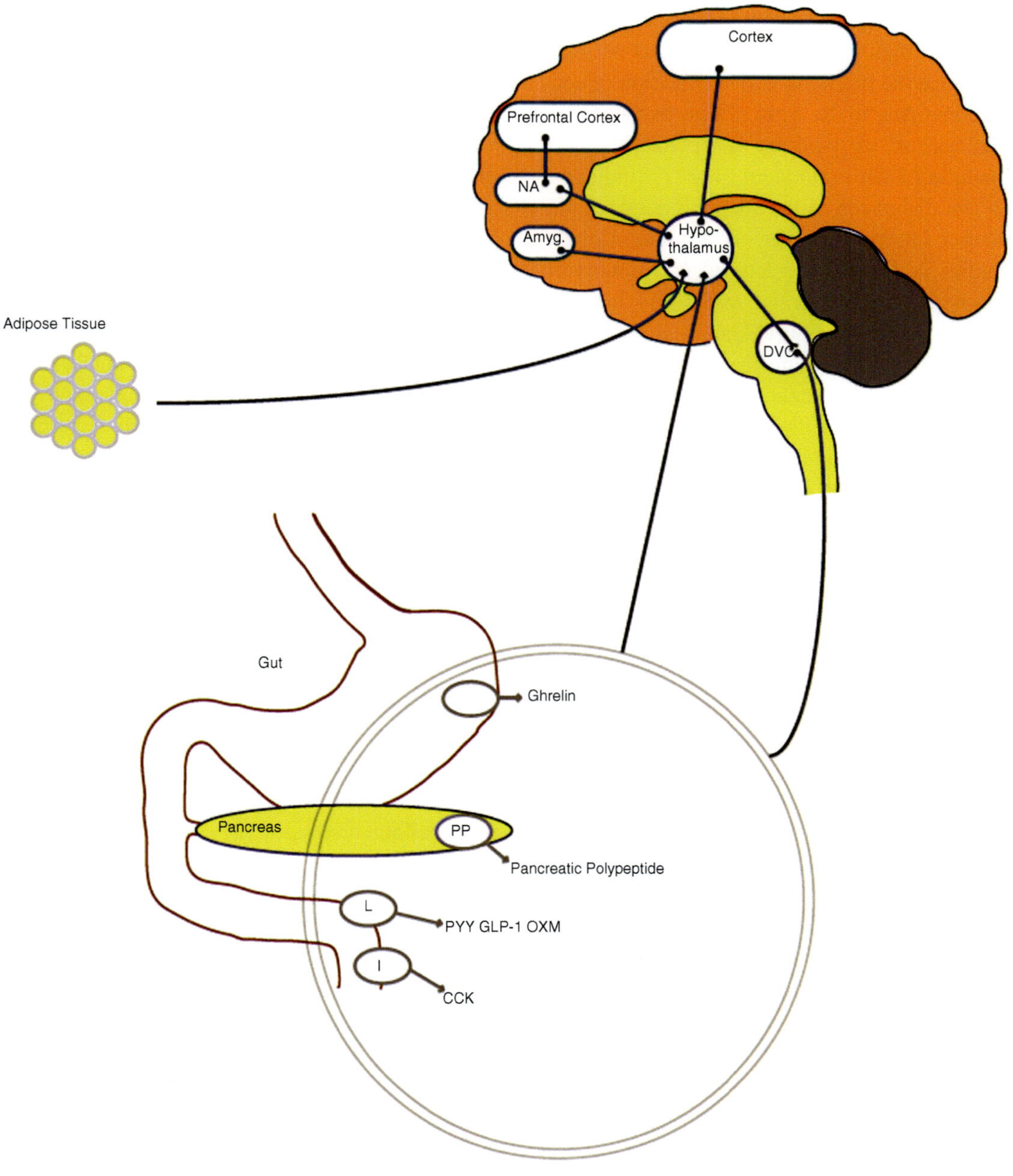

Fig. 19.1 Peripheral signals influence the hypothalamus. Neural projections between the hypothalamus, brainstem, cortex, and reward centers influence food intake. (From Simpson K, Bloom S [16]. Reprinted with permission from Elsevier)

Gastric/Brain Axis and Food Intake

The muscular layers of the stomach house intramuscular arrays in the outer muscular layer and act as stretch receptors and likely mediators of satiation due to their connection with vagal afferents [20, 26]. There are myriad neuroendocrine and exocrine factors involved in the start and cessation of a meal [27–29]. One mechanism that is believed to influence meal termination is via distension of the stomach and subsequent activation of gastric mechanoreceptors [27]. Mechanoreceptors, once stimulated, transport their signal along the vagus nerve, and influence the initiation and termination of a meal by conveying to the current digestive state to the nucleus of the solitary tract located in the medulla of the brain stem [4, 27]. Studies have shown distension of the stomach does not affect hunger satiety. However, the limitation of these studies is distension occurred 10 minutes after meals, with the average meal only lasting 12 minutes while an individual is alone [30–34]. Distension of the stomach which contains food will lead to lead to meal termination. The signals are then relayed to other feeding-related areas of the brain, including the hypothalamus [4, 35, 36] and either activate or inhibit orexigenic signals based on the cumulative effect of the brain and gastric inputs [27]. This leads to a feeling of either hunger or fullness in the body, and an alteration in the consumption of food [18, 19, 27, 36–38]. Neuroimaging that examines gastric distention provides potentially valuable information regarding the vagal afferent pathways to visceral cortical areas. Studies in these areas have focused on activation of neural areas associated with painful versus not painful gastric distension [38, 39]. Along with activation of cerebral networks important for food processing, stomach distension also interacts with gut-secreted peptides [22, 40].

During chronic distension of the stomach wall, levels of ghrelin, a hunger-inducing hormone, initially drop, and contribute to satiety [7]. In experiments with healthy subjects receiving either an intragastric load or a continuous intraduodenal infusion of glucose or a mixed liquid meal, the stomach appears to be important in the short-term control of appetite [41]. Results suggest that gastric and intestinal signals interact to mediate early fullness and satiation, likely via interactions of the secretion of ghrelin, leptin, glucagon-like peptide-1 (GLP-1), and peptide YY (PYY) [41]. Animal studies also support these concepts [37–39] and suggest that a combination of gastric signals and intestinal nutrient stimulation is necessary to elicit optimal satiation and adequate control of eating [41].

Studies dating back 50 years have demonstrated that the behavioral response to gastric distension nearly always includes a reduction in food intake [27, 42], whether this distension is due to ingestion of food [27, 43], or acute intragastric balloon inflation. Normal weight humans exhibited a marked decrease in food intake after acute balloon inflation [34], and studies of obese humans who received chronic balloons as a weight-loss therapy showed weight reduction during the first three months [27]. Modulation of neural and hormonal feedback signaling has been suggested as the basis of intragastric balloons for weight loss, although varying results have been found for ghrelin and for other peptides that are modulated [7, 44, 45]. One possible factor contributing to these variations could be the measurement of total ghrelin and the inactive form of this peptide, as well as changes in body weights and reduced food intake which affect ghrelin levels [7, 42]. When balloons are placed chronically, there is at least a short-term weight loss for three to six months, but there is a lack of long-term efficacy [7, 46, 47]. This may be due to physiological or behavioral adaptations along with divergence between gastric pressure and volume with balloon distension [27, 30].

Weight Loss Strategies and Risks

Recidivism is recognized after all approaches to weight loss. Failure is seen with dietary, behavioral, pharmacological, and surgical interventions for weight loss. A variation of diets, which includes Mediterranean, low fat, and calorie restriction (including both low calorie and very low calorie), resulted in a weight reduction of 5–7.8%, but had a rebound weight gain of 41–61% [48]. The weight regain is due to metabolic adaptation and loss of adherence. Pharmacological approaches for weight loss use medications such as phentermine and extended release topiramate, lorcaserin, combination of bupropion and naltrexone, liraglutide, and orlistat. These medications result in only 5–10% loss of body weight in the most successful patients, and the weight tends to be regained once the medication is stopped [49]. A hindrance to adherence to these medications are the side effects which include, but are not limited to, dry mouth, paresthesia, constipation, dysgeusia, insomnia, and disturbances in cognition, attention, concentration, and memory [48, 49]. Numerous other side effects are associated with each individual drug.

Bariatric surgery was first described in 1969 and is considered the gold standard for morbid obesity [50]. Ileal transposition in 1982 removed a section of the terminal ileum and incorporated it into the duodenum, which was designed to allow ingested nutrients to have earlier contact with ileal cells, to induce the release of GLP-1 and peptide YY, two hormones involved in satiety. Due to associated complications, this is no longer performed. Current methods of bariatric surgery include the laparoscopic banding, which has a mean weight reduction of 15–20%, Roux-en-Y gastric bypass (mean reduction of 25%), and vertical sleeve gastrectomy (mean reduction is 30%) [26]. Complications of these surgeries can include reflux, anastomotic leaks, internal bowel herniation, obstruction, and perforation, nutritional deficiencies, and dumping syndrome. Removal of lap bands is common due to intolerance of nausea and vomiting. Although bariatric surgery is considered the "standard of care" for treatment of severe obesity, long-term efficacy data have shown that more than 20% of patients regain weight and have a recrudescence of obesity-related comorbidities [49]. Protein and nutritional deficiencies and their long-term sequelae in "successful" gastric bypass patients are often understated. The nutritional deficiencies may represent kwashiorkor (Fig. 19.2). Protein malnutrition remains the most severe nutritional complication associated with bariatric surgery [51]. Protein malnutrition is associated with malabsorptive procedures, causing a hospitalization rate of 1% per year, and leads to significant morbidity and poor outcomes [51]. Due to these factors, as few as 1% of patients eligible for these procedures choose to undergo one of them.

Intragastric balloons (IGB) were then developed as a less invasive way for weight loss. Intragastric balloons have been explored as a treatment for obesity since 1985 and were thought to provide an alternative for patients who declined or were not fit for bariatric surgery. A Cochrane review concluded that there are little data to support intragastric balloons' efficacy for weight loss when compared to conventional medical management [48, 52]. These balloons are filled with liquid or gas and cause a space occupation in the stomach to reduce gastric volume and improve satiety. IGB are endoscopically placed in the stomach under sedation. Numerous balloons have been developed since the first IGB was created. Initial reports found some clinical efficacy, but this was short lived, as the effectiveness for weight loss decreased over time as a result of gastric adaptation [53, 54]. Most IGB have reported side effects such as nausea, vomiting, and gastric mucosal damage, thus IGB have not been widely accepted and are a second-line option for patients who are unable to have bariatric surgery [53]. Other methods include Gelesis pill, vagal nerve stimulation and endoscopic methods, such as endoscopic sleeve gastroplasty, Aspire Assist, TransPyloric Shuttle by BaroNova, and the Full Sense Bariatric Device.

Gelesis is a Boston biotech company that created a hydrogel capsule from blend of cellulose and citric acid. The capsule breaks apart in the stomach exposing the matrix, which can absorb 100 times its weight to create space occupation in the stomach. A double-blind placebo-controlled study found that Gelesis weight loss aid participants lost 6.4% of their baseline weight versus 4.4% in the placebo group. Side effects include GI upset such as diarrhea, bloating, abdominal pain, and gas. The price point has not been established [55].

Vagal nerve stimulation was examined in a clinical trial of 233 patients. After 12 months, the experimental group lost an average of 8.5% more excess weight than the control group [56]. However, the experimental group did not meet the primary outcome of a significantly greater percentage of excess weight loss, defined as >10%, compared to the control group. Even though this standard was not met, the FDA Advisory Committee found that 18-month data from the study were supportive of sustained

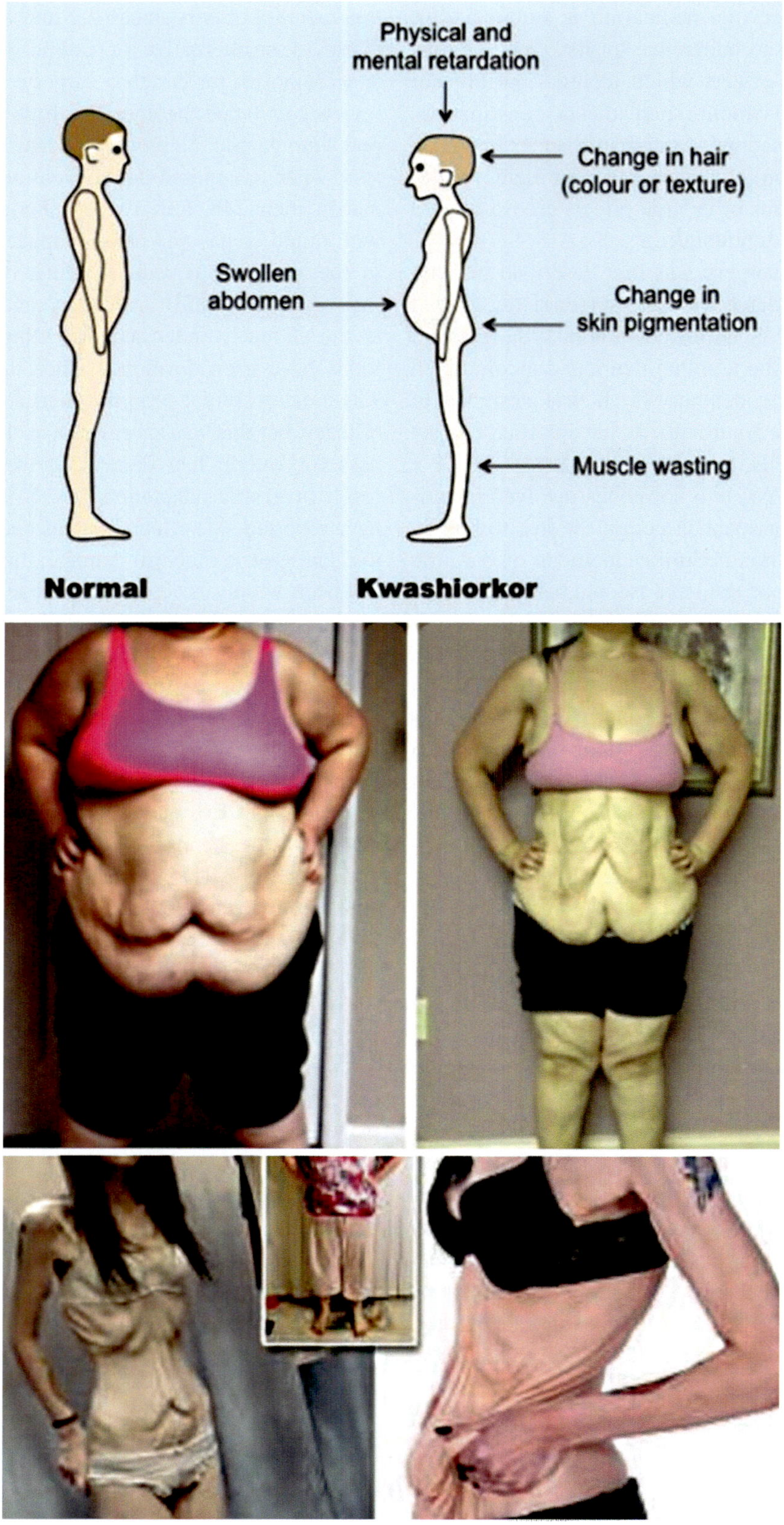

Fig. 19.2 Kwashiorkor description (top panel) and bariatric surgery patient (bottom panels)

weight loss and agreed that the benefits of the device outweighed the risks in patients who met the indication criteria [56]. The approval was based on an FDA-sponsored survey indicating that patients would accept risks associated with the device [56].

Endoscopic methods for weight loss include endoscopic sleeve gastroplasty, which utilized a full-thickness suture to reduce the size of the stomach [57]. Complications from the procedure include nausea, pain, leaks, perforation, perigastric inflammatory fluid collection, splenic laceration, and bleeding [58]. The AspireAssist is a device that placed a tube into the patient's stomach to allow for drainage of the stomach contents after a meal. Drainage of stomach contents is only possible if the patient chews thoroughly and eats slowly [59]. Long-term results of this device are still unknown, and complications include nausea, leaks, perforation, peritonitis, stoma infection, gastric ulceration, and bleeding [59]. BaroNova's TransPyloric Shuttle is placed endoscopically and is designed to slow the passage of food to make the patient feel full sooner and stay full longer. EndoBarrier is a 65-cm long Teflon-coated duodenal jejunal bypass sleeve, which relies on malabsorption for weight loss by allowing undigested food to reach the jejunum. The device was removed from 10.9% of patients in one study due to adverse events [59]. Full Sense Bariatric Device is an esophageal stent connected to a gastric disk via a strut. It is designed to stay in the gastric cardia, in theory, to produce feelings of satiety. Additional procedures being studied include duodenal mucosal resurfacing, to rest the diseased duodenal enteroendocrine cells and self-assembling magnets, which are attempting to divert bile and nutrients to the terminal ileum.

While the aforementioned approaches have demonstrated short-term results, in the absence of unintended surgically induced malabsorption (which is undesirable) or behavioral modification, they lack long-term efficacy. This is because existing techniques do not facilitate noninvasive postoperative adjustment, due to the body's natural adaptation to the surgical and endoscopic changes made. Furthermore, the cornerstone of successful treatment (i.e., behavioral therapy and positive reinforcement) is not incorporated. A study by Spring et al. supports the need for reinforcement and illustrated how mobile technology was of benefit, by demonstrating that remote coaching with mobile technology has a positive impact in overall adoption and maintenance of multiple healthy behavior changes [60]. As a result, both current surgical and endoscopic groups suffer from nonsustained weight loss due to the body's natural adaptation to the changes made, as well as additional complications.

Why There Is a Need for a New Approach

Considering historical evolution of obesity and the recent change in the food industry, which promotes high-caloric and highly addictive food causing failure of the appetite control centers essentially resulting in food addiction, it is easy to see why the current treatments for obesity have been unsuccessful and/or aggressive. An ideal device for obesity management would utilize the existing neurohormonal pathways described above and reinforce the natural physiology of eating, which is intermittent distension, as opposed to some of the currently available products which use chronic distension, restrictive, or obstructive procedures. It has also been theorized that unless the patient is actively involved with treatment of their obesity, long-term efficacy results would be minimal.

These requirements lead to the innovation of Endoscopic Magnetic Appetite Control System (EMACS) by Appetec INC. utilizing magnets. EMACS is an endoscopically placed, free-floating expandable silicone stent with an internal magnet that is manipulated by an external magnet (Fig. 19.3). The external magnet is manipulated by the patient on demand and supervised with an integrated platform. EMACS is minimally invasive, has the potential for use in young adults where food addiction potentiates, and empowers the patient to curb their appetite. Additionally, the device provides positive reinforcement and integrated behavioral therapy that is not seen in other current weight loss methods.

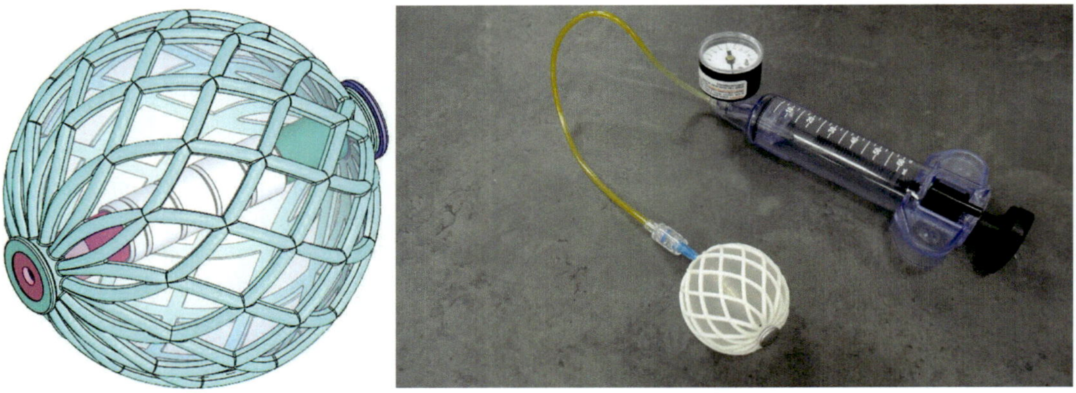

Fig. 19.3 Free floating stent balloon with internal magnet

The EMACS is advantageous over existing technology in three fundamental ways: **(I)** It is significantly smaller in size compared to existing gastric balloons (92 cc, 5.6 cm in diameter), yet large enough not to pass pyloric channel and is far less likely to cause symptoms and complications associated with chronic distention of existing balloons (750–900 cc). It is comparable in size to transpyloric shuttle device [44]. **(II)** It is used intermittently and on-demand, thereby reducing the likelihood of adaptation by the body. **(III)** The external component of the device is linked with a behavioral modification platform. Without this platform, the device is inoperable. This introduces behavioral modification as a component of treatment and can be used prior to placement of the device to select patients likely to be compliant. Furthermore, once the device has been removed after 6–12 month, patients can continue to use the behavioral platform to promote long-term behavioral modification and efficacy.

There are three major components in EMACS: an external magnet, an intragastric stent magnet device, and the platform for a patient to interact with and to monitor one's progress. This system allows the patient to manipulate the stomach intermittently and on demand, which is unlike any currently available intragastric balloon. Secondly, since the intragastric stent magnet device is controlled by the patient, it minimizes discomfort to the patient as distension only occurs when the subject feels hungry or at mealtimes. More importantly, patient control of the device allows this intragastric balloon to overcome the challenge of adaptation current balloons face. This makes the device more sustainable and because it is transient, it is less likely to cause mucosal damage. Additionally, it allows the patient to determine which part of the stomach is best manipulated, for example, the gastric body versus fundus. Lastly, the patient interaction with the platform has a significant opportunity to modify behavior. The platform introduces behavioral modification which can be used prior to placement of the device to select patients likely to be compliant. Furthermore, once the device has been removed after 6–12 month, patients can continue to use the behavioral platform to promote long-term behavioral modification and efficacy.

Since the strength required for the external magnet is quite substantial and can potentially cause injury if the user is accidentally trapped by the attraction between the strong magnet and another magnetic surface, such as steel, we have developed two design concepts for the external magnet to minimize the risks (Fig. 19.4). In the first design, the external magnet is a strong permanent magnet enclosed in a plastic case with magnetic shielding sheet embedded, except for its operating surface. The operating surface is covered by force absorbing material, such as Sorbothane®. The plastic case is designed with a variable spacer to maintain a safe distance between the external magnet and the intragastric

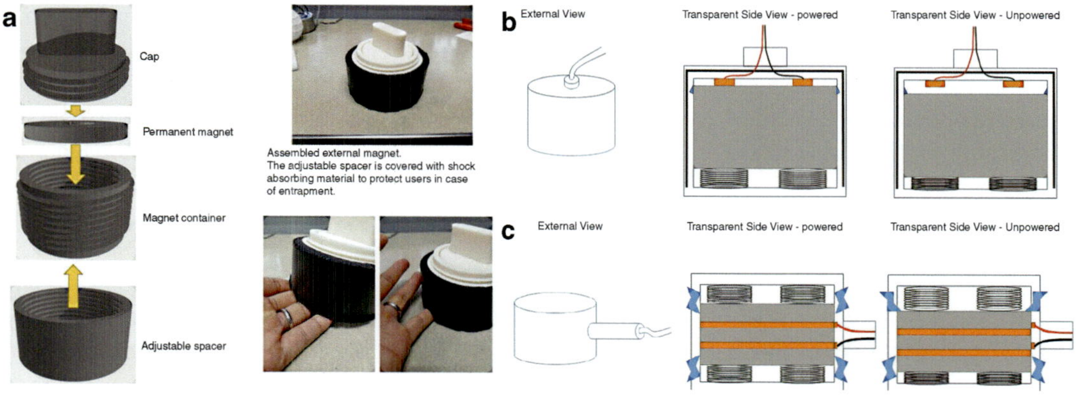

Fig. 19.4 (**a**) External magnet casing and adjustable spacer. (**b**, **c**) Designs of electromagnet housing with emergency shut-down feature for safety. The upper diagram (**b**) is a design for single pole magnet. The lower diagram (**c**) is for bipolar magnets

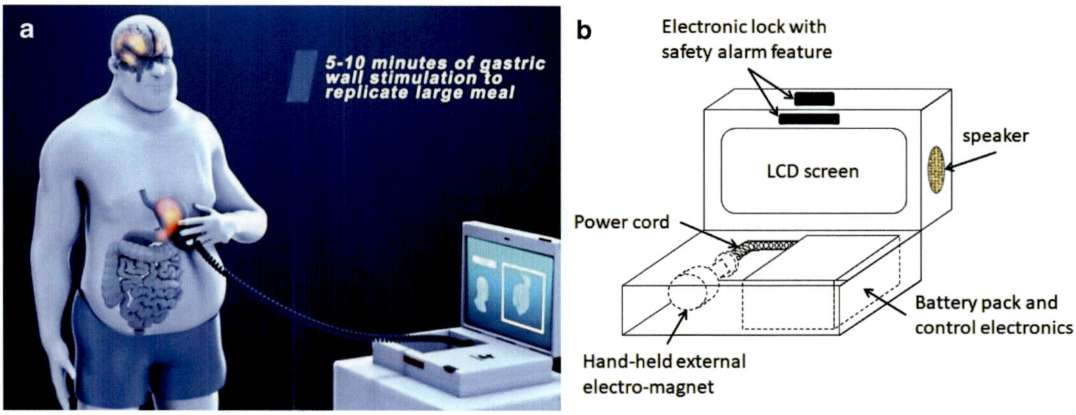

Fig. 19.5 (**a, b**) The magnet case that houses the EMACS platform. This diagram presents the design for housing an electromagnet. For the permanent magnet version, the battery pack may be reduced, and power cord replaced by a spiral cord to attach the magnet to the case

device, as well as with other magnetic surfaces [61]. The second version is an electromagnet. To achieve the strongest possible electromagnet with the least required electric current (to increase battery life and minimize ohmic heating), the materials used for the core of the electromagnet need to have high permeability and high saturation field. Electric metals, commonly found in high power transformers, are often used for this purpose [61]. When the electromagnet is powered, it can be equally strong as the permanent magnet if not stronger. To minimize potential operational risk, not just a layer of force absorbing material is added to the operating surface, the electromagnet is also equipped with an emergency shut-down mechanism in case of accidental entrapment. A manual reset is required to power the magnet again.

The platform would be embedded in a small magnet case, about the size of a personal computer case. The case is designed to carry and operate a handheld external magnet connected by a cord to the case for the capture and manipulation of the intragastric magnet (Fig. 19.5). The magnet case includes an LCD screen to display system information and monitor patient progress. The controller unit for the electromagnet monitors the operation time and cuts the power when the time limit is reached (in this version of an external electromagnet). The central platform will have the ability to incorporate artificial intelligence to optimize diet, exercise, and behavioral modification and be further managed by a healthcare provider via internet connection. These added features should significantly enhance the long-term efficacy of the device.

Developmental Approach of EMACS

EMACS is currently in the prototype development and animal testing stage. The developmental process from rough sketch to prototype development and experimental design has had to consider the following:

- Historical use and safety of magnets in the GI tract [62]
- Practicality and safety of the magnetic forces required to operate the system
- Ease of endoscopic placement and removal
- Durability and functionality of the system within the GI tract
- Experimental design in appropriate animal model to test safety and explore the mechanism of action

Magnets in the GI Tract

Magnets in cattle have been used since the 1950s. Two-and-a-half- to three-inch alnico bar magnets were placed in the stomachs of cattle to control bovine traumatic gastritis [63]. In humans, magnets were first used in 1957 to safely retrieve foreign bodies from the stomach and esophagus [59]. Magnetically actuated capsule systems have been extensively studied in the literature [53, 64–67]. These systems utilize permanent magnets in a capsule system and an external magnetic field, which is used to control the capsule locomotion [53]. The development of magnet-assisted capsule endoscopy (MACE) systems occurred in 2009, with additional experiments in 2010 and 2013. The development of magnetic capsule manipulation allows capsules to be steered so areas of the gastrointestinal tract that are being passed too quickly or large cavities can be thoroughly examined [68]. These trials include the given image system, which creates a maximum magnetic force between capsule and magnet of 256 g/cm^2 (25.1 kPa). The Olympus and Siemens system, developed in 2010, uses a magnetic field of up to 200 mT, and a MicroCam-Navi, which has a pressure of 30.3 kPa [66, 67]. These studies note that magnetic strength drops exponentially with distance, and that the external magnet can initiate capsule movement on a vertical plane at ~8cm [69]. The 2013 trial consisted of the use of a Microcam-Navi device on twenty-six subjects, a median procedure time of 24 minutes, with five positions requiring the internal magnet be held in a stagnant position by the external magnet for one minute [66]. In these studies, no serious adverse effects were reported. Nor were there reports of any evidence of mucosal injury.

Additional magnetic devices include the Gabriel Blue Tube and the Levita Magnetic Surgical System, both of which are FDA approved [70]. The Gabriel Blue Tube consists of three handheld N42 magnets: 7, 5, and 3 lbs. We calculated the resultant gastric mucosa pressures to be up to 150 kPa [71, 72]. There have been no reports of mucosal damage in published trials or in postmarketing. The Levita Magnetic Surgical System utilizes a trocar with a magnetic detachable tip and a large magnet controller that is maneuvered across the abdomen, which applies pressures of up to 250 kPa based on a standard N42 magnet [73]. Frequently when magnets are used in devices, the manufacturer focuses on the strength of the magnetic field. When two magnets are used in a system, it is imperative that the magnetic force between the two magnets and the resultant pressure on any tissue is known.

Practicality and Safety of the Magnetic Forces Required to Operate the System

Surprisingly, there was scant information in the literature regarding the variability of the distance between the skin and the stomach in human subjects. Given that the size of the introducer needle for percutaneous endoscopic gastrostomy (PEG) placement is the same for all subjects, we suspected that there would be small variability across a wide BMI range.

Trans-gastric magnetic capture is an existing and utilized concept. In the development of Microcam-Navi, computed tomography (CT) was undertaken and estimated the skin surface to the proximal and distal stomach to be 16.5cm and 9.0cm. These measurements were taken from the skin to the center of the distal and proximal stomach, not to the stomach mucosa.

Using Human Patients, Our Team Determined

Variability of the Abdominal Wall Over a Wide Range of BMI

To create our device, we needed to determine the distance from the skin surface to the inner gastric mucosa of the antrum and fundus to determine a range of operation of the trans-gastric magnetic device. We analyzed 114 CT scans of the abdomen, with and without standard contrast to assess fundus and antrum measurements with regard to BMI, contrast status, and sex. The patient characteristics were taken from medical charts. Continuous measures were reported as means and standard deviations (SD) or medians and interquartile ranges (IQR). Categorical measures were reported as frequencies and percentages. Spearman's rank order correlation was used to assess the relationship between BMI and fundus and antrum measurements. The Kruskal–Wallis test was used to compare fundus and antrum measurements by BMI categories. The Mann–Whitney U test was used to compare fundus and antrum measurements by contrast status and sex. A p-value < 0.05 was used to define statistical significance for all tests conducted. SAS software version 9.4 was used for all analyses.

Among the sample of patients, the mean age was 50 years, 66% were female, the median BMI measurement was 29.50 kg/m^2, the median fundus measurement was 59.80 mm, and the median antrum measurement was 37.00 mm (Table 19.1). A statistically significant correlation was shown between BMI and both fundus and antrum measurements (both p < 0.0001, Table 19.2). There was a moderately positive relationship between BMI and fundus measurement (rho=0.48) and BMI and antrum measurement (rho=0.58). When making comparisons by BMI categories, both the fundus measurement and antrum measurement were significantly different by category (both p<0.0001, Table 19.3). Post-hoc comparisons revealed that the fundus measurement was significantly different between the ≤30 kg/m^{2}and the

Table 19.1 Descriptive characteristics of patients (N=113 patients, N=114 procedures[a])

Characteristic	
Age (years)	
Mean (±SD)	50.01 (±18.48)
Sex, n (%)	
Male	38 (33.63)
Female	75 (66.37)
Contrast, n (%)	
Yes	53 (46.49)
No	61 (53.51)
BMI (kg/m^2)	
Median (IQR)	29.50 (25.00, 35.00)
BMI Categories, n (%)	
≤30	65 (57.02)
31–39	36 (31.58)
≥40	13 (11.40)
Fundus (mm)	
Median (IQR)	59.80 (36.50, 95.00)
Antrum (mm)	
Median (IQR)	37.00 (28.10, 47.10)

IQR interquartile range, *SD* standard deviation

[a]Note: There were 113 total patients but 114 procedures because one patient had two procedures. N = 113 for age and sex results; N = 114 for contrast, BMI, fundus, and antrum results

Table 19.2 Correlation between BMI and fundus and antrum measurements (N = 114)

	Spearman's rho	p-value[a]
BMI (kg/m^2) and fundus (mm)	0.48	<0.0001
BMI (kg/m^2) and antrum (mm)	0.58	<0.0001

[a]p-value derived from the Spearman's rank order correlation test

Table 19.3 Comparison of fundus and antrum measurements by BMI categories (N=114)

	BMI ≤ 30 kg/m^2 n = 65	BMI 31–39 kg/m^2 n = 36	BMI ≥ 40 kg/m^2 n = 13	p-value[a]
Fundus (mm)				
Median (IQR)	47.80 (32.00, 78.90)	60.90 (46.85, 92.70)	115.40 (110.30, 123.00)	<0.0001[b]
Antrum (mm)				
Median (IQR)	33.00 (25.00, 39.50)	38.70 (30.30, 48.35)	67.40 (52.90, 82.50)	<0.0001[c]

IQR interquartile range
[a]p-value derived by the Kruskal-Wallis test
[b]Post-hoc tests indicate the following pairwise comparisons are significant at the 0.05 level:
BMI ≤30 kg/m^{2}and BMI ≥40 kg/m^2
BMI 31–39 kg/m^{2}and BMI ≥40 kg/m^2
[c]Post-hoc tests indicate the following pairwise comparisons are significant at the 0.05 level:
BMI ≤30 kg/m^{2}and BMI 31–39 kg/m^2
BMI ≤30 kg/m^{2}and BMI ≥40 kg/m^2
BMI 31–39 kg/m^{2}and BMI ≥40 kg/m^2

≥40 kg/m^{2}groups, and the 31–39 kg/m^{2}and the ≥40 kg/m^{2}groups. It was not significantly different between the ≤30 kg/m^{2}and BMI 31–39 kg/m^{2}groups. Post-hoc comparisons revealed that the antrum measurement was significantly different between the ≤30 kg/m^{2}and the 31–39 kg/m^{2}groups, the ≤30 kg/m^{2}and the ≥40 kg/m^{2}groups, and the 31–39 kg/m^{2}and the ≥40 kg/m^{2}groups.

Fundus and antrum measurements were compared by sex for each BMI category (Table 19.4). There were no significant differences in measurements between males and females, except for the antrum measurement in the 31–39 kg/m^2 category (36.30 mm vs. 44.20 mm, p=0.028). Antrum measurements were also compared by sex for patients who had a BMI between 20 and 45 kg/m^2, and there were no significant differences between males and females (Table 19.5).

There was a significant difference in fundus and antrum measurements by contrast status (Table 19.6). The median fundus measurement for those with contrast was smaller than the median fundus measurement for those without contrast (42.60 mm vs. 89.60 mm, p<0.0001). The median antrum measurement was smaller for those with contrast compared to those without contrast (33.00 mm vs. 39.50 mm, p=0.033).

In summary, despite the expected positive correlation between the measured distance from the stomach to the skin surface and BMI, we found that the change in distance is small in the antrum, but not in the fundus, across a wide BMI range with or without contrast. This provides an ideal location for capture of intragastric devices that use trans-gastric manipulation due to the short and stable distance from the internal gastric

Table 19.4 Comparison of fundus and antrum measurements by sex per BMI category (N = 114)

	BMI ≤ 30 kg/m^2		
	Male ***n* = 24**	**Female** ***n* = 41**	***p*-value**[a]
Fundus (mm)			
Median (IQR)	67.45 (35.50, 82.60)	44.30 (30.30, 60.50)	0.15
Antrum (mm)			
Median (IQR)	31.75 (26.70, 41.50)	34.10 (22.80, 38.90)	0.57
	BMI 31–39 kg/m^2		
	Male ***n*=12**	**Female** ***n*=24**	***p*-value**[a]
Fundus (mm)			
Median (IQR)	60.35 (28.25, 99.25)	60.90 (53.15, 86.70)	0.61
Antrum (mm)			
Median (IQR)	36.30 (22.90, 38.70)	44.20 (31.40, 52.05)	0.028
	BMI ≥ 40 kg/m^2		
	Male ***n*=2**	**Female** ***n*=11**	***p*-value**[a]
Fundus (mm)			
Median (IQR)	142.15 (137.80 146.50)	113.60 (96.50, 122.90)	0.060
Antrum (mm)			
Median (IQR)	85.00 (84.00, 86.00)	56.70 (52.60, 71.80)	0.12

IQR interquartile range
[a]p-value derived by the Mann-Whitney U test

mucosa to the abdominal wall [74]. Subsequent to the capture of the intragastric device, the body and fundus would be readily amenable to stimulation and distension.

Table 19.5 Comparison of antrum measurement by sex for BMI 20–45 kg/m^2(N=103)

	Male n=36	Female n=67	p-value[a]
Antrum (mm)			
Median (IQR)	34.65 (26.70, 41.20)	38.60 (31.30, 49.00)	0.058

IQR interquartile range
[a]p-value derived by the Mann-Whitney U test

Table 19.6 Comparison of fundus and antrum measurements by contrast categories (N=114)

	Contrast n=53	No Contrast n=61	p-value[a]
Fundus (mm)			
Median (IQR)	42.60 (30.40, 50.20)	89.60 (71.30, 103.80)	<0.0001
Antrum (mm)			
Median (IQR)	33.00 (23.50, 42.20)	39.50 (31.40, 51.50)	0.0033

IQR interquartile range
[a]p-value derived by the Mann-Whitney U test

Calculated Pressure Ranges That Would Be Generated by the Proposed Internal and External Magnets

To identify and optimize the configuration in which the external magnet would produce enough pulling force on the internal magnetic intragastric device, we employed a theoretical model called the Gilbert model (Fig. 19.6) to calculate the expected magnetic force between the two over a range of distance from 2 to 8 cm with 0.5 cm interval. The dimension of the internal device is a cylinder of 9.5mm (OD) x 19mm (length) and is similar to a PillCam device. The size of the external magnet is determined by two criteria. One is to produce a pulling force ~2 N (equivalent to the weight of roughly 200 g) at 5 cm distance, and the other is to be as lightweight as possible. Using the physical parameters (surface magnetization, mass density, etc.) of N42 grade magnets for both the internal and external magnet, the Gilbert model calculations suggest the external magnet to be a disk of 6.35 cm (OD) x 1.27 cm (thickness), which is about the lightest weight possible to produce ~2 N of force. Bench tests were then conducted to measure the magnetic force between the two magnets by attaching the internal magnet to a force sensor while being pulled by the external

Fig. 19.6 Gilbert Model equation integrates for the cylindrical coordinate system, where + denotes the north pole face, – denotes the south pole face, index 1 indicates the hand-held magnet, index 2 indicates the magnetic pill, and A denotes surface integration over the area of the pole faces

$$F_m = \frac{1}{4\pi\mu_0}\left(\int_{A_1^+}\int_{A_2^+}\frac{q_{m,1^+}\,q_{m,2^+}}{|r_{1^+2^+}|^2}dA_2^+\,dA_1^+ + \int_{A_1^-}\int_{A_2^+}\frac{q_{m,1^-}\,q_{m,2^+}}{|r_{1^-2^+}|^2}dA_2^+\,dA_1^- + \int_{A_1^+}\int_{A_2^-}\frac{q_{m,1^+}\,q_{m,2^-}}{|r_{1^+2^-}|^2}dA_2^-\,dA_1^+ + \int_{A_1^-}\int_{A_2^-}\frac{q_{m,1^-}\,q_{m,2^-}}{|r_{1^-2^-}|^2}dA_2^-\,dA_1^-\right).$$

magnet at ½-cm intervals for an 8-cm distance. Reliability of the Gilbert model calculation was affirmed by the bench test data and the greatest difference between the two is less than 15%. Given the nonideal magnetization of the N42 magnets and the uncertainty in distance measurements, this level of discrepancy is expected.

Once the magnetic force profile between 2-cm and 8-cm distance was established, the induced pressure was determined by first finding the contact area between the intragastric device and the gastric mucosa. Since the internal magnet is located at the center of an intragastric balloon of diameter 6.5 cm, the area of contact the balloon makes with the gastric mucosa is similar to a circle with diameter ~2.5 cm. The magnet-induced pressure is then calculated by dividing the above-measured force by this contact area ($P = F/A$, the definition of pressure) [75].

Compare the Calculated Pressure Range to Known Gastric Wall Pressure Profiles Found in Endoscopy, Surgery, or With Other Medical Equipment in Clinical Use

In humans, vomiting can produce pressures of 38.65 kPa. In animal studies using rats, pressures of 50 kPa have been reported as safe on thigh muscle tissue after compressive loading. Peg tube bumpers, when tight, are reported to cause gastric mucosa ulcerations after 7 days, and when measured in actual patients by us had acute pressures from 10 to 27 kPa. Similarly, in laboratory tissue models compressed by peg tube bumpers, we were able to produce pressures of 30, 70, and 248 kPa with tissue thicknesses of 0.8, 1.05, and 1.3 cm, respectively. Pressures of 19.3–26.2 kPa were used with the Olympus CV 160 Evis Exera to open the stomach during endoscopy (Fig. 19.7).

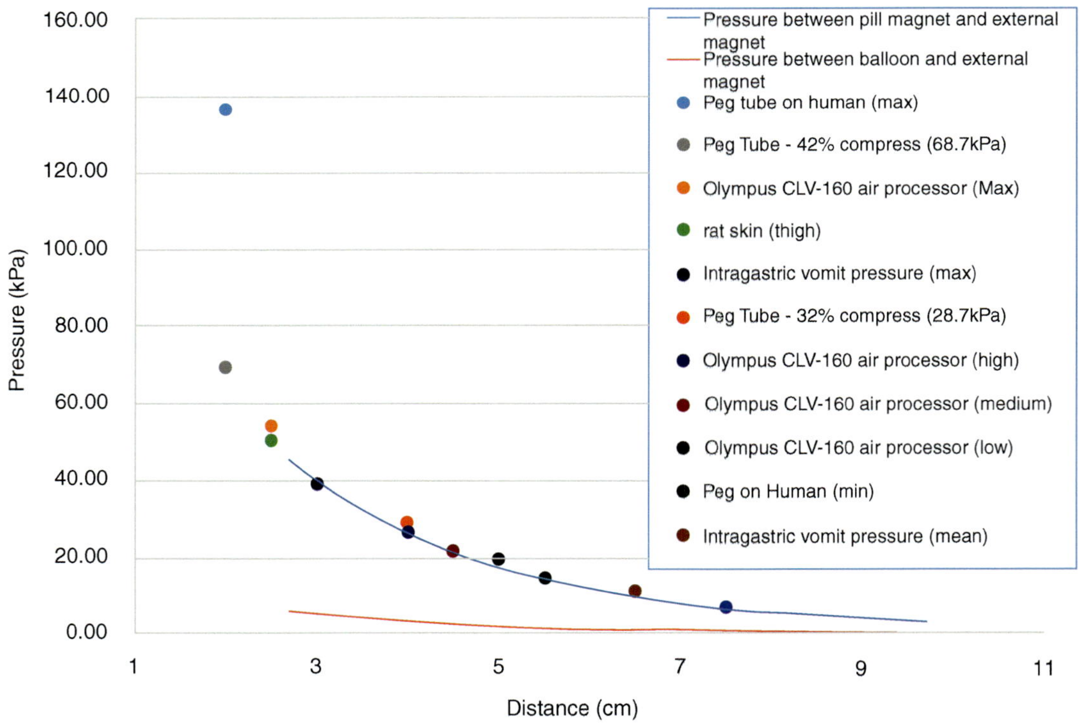

Fig. 19.7 Measured magnet induced pressure between handheld magnet (63.5mm x 50.8mm) and internal magnet (pill magnet 9.5mmx19mm) versus distance as compared to historical and experimental trans-gastric pressures. The pressure between handheld external magnet and a magnet-containing balloon is also shown for comparison. Note the cutoff at 3 cm which represents the shortest hypothetical distance between the internal magnet positioned inside the balloon and the skin surface

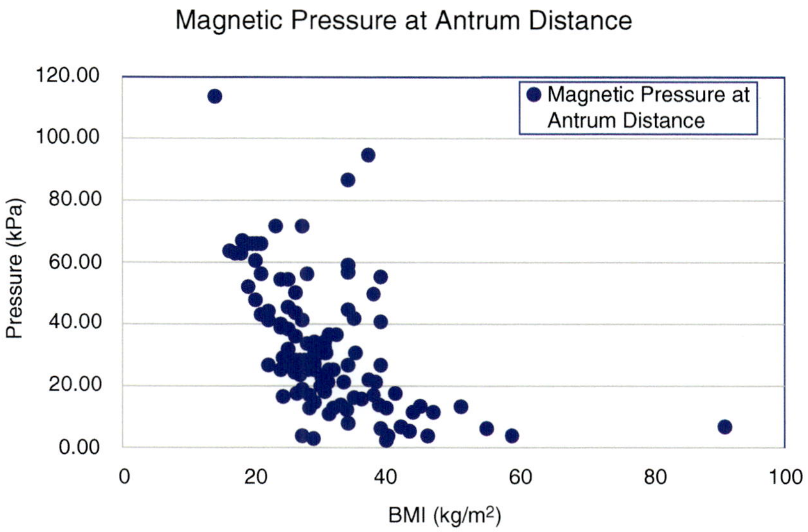

Fig. 19.8 Expected magnetic force relative to distance of the antrum/fundus to abdominal skin surface relative to BMI in 114 sequential patients, with a wide BMI range, who had undergone CT imaging with measured shortest skin to antral mucosa and skin to fundal mucosa

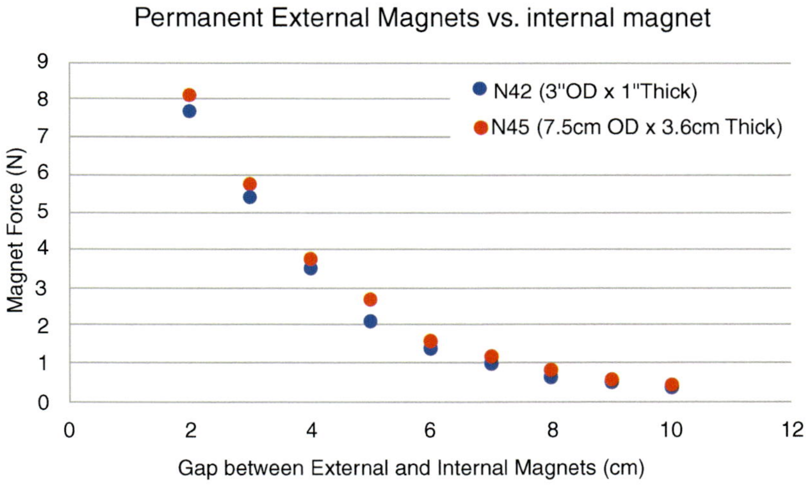

Fig. 19.9 The force between the magnetic intragastric balloon and two similar external magnets. The balloon can be moved and captured by the N42 external magnet at a distance of more 10 cm away from the external magnet

Also, recent publications show pressures of 200–600 kPa with graspers on the gastric wall during laparoscopic surgery [75–77].

Using Gilbert formula and hypothetical magnet sizes (cylinder of 3.1 cm in diameter and 19mm in length and external magnet is a disk of 6.35cm in diameter and 1.27cm in thickness), we calculated the hypothetical gastric wall pressures between the two magnets in the 114 patients in which we had CT data (Fig. 19.8). The size and strength of the magnets were calculated such that they conformed to anatomical use. As can be seen, there is a wide range of operability of 20–55.

Due to the large contact area between the intragastric balloon and the gastric mucosa, it allows the use of even stronger magnets than currently proposed to generate larger forces for capture if needed for patients with larger BMI, but minimal surface pressures < 20kPa. Our current prototype consists of an internal magnet 3.1 cm mm in diameter and 19 mm long and the external magnet is 3" in diameter and 1" thick. Capture readily occurs at less than 16 cm (Fig. 19.9). The pressure profile for this external magnet and an additional larger magnet are shown in the attached graph (Fig. 19.10).

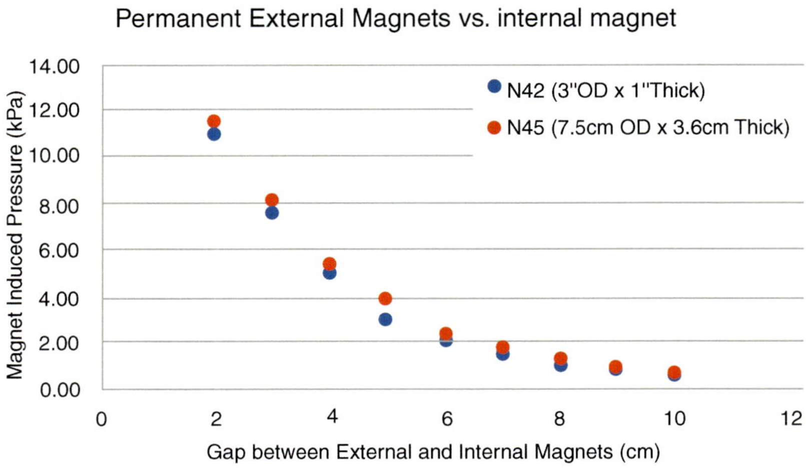

Fig. 19.10 The pressures induced by the force between the magnetic intragastric balloon and two similar external magnets, respective, based on the data in Fig. 19.9

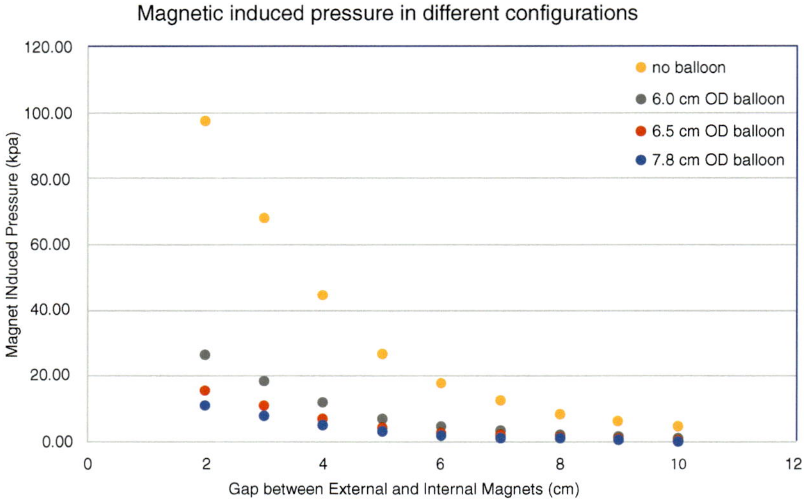

Fig. 19.11 Gap between internal and external magnets vs pressure

Our balloon stent currently is at a diameter of 6.5cm. The magnetic force and pressures generated are represented in the diagrams below depending on the size of the sphere (Fig. 19.11). It should be noted that the minimum distance between gastric mucosa and abdominal wall surface is estimated to be ~3cm [73, 78].

Endoscopic Placement and Removal

The intragastric portion of the device has to be delivered and removed relatively easily and remain intact in the gastric environment for 6 months or longer. The intragastric device contains the stent, a balloon, and a shaft on which the internal magnet is housed. Prior to deployment, the balloon is completely deflated, and the stent and its delivery components are wrapped in a cover sheet with a diameter of 18 cm so that it can easily pass the esophagus into the stomach. The device is inserted endoscopically through the esophagus with the help of a guidewire and an option to use an overtube, if needed. Also accompanying the guidewire is an inflation tube that is inserted into the device through a check valve. When the device enters the stomach, the device will first be released from the sheet cover, followed by removal of the guidewire. Our current prototypes have options of bioabsorbable cover sheet or traditional retrievable cover sheet. Once the balloon is free from the cover sheet, it will be inflated to expand the stent to the full size followed by the removal of the inflation tube. The placement of the intragastric device is now complete and the endoscope will be removed. The whole procedure is under endoscopic monitoring to ensure proper placement of the device.

To remove the intragastric device, an endoscope is placed. The balloon must be deflated first. Forceps are inserted through the endoscope under direct vision and the balloon is captured, punctured, and air is released. The deflation could be enhanced with the aid of a suction catheter and a pump. When the balloon is deflated, a collar on the center shaft will be accessible for placement of a suture snare to assist in removal of the device. Then the device will be pulled out of the stomach by pulling the endoscope, suture wire, and the deflated stent balloon as a system. Since the balloon is punctured and no longer pressurized, as the device exits the stomach and enters the esophagus, it will collapse and conform to the size of the esophagus. Alternatively, an overtube can also be used in this procedure to assist removal.

Durability and Functionality of the System Within the GI Tract

Since the intragastric device is intended to stay in the stomach for 6 months to one year, the materials must be durable so that the integrity and the functionality of the device can be maintained at all times. To endure the hostile environment in the stomach, with acid and movements, the material used to make the stent and balloon must be not only biocompatible, but also acid-resistant and shear-resistant. We choose to use silicon for this application due to prior approval for usage in similar conditions. It is also flexible enough to endure substantial shape change during implementation (inflated), in-operation (squeezed and compressed), and removal (deflated).

The internal magnet is slid on a sliding tube that goes through the center of the balloon and stent. The tube is joined to the stent/balloon structure on both ends with check valves allowing the guidewire and inflation tube to go through. The sliding movement of the internal magnet is limited to the center third of the tube. This arrangement is to allow force, when attracted by the external magnet, to be more uniformly distributed over a bigger contact area between the intragastric device and the esophageal surface, instead of concentrated at the check valve. The stent frame can be broken apart with endoscopic tools if needed. This will safeguard against inadvertent balloon rupture or deflation with potential bezoar formation.

Animal Studies

It has been interesting that most interventions in the field of bariatric surgery or endoscopy have been made without detailed attention to underlying potential mechanism of action. The potential mechanisms for neurohormonal pathways that could be affected and utilized by EMACS have been discussed earlier. We have proposed the following animal protocol that would not only establish the safety of the device in an animal model but at least provide insight into possible mechanism of action. We are also aware that the cornerstone of our device, that is, incorporation of behavior modification to change eating habits, will not be applicable in an animal model, especially swine. However, the swine stomach is similar in size and shape to a human stomach. The pig anatomy makes it ideal for magnetic capture and the distance from skin to gastric wall is ~5 cm [57]. Pigs in the 20–50 kg range have been used in previous bariatric studies [58]. Mini pigs will be used to determine feasibility of placement, durability, and removal of the device. Also, the mini pigs will be used to determine the proposed efficacy of the device by monitoring the effect of the device on pig growth, weight, and the impact on GI hormones involved in satiety. Mini pigs weighing 20 kg at the onset of the study on a feed to grow diet normally weigh 50 kg after 6 months. The rationale for mini pigs is shorter stature and shorter distance between their abdomen and the ground, allowing for the use of external magnets at the bottom of a special cage (Fig. 19.12).

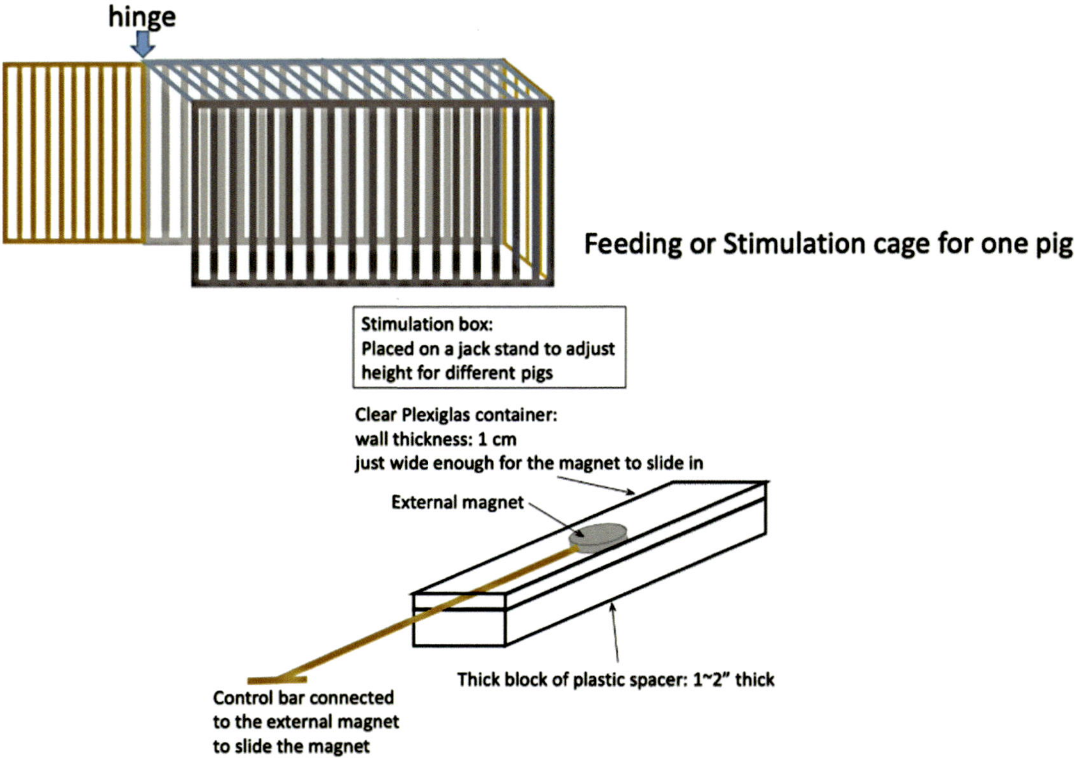

Fig. 19.12 Animal cage to allow for the use of external magnets during animal studies

Initially, two pigs weighing 20kg and 50kg, respectively, will be used. Technical aspects related to sedation, anesthesia, blood draw, removal, and magnetic capture will be tested and practiced on these two pigs, ahead of planned animal studies. Twelve pigs, six males and six females, weighing 20kg will be housed in a group stall.

1. Six male and six female mini pigs will have anatomical measurements including weight, height, and distance of the abdomen to ground. Lab values (CBC, chemistry, and gut peptides) will be obtained. The device will be placed endoscopically, expanded, and released in the stomach in eight pigs (four male), with four non device pigs serving as controls who will have sham endoscopy. The pigs will be housed together (flooring will be elevated such that it will minimize the risk of pica) and will only have access to water.
2. At specific hours each day, individual pigs will be taken to special individual experimental cages (Fig. 19.12) where they will be fed twice daily. The cage is designed so the pig is relatively immobile. The magnetic simulation will be done by the technician using an external magnet under a clear plexiglass floor. The size, height, and distance of the external magnet will be adjusted according to pig size to simulate magnetic pressures comparable to a human subject by rubbing an external magnet on the surface of the abdomen. Different sized cages corresponding to different time intervals in the study will be used.
3. Each month baseline feeding duration in pigs will be measured and is expected to be 9–11 minutes [4, 60]. Five minutes of gastric stimulation simultaneous with normal feeding time will be performed at the onset of feeding alternating with the midpoint of feeding in a counterbalanced crossover fashion with a

switch at 3 months. The technician will ensure that the magnet movement corresponds to the anatomical element of the pig stomach.

4. Food consumption will be measured by the MBRose individual feed Intake monitor [61], and the pig will be returned to the group stall.
5. The magnet will be detected weekly in the experimental group via a metal detector. If not detected, the pig will undergo further imaging.
6. At 1, 3, and 6 months, the pigs will undergo baseline fasting peptide measurement and then upper endoscopy for visualization of the GI tract with assessment, by biopsy (H&E staining) of any damage to the esophagus and stomach.
7. After endoscopic examination is completed, a 200-cc liquid meal via an OG tube while the pig is intubated is given and a 5-minute magnetic stimulation will be given by a handheld magnet. Peptide levels will be measured at 0, 15, 30, and 60 minutes.
8. Control pigs will have identical protocols without the magnetic stimulation using a simulated nonmagnetic device (placebo). At 6 months, the device is collapsed by air suction and removed endoscopically.
9. Two weeks after the last endoscopy, the pigs will be euthanized per IACUC guidelines and gross and microscopic (H&E) visualization of the stomach will be done.

Conclusion and Future

Obesity and its complications are now the leading cause of morbidity and mortality worldwide. It is unlikely that the food industry will take a meaningful and active role in combating obesity anytime soon. New innovations are required to help modify human behavior with respect to control of appetite and food. Magnets can provide a safe and effective way to simulate the pathways that are activated upon eating in an effort to provide the patients a tool to help reinforce behavior modification. The proposed device, EMACS, has been designed to accommodate this need and in 3 years.

References

1. Begley S. Fat and getting fatter: U.S. obesity rates to soar by 2030. Reuters. Published 18 Sept 2012. https://www.reuters.com/article/us-obesity-us/fat-and-getting-fatter-u-s-obesity-rates-to-soar-by-2030-idUSBRE88H0RA20120918.
2. Hruby A, Hu FB. The epidemiology of obesity: a big picture. Pharm Econ. 2015;33(7):673–89. https://doi.org/10.1007/s40273-014-0243-x.
3. Wang Y, Beydoun MA, Liang L, Caballero B, Kumanyika SK. Will all Americans become overweight or obese? estimating the progression and cost of the US obesity epidemic. Obesity (Silver Spring). 2008;16(10):2323–30. https://doi.org/10.1038/oby.2008.351.
4. Kentish SJ, O'Donnell TA, Frisby CL, Li H, Wittert GA, Page AJ. Altered gastric vagal mechanosensitivity in diet-induced obesity persists on return to normalchow and is accompanied by increased food intake. Int J Obes 2005. 2014;38(5):636–42. https://doi.org/10.1038/ijo.2013.138.
5. Abdelaal M, le Roux CW, Docherty NG. Morbidity and mortality associated with obesity. Ann Transl Med. 2017;5(7) https://doi.org/10.21037/atm.2017.03.107.
6. Roth J, Qiang X, Marbán SL, Redelt H, Lowell BC. The obesity pandemic: where have we been and where are we going? Obes Res. 2004;12(Suppl 2):88S–101S. https://doi.org/10.1038/oby.2004.273.
7. Mohammed MA, Anwar R, Mansour AH, Elmasry E, Othman G. Effects of intragastric balloon versus conservative therapy on appetite regulatory hormones in obese subjects. Trends Med Res. 2014;9(2):58–80. https://doi.org/10.3923/tmr.2014.58.80.
8. Meldrum DR, Morris MA, Gambone JC. Obesity pandemic: causes, consequences, and solutions-but do we have the will? Fertil Steril. 2017;107(4):833–9. https://doi.org/10.1016/j.fertnstert.2017.02.104.
9. Swinburn BA. Obesity prevention: the role of policies, laws and regulations. Aust New Zealand Health Policy. 2008;5(1):12. https://doi.org/10.1186/1743-8462-5-12.
10. Davy B, Jahren H. New markers of dietary added sugar intake. Current Opinion in Clinical Nutrition and Metabolic Care. 2016;19:1. https://doi.org/10.1097/MCO.0000000000000287.
11. Christakis NA, Fowler JH. The spread of obesity in a large social network over 32 years. N Engl J Med. 2007;357(4):370–9. https://doi.org/10.1056/NEJMsa066082.
12. Kral TVE, Roe LS, Rolls BJ. Combined effects of energy density and portion size on energy intake in women. Am J Clin Nutr. 2004;79(6):962–8. https://doi.org/10.1093/ajcn/79.6.962.
13. Milanski M, Arruda AP, Coope A, et al. Inhibition of hypothalamic inflammation reverses diet-induced insulin resistance in the liver. Diabetes. 2012;61(6):1455–62. https://doi.org/10.2337/db11-0390.

14. Milanski M, Degasperi G, Coope A, et al. Saturated fatty acids produce an inflammatory response predominantly through the activation of TLR4 signaling in hypothalamus: implications for the pathogenesis of obesity. J Neurosci. 2009;29(2):359–70. https://doi.org/10.1523/JNEUROSCI.2760-08.2009.
15. De Souza CT, Araujo EP, Bordin S, et al. Consumption of a fat-rich diet activates a proinflammatory response and induces insulin resistance in the hypothalamus. Endocrinology. 2005;146(10):4192–9. https://doi.org/10.1210/en.2004-1520.
16. Simpson KA, Bloom SR. Appetite and Hedonism: Gut Hormones and the Brain. Endocrinology and Metabolism Clinics of North America. 2010;39(4): 729–43. https://doi.org/10.1016/j.ecl.2010.08.001.
17. Cummings DE, Overduin J. Gastrointestinal regulation of food intake. J Clin Invest. 2007;117(1):13–23. https://doi.org/10.1172/JCI30227.
18. Wang G-J, Tomasi D, Backus W, et al. Gastric distention activates satiety circuitry in the human brain. NeuroImage. 2008;39(4):1824–31. https://doi.org/10.1016/j.neuroimage.2007.11.008.
19. Ly HG, Dupont P, Van Laere K, Depoortere I, Tack J, Van Oudenhove L. Differential brain responses to gradual intragastric nutrient infusion and gastric balloon distension: A role for gut peptides? NeuroImage. 2017;144:101–12. https://doi.org/10.1016/j.neuroimage.2016.09.032.
20. Raynor HA, Champagne CM. Position of the academy of nutrition and dietetics: interventions for the treatment of overweight and obesity in adults. J Acad Nutr Diet. 2016;116(1):129–47. https://doi.org/10.1016/j.jand.2015.10.031.
21. Berthoud H-R, Münzberg H, Morrison CD. Blaming the brain for obesity: Integration of hedonic and homeostatic mechanisms. Gastroenterology. 2017;152(7):1728–38. https://doi.org/10.1053/j.gastro.2016.12.050.
22. Ritter RC. Gastrointestinal mechanisms of satiation for food. Physiology & Behavior. 2004;81(2):249–73. https://doi.org/10.1016/j.physbeh.2004.02.012.
23. Stice E, Spoor S, Bohon C, Veldhuizen MG, Small DM. Relation of reward from food intake and anticipated food intake to obesity: a functional magnetic resonance imaging study. J Abnorm Psychol. 2008;117(4):924–35. https://doi.org/10.1037/a0013600.
24. Geiger BM, Behr GG, Frank LE, et al. Evidence for defective mesolimbic dopamine exocytosis in obesity-prone rats. FASEB J. 2008;22(8):2740–6. https://doi.org/10.1096/fj.08-110759.
25. Volkow ND, Wang G-J, Telang F, et al. Low dopamine striatal D2 receptors are associated with prefrontal metabolism in obese subjects: possible contributing factors. Neuroimage. 2008;42(4):1537–43. https://doi.org/10.1016/j.neuroimage.2008.06.002.
26. Dixon JB, Lambert EA, Lambert GW. Neuroendocrine adaptations to bariatric surgery. Mol Cell Endocrinol. 2015;418(Pt 2):143–52. https://doi.org/10.1016/j.mce.2015.05.033.
27. Hargrave SL, Kinzig KP. Repeated gastric distension alters food intake and neuroendocrine profiles in rats. Physiol Behav. 2012;105(4):975–81. https://doi.org/10.1016/j.physbeh.2011.11.006.
28. Woods SC, D'Alessio DA. Central control of body weight and appetite. J Clin Endocrinol Metab. 2008;93(11 Suppl 1):S37–50. https://doi.org/10.1210/jc.2008-1630.
29. Maljaars J, Peters HPF, Masclee AM. Review article: The gastrointestinal tract: neuroendocrine regulation of satiety and food intake. Aliment Pharmacol Ther. 2007;26(Suppl 2):241–50. https://doi.org/10.1111/j.1365-2036.2007.03550.x.
30. Lepionka L, Malbert CH, Laplace JP. Proximal gastric distension modifies ingestion rate in pigs. Reprod Nutr Dev. 1997;37(4):449–57. https://doi.org/10.1051/rnd:19970406.
31. Pappas TN, Melendez RL, Debas HT. Gastric distension is a physiologic satiety signal in the dog. Digest Dis Sci. 1989;34(10):1489–93. https://doi.org/10.1007/BF01537098.
32. Lepionka L, Malbert CH. Perprandial changes in gastric wall tension control ingestion in pigs. Reprod Nutr Dev. 1997;37(3):351–1. https://doi.org/10.1051/rnd:19970341.
33. Oesch S, Rüegg C, Fischer B, Degen L, Beglinger C. Effect of gastric distension prior to eating on food intake and feelings of satiety in humans. Physiology & Behavior. 2006;87(5):903–10. https://doi.org/10.1016/j.physbeh.2006.02.003.
34. Geliebter A. Gastric distension and gastric capacity in relation to food intake in humans. Physiology & Behavior. 1988;44(4–5):665–8. https://doi.org/10.1016/0031-9384(88)90333-2.
35. Stephan E, Pardo JV, Faris PL, et al. Functional neuroimaging of gastric distention. J Gastrointest Surg. 2003;7(6):740–9. https://doi.org/10.1016/s1091-255x(03)00071-4.
36. Konturek SJ, Konturek JW, Pawlik T, Brzozowki T. Brain-gut axis and its role in the control of food intake. J Physiol Pharmacol. 2004 Mar;55(1 Pt 2): 137–54.
37. Oudenhove LV, Vandenberghe J, Dupont P, et al. Cortical deactivations during gastric fundus distension in health: visceral pain-specific response or attenuation of 'default mode' brain function? A H215O-PET study. Neurogastroenterology & Motility. 2009;21(3):259–71. https://doi.org/10.1111/j.1365-2982.2008.01196.x.
38. Geeraerts B, Oudenhove LV, Dupont P, et al. Different regional brain activity during physiological gastric distension compared to balloon distension: a H215O-PET study. Neurogastroenterology & Motility. 2011;23(6):533–e203. https://doi.org/10.1111/j.1365-2982.2010.01642.x.
39. Vandenbergh J, DuPont P, Fischler B, et al. Regional brain activation during proximal stomach distention in humans: A positron emission tomography study. Gastroenterology. 2005;128(3):564–73. https://doi.org/10.1053/j.gastro.2004.11.054.

40. Delzenne N, Blundell J, Brouns F, et al. Gastrointestinal targets of appetite regulation in humans. Obesity Reviews. 2010;11(3):234–50. https://doi.org/10.1111/j.1467-789X.2009.00707.x.
41. Steinert RE, Meyer-Gerspach AC, Beglinger C. The role of the stomach in the control of appetite and the secretion of satiation peptides. American Journal of Physiology-Endocrinology and Metabolism. 2012;302(6):E666–73. https://doi.org/10.1152/ajpendo.00457.2011.
42. Share I, Martyniuk E, Grossman MI. Effect of Prolonged Intragastric Feeding on Oral Food Intake in Dogs. American Journal of Physiology-Legacy Content. 1952;169(1):229–35. https://doi.org/10.1152/ajplegacy.1952.169.1.229.
43. Paintal AS. A study of gastric stretch receptors; their role in the peripheral mechanism of satiation of hunger and thirst. J Physiol (Lond). 1954;126(2):255–70. https://doi.org/10.1113/jphysiol.1954.sp005207.
44. Mion F, Napoléon B, Roman S, et al. Effects of intragastric balloon on gastric emptying and plasma ghrelin levels in non-morbid obese patients. Obes Surg. 2005;15(4):510–6. https://doi.org/10.1381/0960892053723411.
45. Martinez-Brocca MA, Belda O, Parejo J, et al. Intragastric balloon-induced satiety is not mediated by modification in fasting or postprandial plasma ghrelin levels in morbid obesity. Obes Surg. 2007;17(5):649. https://doi.org/10.1007/s11695-007-9109-z.
46. Shiiya T, Nakazato M, Mizuta M, et al. Plasma ghrelin levels in lean and obese humans and the effect of glucose on ghrelin secretion. J Clin Endocrinol Metab. 2002;87(1):240–4. https://doi.org/10.1210/jcem.87.1.8129.
47. Sander B, Arantes VN, Alberti L, Neto MG, Grecco E, Souza TF. 550 Long-term effect of intragastric balloon in the management of obesity. Gastrointestinal Endoscopy. 2017;85(5, Supplement):AB83. https://doi.org/10.1016/j.gie.2017.03.113.
48. Ruban A, Stoenchev K, Ashrafian H, Teare J. Current treatments for obesity. Clin Med (Lond). 2019;19(3):205–12. https://doi.org/10.7861/clinmedicine.19-3-205.
49. Kumar RB, Aronne LJ. Review of multimodal therapies for obesity treatment: Including dietary, counseling strategies, and pharmacologic interventions. Techniques in Gastrointestinal Endoscopy. 2017;19(1):12–7. https://doi.org/10.1016/j.tgie.2016.11.003.
50. Gandarillas M, Hodgkinson SM, Riveros JL, Bas F. Effect of three different bariatric obesity surgery procedures on nutrient and energy digestibility using a swine experimental model. Exp Biol Med (Maywood). 2015;240(9):1158–64. https://doi.org/10.1177/1535370214567635.
51. Lupoli R, Lembo E, Saldalamacchia G, Avola CK, Angrisani L, Capaldo B. Bariatric surgery and long-term nutritional issues. World J Diabetes. 2017;8(11):464–74. https://doi.org/10.4239/wjd.v8.i11.464.
52. Moura D, Oliveira J, Moura EGHD, et al. Effectiveness of intragastric balloon for obesity: A systematic review and meta-analysis based on randomized control trials. Surgery for Obesity and Related Diseases. 2016;12(2):420–9. https://doi.org/10.1016/j.soard.2015.10.077.
53. Do TN, En T, Seah T, Yu HK, Phee SJ. Development and Testing of a Magnetically Actuated Capsule Endoscopy for Obesity Treatment. PLoS one. 2016;11(1):1–24. doi:https://doi.org/10.1371/journal.pone.0148035
54. Dumonceau J-M. Evidence-based review of the Bioenterics intragastric balloon for weight loss. Obes Surg. 2008;18(12):1611–7. https://doi.org/10.1007/s11695-008-9593-9.
55. New weight loss pill that expands in your stomach: is it safe? Healthline. Published 19 Apr 2019. https://www.healthline.com/health-news/plenty-weight-loss-pill. Accessed 13 Aug 2020.
56. Newly approved weight loss device blocks the vagus nerve. EndocrineWeb. https://www.endocrineweb.com/professional/obesity/newly-approved-weight-loss-device-blocks-vagus-nerve. Accessed 13 Aug 2020.
57. Bazerbachi F, Vargas Valls EJ, Abu Dayyeh BK. Recent Clinical Results of Endoscopic Bariatric Therapies as an Obesity Intervention. Clin Endosc. 2017;50(1):42–50. https://doi.org/10.5946/ce.2017.013.
58. Sharaiha R. Managing Obesity With Endoscopic Sleeve Gastroplasty. Gastroenterol Hepatol (N Y). 2017;13(9):547–9.
59. Norén E, Forssell H. Aspiration therapy for obesity; a safe and effective treatment. BMC Obes. 2016;3 https://doi.org/10.1186/s40608-016-0134-0.
60. Spring B, Schneider K, McFadden HG, et al. Multiple Behavior Change in Diet and Activity: A Randomized Controlled Trial Using Mobile Technology. Arch Intern Med. 2012;172(10):789–96. https://doi.org/10.1001/archinternmed.2012.1044.
61. Vibration: origins, effects, solutions | Galen Carol Audio | Galen Carol Audio. https://www.gcaudio.com/tips-tricks/vibration-origins-effects-solutions/. Accessed 13 Aug 2020.
62. Equen M, Roach G, Brown R, Bennett T. Magnetic Removal of Foreign Bodies from the Esophagus, Stomach, and Duodenum. AMA Arch Otolaryngol. 1957;66(6):698–706. https://doi.org/10.1001/archotol.1957.03830300078007.
63. The use of magnets in the control of traumatic gastritis of cattle. - Abstract – Europe PMC. https://europepmc.org/article/med/13366840. Accessed 13 Aug 2020.
64. Yim S, Sitti M. Shape-Programmable Soft Capsule Robots for Semi-Implantable Drug Delivery. IEEE Transactions on Robotics. 2012;28(5):1198–202. https://doi.org/10.1109/TRO.2012.2197309.
65. Lien G, Liu C, Jiang J, Chuang C, Teng M. Magnetic Control System Targeted for Capsule Endoscopic Operations in the Stomach—Design, Fabrication, and in vitro and ex vivo Evaluations. IEEE Transactions

on Biomedical Engineering. 2012;59(7):2068–79. https://doi.org/10.1109/TBME.2012.2198061.
66. Rahman I, Afzal NA, Patel P. The role of magnetic assisted capsule endoscopy (MACE) to aid visualisation in the upper GI tract. Computers in Biology and Medicine. 2015;65:359–63. https://doi.org/10.1016/j.compbiomed.2015.03.014.
67. Keller J, Fibbe C, Volke F, et al. Remote magnetic control of a wireless capsule endoscope in the esophagus is safe and feasible: results of a randomized, clinical trial in healthy volunteers. Gastrointestinal Endoscopy. 2010;72(5):941–6. https://doi.org/10.1016/j.gie.2010.06.053.
68. Gottlieb KT, Banerjee S, Barth BA, et al. Magnets in the GI tract. Gastrointestinal Endoscopy. 2013;78(4): 561–7. https://doi.org/10.1016/j.gie.2013.07.020.
69. Rahman I, Kay M, Bryant T, et al. Optimizing the performance of magnetic-assisted capsule endoscopy of the upper GI tract using multiplanar CT modelling. Eur J Gastroenterol Hepatol. 2015;27(4):460–6. https://doi.org/10.1097/MEG.0000000000000312.
70. Gabriel S, Thompson WM, Bhar A, Swadene L, Ashley D. Development and Technology Transfer of the Syncro Blue Tube (Gabriel) Magnetically Guided Feeding Tube. Macon: Syncro Medical Innovations, Inc.; 2017. https://apps.dtic.mil/sti/citations/AD1038950. Accessed 14 Aug 2020.
71. Gabriel SA, McDaniel B, Ashley DW, Dalton ML, Gamblin TC. Magnetically guided nasoenteral feeding tubes: a new technique. Am Surg. 2001;67(6):544–8; discussion 548–549.
72. Gabriel SA, Ackermann RJ. Placement of nasoenteral feeding tubes using external magnetic guidance. Journal of Parenteral and Enteral Nutrition. 2004;28(2):119–22. https://doi.org/10.1177/0148607104028002119.
73. Rivas H, Robles I, Riquelme F, et al. Magnetic Surgery. Ann Surg. 2018;267(1):88–93. https://doi.org/10.1097/SLA.0000000000002045.
74. Pressure. http://hyperphysics.phy-astr.gsu.edu/hbase/press.html#pre. Accessed 8 Mar 2020.
75. Nakayama S, Hasegawa S, Nagayama S, et al. The importance of precompression time for secure stapling with a linear stapler. Surg Endosc. 2011;25(7):2382–6. https://doi.org/10.1007/s00464-010-1527-7.
76. Cartmill JA, Shakeshaft AJ, Walsh WR, Martin CJ. High Pressures Are Generated at the Tip of Laparoscopic Graspers. Australian and New Zealand Journal of Surgery. 1999;69(2):127–30. https://doi.org/10.1046/j.1440-1622.1999.01496.x.
77. Shakeshaft AJ, Cartmill JA, Walsh WR, Martin CJ. A curved edge moderates high pressure generated by a laparoscopic grasper. Surg Endosc. 2001;15(10):1232–4. https://doi.org/10.1007/s00464-001-0036-0.
78. Rapaccini GL, Aliotta A, Pompili M, et al. Gastric wall thickness in normal and neoplastic subjects: a prospective study performed by abdominal ultrasound. Gastrointest Radiol. 1988;13(1):197–9. https://doi.org/10.1007/BF01889058.

Future/Research in Magnetic Surgery

20

Michel Gagner

Can one determine the course of the future? I like the quote of Henri Bergson, "The idea of the future, pregnant with an infinity of possibilities, is thus more fruitful than the future itself, and this is why we find more charm in hope than in possession, in dreams than in reality."

Let us explore recent efforts of the last decade to review where the endeavours are progressing. The use of magnets for loss of domain has been looked at in a short porcine video experiment using either endoluminal magnets or use of metallic expandable stents in 2011 [1]. We have not heard any further substantial developments from either the Strasbourg team on this or from the UCSF team, excepting a few anecdotal cases from UCSF in very selective indications. In fact, the Strasbourg team did publish a year later on the latter technique of submucosal endoscopic myotomies of the oesophagus, some in spiral shapes, without the collaboration of the UCSF but instead with Stanford University, a competitor in California. Just 13 miles apart and 21 minutes by car, which leads me to believe that they would rather use the endoscopic technique and found it more promising for paediatric patients in this ex vivo model, than magnetic lengthening [2].

But if we go back to Dr. Michael Harrison's seven human cases [3, 4], both published in 2017 (one with five patients and the other with two), we find the use of his designed magnets for the intestine with open surgery, as the original designs were neither endoscopic nor laparoscopic friendly. These "Harrison rings" were placed in the lumen of each small bowel, brought together to form a side-to-side or end-to-end anastomosis, depending on the case. Magnet movements were monitored with consecutive radiographs until they were expelled in the stools. Those first five patients had severe systemic disease and underwent intricate open urinary reconstruction operations, with the magnets employed to restore small bowel continuity after isolation of an ileum portion. All magnets were without obstruction, ache, or complications, including leaks, haemorrhage, or stenosis at median follow-up of 13 months [3]. For the other paediatric patients, magnets were applied for a diverting loop ileostomy due to malignant bowel obstruction, and for the adolescent, to restore a diverting ileostomy; however, the magnetic rings were navigated with fluoroscopy and each tied with sutures that exited the stoma, which were pulled when patency was achieved. The procedural time took <20 minutes, and there were no complications, with passage of stool by the fourth and fifth days. Magnets were removed 14 and 15 days post-operatively, without suggestion of any leaks [4]. Eight years prior, porcine comparisons with stapled and hand-sewn compression anastomosis were done to confirm safety and to substantiate the human application [5]. However, pigs have different intestinal wall

M. Gagner (✉)
Hôpital du Sacré-Cœur de Montréal, Montréal, QC, Canada

Chief of Surgery, Westmount Square Surgical Center, Westmount, QC, Canada

M. Gagner (ed.), *Magnetic Surgery*, https://doi.org/10.1007/978-3-030-73947-8_20

thicknesses, which are generally thinner than humans. As described before in other chapters, the two neodymium–iron–boron magnets were incorporated to polytetrafluoroethylene (PTFE) mouldings, and tested two types of compression, one uniform and the other with gradient. Sixteen pigs underwent open surgery with formation of a magnetic side-to-side anastomosis: 8 uniform and 8 with a gradient. Each also had a stapled anastomosis, and five had hand-sewn anastomosis [5]. All magnetic devices fashioned patent anastomoses without leaks, but one stapled anastomosis occasioned a contained leak. There were no statistically significant differences in the mechanical integrity of all different types of anastomoses. The gradient compression seemed to provide faster anastomotic patency (67% vs. 33% at 1 week), presumably from central necrosis. There were no strictures and histology established mucosal and serosa apposition across the magnetic anastomosis; it was declared safe and effective [5].

The earlier work of Leroy et al. in Strasbourg established the feasibility of lower colorectal anastomosis in the porcine model [6]. Again using 15 of 16 swine, 10 of which underwent side-to-side anastomoses and 5 of which underwent end-to-side connections. Once more, the Harrison rings were not designed for laparoscopic surgery, and colorectal anastomoses were performed using a hybrid NOTES technique. The mean operating time was brief at 71 minutes. Burst pressure at 10 days was greater than 95 mmHg in both groups. Inflammation and fibrosis were analogous between magnetic and stapled anastomoses. A minimal compression force of 4 N appeared to be prerequisite for consistent magnetic anastomoses [6].

Indeed, radio frequency is a potential addition in compression anastomosis, as the healing of these tissue connections happens over a few days, dependent on the force of the two magnets and their proper alignments. One idea to obtain alignment knowledge is to tag the magnets with a miniaturized battery-less radio frequency identification (RFID) to wirelessly telemeter the pressure status [7]. Jiang and colleagues have designed multilayer circular spiral coil with diameters of 10, 15, 19, and 27 mm to support what they called "magnamosis". According to the authors, there is no degradation with saline immersion or when placed adjacent to rare-earth magnets, and operating distance of the RFID tags is >10 cm in a 20 Å ~ 22 cm^2 area [7]. More recently, similar tags have been used in laparoscopic surgery for tumour identification and making the laparoscopic stapling with adequate margins, even at distance at which the RFID tag was within 10 mm. These latest published studies indicate the feasibility of the clinical application of RFID tag as a marker for identifying the proper site of variable gastrointestinal tumours [8, 9].

Endoscopic delivery has been worked on for some time, as our group worked on this since 2007. Our concept of proximal and distal endoscopy for GI anastomosis has been submitted to the patent office at that time. Others in the USA have used magnetic retraction during endoscopy [10]. In an experimental 2009 study using our patented concept, Gonzalez et al. used eight pigs under general anaesthesia underwent colonoscopy to deliver a magnetic ring (again, made for open surgery) to the hepatic flexure, while simultaneous upper endoscopy delivered the other magnetic ring into the duodenum using a variation of techniques. The two magnetic rings were brought into magnetic juxtaposition under laparoscopic guidance [11]. It confirmed that our intellectual property from Endo Metabolic Solutions (EMS) was indeed the right concept. The rings, using a guide wire and balloon appliance, were apparently redesigned to include a shell with an indentation to adapt an endoscopic snare. Laparoscopic visualization was necessary as the localization endoscopically could not be assured, and the magnets collaged without interference of intervening tissues. The duodenocolonic anastomosis, a concept that I had created several years earlier, came to fruition again. Final histological examinations revealed comprehensive healing in as early as 7 days.

A single pig was subjected to an experimental design, creating a transgastric access to the peritoneal cavity, placing the upper magnetic ring in the proximal bowel by enterotomy, followed by a transrectal access to dissect the sigmoid, resecting and extracting transrectally, and delivering the distal magnetic ring for apposition [12]. An elaborate natural orifice technique was obtained for this segmental colectomy performed in 139 minutes, but most likely would increase unnecessary risks of leakages in humans. The post-operative course was uneventful and magnetic rings were expelled in the faeces quite early on post-operative day 5. Endoscopic examination at post-operative day 14 revealed a patent anastomosis, and necropsy revealed a burst pressure of 198 mm Hg, without abscesses or peritonitis [12].

A similar experiment was published, stating the same message, using a "3D METRIS" system which consisted of a tube (1.2 m long and 2.2 mm in diameter) that fits into the operating channel of a conventional endoscope and holds seven 8 × 1 mm electromagnetic probes allocated on its length [13]. These probes are traced by a commercially obtainable magnetic tracking system (Aurora, Northern Digital Inc., Waterloo, Ontario, Canada), which then produces a three-dimensional rendering of the endoscope position. Two endoscopes were advanced in an anaesthetized pig, one inside the stomach and the other from the rectum. Both endoscopes were armed with a magnetic ring attached with a simple snare, but again, this was not completely endoscopic as it required a laparoscopic surveillance. The tracking system "helped" steered both tips of endoscopes within 2 cm to a "rendezvous" location between the colon and stomach. Although the authors stated that necropsy revealed secure magnetic rings without entrapment of bowel wall, mesentery, or omental fat, this may materialize in the future, as 2 cm is a sizeable distance [13].

Finally, the efforts from Thompson et al. by using segmental magnets have been recently published [14, 15]. Although they state that they have developed a technology based on miniature self-assembling magnets, this is a reproduction of our prior patent describing the same assembly of small magnets in the channel of a flexible endoscope to create larger calibre anastomoses. They have used a swine model to attempt endoscopic jejunoileal connection using magnets in eight Yorkshire pigs. Still, despite the aim to perform total endoscopy, surgical assistance was required and an enterotomy was created through which the ileal magnet was inserted using a modified laparoscopic delivery tool. Magnets were manually coupled. Pigs underwent serial endoscopies for anastomosis assessment. Of course, with manual assistance, the success of coupling the magnets was at 100%. After 3 months, the jejunoileal connections of up to 30 mm created were still patent and leak-free. The magnets were expelled by day 12. At 3-month necropsy, adhesions were minimal and burst pressure testing confirmed superior integrity of anastomotic tissue, nearly as strong as normal intestines. Histology showed full epithelialization across the anastomosis with no evidence of submucosal fibrosis or inflammation [14, 15].

Strong from this small experiment but unable to perform a complete endoscopic procedure, Machytka et al., from the Surgical department of the University Hospital in Ostrava in the Czech Republic, went to a human pilot study designed to evaluate the technical feasibility, safety, and clinical performance of their incisionless magnetic anastomosis to create a jejunal-ileal bypass, according to the institution's ethics committee April 17, 2014 [16]. The four last authors are stockholders of GI Windows, the company based in West Bridgewater Massachusetts that sponsored this trial. Key in this trial is the limit imposed of 40 minutes for assembly of the magnets, at which point it was decided to take over by laparoscopy. Of the 14 patients, three withdrew consent, one was removed for pulmonary problems, and the magnets could not be apposed in two. The authors reported they were able to perform this in 10 patients principally treated for obesity, type 2 diabetes mellitus, and prediabetes, and all underwent general anaesthesia. With laparoscopic supervision, small magnets were delivered through the working channel of a colonoscope, with an average duration of 115 minutes, just below 2 hours. This of course, established the difficulty of a complete endoscopic procedure not knowing with 100% certainty where the tip of the endoscope is in the bowel, as jejunoileal bypasses have been abandoned in the past for creating hepatic failures as a mistake in judgement of the exact location of the anastomosis could create this situation in patients. They reported that the upper magnet was 50–100 cm from the Treitz and the lower magnet about 50–100 cm from the ileocecal valve, making a 100 cm channel at minima, or 200 cm at maxima. The procedure was performed laparoscopically in 80% of cases, only in two cases were they able to endoscopically couple the magnets (still under laparoscopic vision), as an antimesenteric position is a must. So, all we can conclude is that this is a laparoscopic procedure and not an endoscopic one, as the authors seems to claim, because gastroenterologists will not be able to do this outside the operating room and will need general surgeons with laparoscopic expertise. Magnets were expelled in 12 days on average, ranging from 8 to 28 days, except one patient where the bowel had been sutured at laparoscopy…retrieved at day 123 by endoscopy. Endoscopic visualization of the anastomosis was obtained at 2, 6, and 12 months, hence at the reach of a natural orifice, and not too deep in the midgut. There were no serious adverse events, and patency was confirmed in all patients at 1 year. Average total weight loss was 14.6% (40% excess weight loss at 12 months), generating a significant decline in glycated haemoglobin levels observed in all diabetic (1.9%) and prediabetic (1.0%) patients, while reducing the use of diabetic drugs. Insulin serum levels went up and serum glucose downward statistically significantly. It is unknown how the large mesenteric window will be managed, as an internal hernia in the future is always possible, resulting in an intestinal obstruction with possible bowel loss from necrosis. Further, the jejunoileal bypass was abandoned more than 40 years ago due to severe nutritional side effects, bacterial overgrowth, and hepatic failures. A follow-up at 12 months is unlikely to catch these problems. It is likely that the "mid" jejunal-ileal bypass will not be a common procedure because of these issues. Indeed, 40% of patients in the present study have recurrent diarrhoea, and many have mineral and vitamins issues already. On the positive side, a side-to-side may have fewer side effects than the classic jejunoileal bypass. There are no IFSO nor ASMBS approval statements for a jejunoileal bypass currently.

This is where we stand now with only very small and limited animal and human experiences recorded in the last decade. What do we need? We need large multicentre studies to establish the safety and feasibility of magnetic compression anastomosis in all kinds of conditions, elective and urgent, with different normal and pathological tissue, similar to what staples and sutures are used. We need to establish a safe and easy delivery via endoscope and need a system of localization within the bowel to know where we are in relationship with the ligament of Treitz and ileocecal valve. Since the material used and the time it remains in the tissue is relatively short, it is unlikely that any form of toxicity will occur; rare cases of allergies are always possible. More reports are coming from China, where vascular biliodigestive and gastrointestinal concepts were presented and published recently. Some examples of these have been presented at the last meeting of the American College of Surgeons in San Francisco in 2019.

The recent efforts of GT Metabolic Solutions Inc. are quite remarkable. The experimental laboratory team (Fig. 20.1) has successfully concluded permeable side-to-side duodeno-ileostomy anastomosis in all porcine animals (Fig. 20.2) without bleeding or leaks, using a new prototype (Fig. 20.3), with successful natural extrusion per anus, without obstruction in all animals in 2020. This will be the basis for a first-in-man (FIM) clinical series in 2021.

The endoscopists, surgical and medical, and gastroenterologists are now on board to perform more bariatric therapeutics, and this is excellent news supported by the ASGE/ASMBS Task Force on Endoscopic Bariatric Therapy [17]. The future is very bright. Let me finish with a quote from Nikola Tesla: *Let the future tell the truth and evaluate each one according to his work and accomplishments. The present is theirs; the future, for which I have really worked, is mine.*

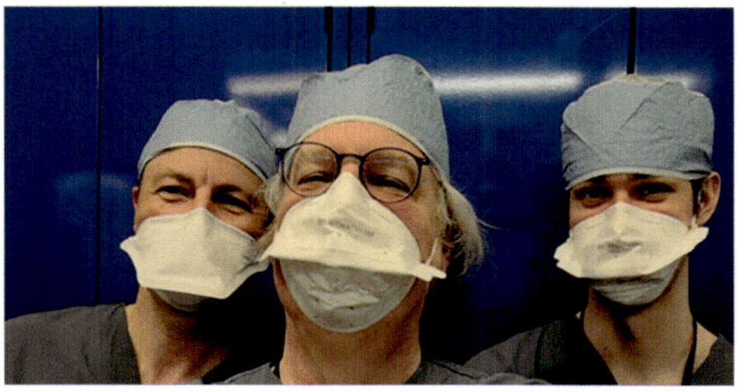

Fig. 20.1 Selfie from the Experimental Laboratory Team. From left to right: Todd Krinke, BAEM, Michel Gagner, MD, FRCSC, FACS, and Maxime Lapointe-Gagner, B.Sc

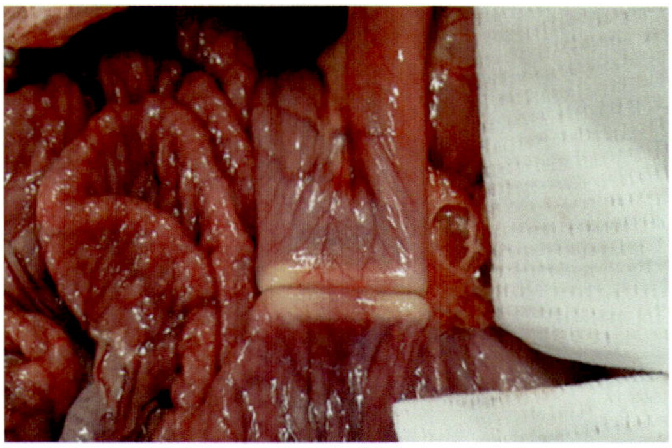

Fig. 20.2 Position of magnets in the duodenal and ileal lumen

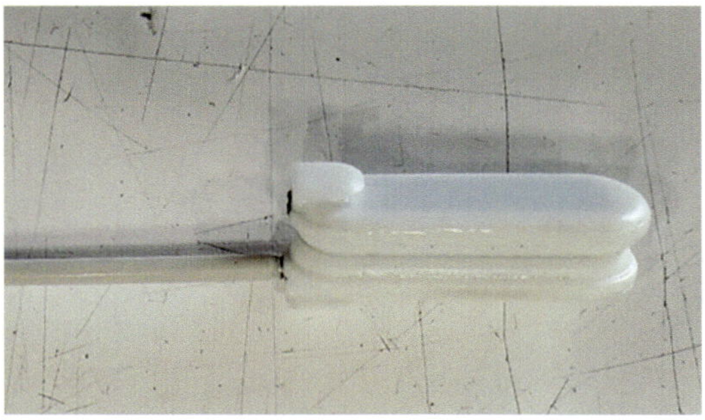

Fig. 20.3 Longitudinal magnets and attached endoscopic catheter for linear duodeno-ileal anastomosis. (From GT Metabolic Solutions, Inc.)

References

1. Perretta S, Wall JK, Dallemagne B, Harrison M, Becmeur F, Marescaux J. Video: two novel endoscopic esophageal lengthening and reconstruction techniques. Surg Endosc. 2011;25(10):3440.
2. Wall J, Perretta S, Diana M, Dhumane P, Haro JI, Dallemagne B, Becmeur F, Krummel T, Marescaux J. Submucosal endoscopic myotomies for esophageal lengthening: a novel minimally invasive technique with feasibility study. Eur J Pediatr Surg. 2012;22(3):217–21.
3. Graves CE, Co C, Hsi RS, Kwiat D, Imamura-Ching J, Harrison MR, Stoller ML. Magnetic compression anastomosis (magnamosis): first-in-human trial. J Am Coll Surg. 2017;225(5):676–681.e1. https://doi.org/10.1016/j.jamcollsurg.2017.07.1062. Epub 2017 Aug 23.
4. Toselli L, Martinez-Ferro M, Cervio G, Kwiat D, Imamura-Ching J, Graves CE, Gaston B, Harrison M. Magnetic compression anastomosis (magnamosis) for functional undiversion of ileostomy in pediatric patients. J Laparoendosc Adv Surg Tech A. 2017;27(12):1314–7.
5. Jamshidi R, Stephenson JT, Clay JG, Pichakron KO, Harrison MR. Magnamosis: magnetic compression anastomosis with comparison to suture and staple techniques. J Pediatr Surg. 2009;44(1):222–8.
6. Wall J, Diana M, Leroy J, Deruijter V, Gonzales KD, Lindner V, Harrison M, Marescaux J. MAGNAMOSIS IV: magnetic compression anastomosis for minimally invasive colorectal surgery. Endoscopy. 2013;45(8):643–8.
7. Jiang H, Chen S, Kish S, Loh L, Zhang J, Zhang X, Kwiat D, Harrison M, Roy S. Miniaturizing RFID for magnamosis. Conf Proc IEEE Eng Med Biol Soc. 2014;2014:638–41.
8. Kojima F, Sato T, Tsunoda S, Takahata H, Hamaji M, Komatsu T, Okada M, Sugiura T, Oshiro O, Sakai Y, Date H, Nakamura T. Development of a novel marking system for laparoscopic gastrectomy using endoclips with radio frequency identification tags: feasibility study in a canine model. Surg Endosc. 2014;28(9):2752–9.
9. Joo HY, Lee BE, Choi CI, Kim DH, Kim GH, Jeon TY, Kim DH, Ahn S. Tumor localization using radiofrequency identification clip marker: experimental results of an ex vivo porcine model. Surg Endosc. 2019;33(5):1441–50.
10. Bruns NE, Glenn IC, Craner DR, Schomisch SJ, Harrison MR, Ponsky TA. Magnetic compression anastomosis (magnamosis) in a porcine esophagus: proof of concept for potential application in esophageal atresia. J Pediatr Surg. 2019;54(3):429–33.
11. Gonzales KD, Douglas G, Pichakron KO, Kwiat DA, Gallardo SG, Encinas JL, Hirose S, Harrison MR. Magnamosis III: delivery of a magnetic compression anastomosis device using minimally invasive endoscopic techniques. J Pediatr Surg. 2012;47(6):1291–5.
12. Leroy J, Perretta S, Diana M, Wall J, Lindner V, Harrison M, Marescaux J. An original endoluminal magnetic anastomotic device allowing pure NOTES transgastric and transrectal sigmoidectomy in a porcine model: proof of concept. Surg Innov. 2012;19(2):109–16.

13. Diana M, Wall J, Perretta S, Dallemagne B, Gonzales KD, Harrison MR, Agnus V, Soler L, Nicolau S, Marescaux J. Totally endoscopic magnetic enteral bypass by external guided rendezvous technique. Surg Innov. 2011;18(4):317–20.
14. Ryou M, Thompson CC. Magnetic retraction in natural-orifice transluminal endoscopic surgery (NOTES): addressing the problem of traction and countertraction. Endoscopy. 2009;41(2):143–8.
15. Ryou M, Aihara H, Thompson CC. Minimally invasive entero-enteral dual-path bypass using self-assembling magnets. Surg Endosc. 2016;30(10):4533–8.
16. Machytka E, Bužga M, Zonca P, Lautz DB, Ryou M, Simonson DC, Thompson CC. Partial jejunal diversion using an incisionless magnetic anastomosis system: 1-year interim results in patients with obesity and diabetes. Gastrointest Endosc. 2017;86(5):904–12.
17. ASGE/ASMBS Task Force on Endoscopic Bariatric Therapy, Ginsberg GG, Chand B, Cote GA, Dallal RM, Edmundowicz SA, Nguyen NT, Pryor A, Thompson CC. A pathway to endoscopic bariatric therapies. Gastrointest Endosc. 2011;74(5):943–53.

Index

M. Gagner (ed.), *Magnetic Surgery*, https://doi.org/10.1007/978-3-030-73947-8

G

H

I

J

L

M

N

GPSR Compliance

The European Union's (EU) General Product Safety Regulation (GPSR) is a set of rules that requires consumer products to be safe and our obligations to ensure this.

If you have any concerns about our products, you can contact us on ProductSafety@springernature.com

In case Publisher is established outside the EU, the EU authorized representative is:

Springer Nature Customer Service Center GmbH
Europaplatz 3
69115 Heidelberg, Germany

Batch number: 10756384

Printed by Printforce, the Netherlands